CLINICAL & NURSING STAFF DEVELOPMENT

Current Competence, Future Focus

SECOND EDITION

D0851450

CLINICAL & NURSING STAFF DEVELOPMENT

Current Competence, Future Focus

SECOND EDITION

Karen J. Kelly-Thomas, PhD, RN,C, CNAA

President, Kelly Thomas Associates
Alexandria, Virginia

Director of Practice and Research, Association of Women's Health,
Obstetric, and Neonatal Nurses (AWHONN)
Washington, DC

Founding Member, National Nursing Staff
Development Organization (NNSDO)

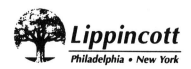

Lippincott
Philadelphia • New York

Acquisitions Editor: Lisa Marshall
Assistant Editor: Sandra Kasko
Project Editor: Gretchen Metzger
Senior Production Manager: Helen Ewan
Senior Production Coordinator: Nannette Winski
Design Coordinator: Nicholas Rook
Indexer: Michael Ferreira

Edition 2

9 8 7 6 5 4 3 2

Library of Congress Cataloging-in-Publications Data

Clinical and nursing staff development : current competence, future
  focus / [edited by] Karen J. Kelly-Thomas. — 2nd ed.
      p.   cm.
    Rev. ed. of: Nursing staff development. c1992.
    Includes bibliographical references and index.
    ISBN 0-397-55416-8 (alk. paper)
    1. Nurses—In-service training.   2. Nursing—Study and teaching (Continuing
  education) I. Kelly-Thomas, Karen J.   II. Nursing staff development.
    [DNLM: 1. Education, Nursing, Continuing.   2. Nursing Staff—education.   3. Clinical
  Competence.   4. Staff Development—methods.
  WY 18.5 C641 1998]
  RT76.N85   1998
  610.73'071'55—dc21
  DNLM/DLC
  for Library of Congress   98-10655
                                                                       CIP

Care has been taken to confirm the accuracy of the information presented and to describe generally accepted practices. However, the authors, editors, and publisher are not responsible for errors or omissions or for any consequences from application of the information in this book and make no warranty, express or implied, with respect to the contents of the publication.

The authors, editors, and publisher have exerted every effort to ensure that drug selection and dosage set forth in this text are in accordance with current recommendations and practice at the time of publication. However, in view of ongoing research, changes in government regulations, and the constant flow of information relating to drug therapy and drug reactions, the reader is urged to check the package insert for each drug for any change in indications and dosage and for added warnings and precautions. This is particularly important when the recommended agent is a new or infrequently employed drug.

Some drugs and medical devices presented in this publication have Food and Drug Administration (FDA) clearance for limited use in restricted research settings. It is the responsibility of the health care provider to ascertain the FDA status of each drug or device planned for use in their clinical practice.

Dedicated to my sister Anne, a.k.a. Jane

and

my grandchildren, Chelsea, Zachary, and Matthew

Foreword

"The times they are a'changin'"—and staff development is changing as well. Karen Kelly-Thomas has assembled an impressive group of contributors in this second edition of her well-known work. These contributors not only acknowledge and describe the changing times in staff development; they seem able to predict the future of the practice.

The first chapter of *Clinical & Nursing Staff Development: Current Competence, Future Focus* sets the stage for the text as a whole, outlining the changes that staff development specialists are experiencing due to the significant and ongoing changes in health care systems. Mergers, acquisitions, re-engineering, downsizing, and other challenges have caused staff development specialists to review their practice and to learn to cope with a myriad of unfamiliar situations. This text has moved away from staff development in acute care settings toward staff development in the variety of locations in which health care services are delivered.

Kelly-Thomas also proposes a new definition of staff development, and a model for viewing the services that staff development specialists provide. Although the term *clinical* represents the major focus of staff development in any setting, what seems to me to be missing is language related to learning; however, learning is addressed in context by Aucoin (Chapter 10) and Schoenly (Chapters 9 and 12). Certainly, the focus on competence assessment and competence development is well placed.

The text provides a range of topics reflecting issues found in contemporary staff development practice. From theory-based to practice applications, staff development specialists at any stage of the novice-to-expert continuum will find in this book information to use in their practice.

Of particular note are the chapters on outcome measurement and strategic thinking—topics of current concern in all specialty areas of nursing practice. Measuring outcomes is essential to answering questions related to the value or worth of staff development in health care, and Sikma (Chapter 8) presents a model that can make outcome measurement workable in most staff development programs. The application of strategic thinking to the curriculum development process through the model presented and subsequently to staff development practice should prove helpful in today's health care arena.

Discussing models of staff development, Brunt (Chapter 2) clearly places the emphasis where it belongs: on outcomes, rather than on the ongoing dilemma of centralized vs. decentralized staff development. The several chapters on competence assessment and competence development mirror contemporary thought and provide guidelines for practice.

The emphasis throughout the text on evaluation and research indicates the increasing sophistication of today's staff development specialist. Even a few years ago, such topics were treated as separate facets of a staff development educator's repertoire, and not very well-developed facets at that.

Yet this book offers something to the novice staff development specialist as well. The chapter on the mandatories clearly will be of assistance in managing required learning activities. The chapter on planning staff development programs is a broad, comprehensive overview with many suggestions to ensure that the planning process is successful.

Novices and experts alike will benefit from the chapters on operations and administration. Even those not in administrative positions will gain perspective on factors such as cost control, resource allocation, and customer service.

Contemporary as well as classic literature is cited throughout. Readers wishing to investigate a topic further may find a plethora of resources. It was good to see the first published data from Kelly-Thomas's dissertation on the intuition of staff development.

I particularly liked the chapter on the environment of learning. Many years of experience have taught me to not underestimate the influence of the environment on learning. Being cognizant of the adverse impact on learning caused by an uncomfortable *classroom* (inadequate lighting, poor acoustics, and hard seats) is relatively easy for the experienced staff development specialist. Being cognizant of the impact on learning caused by an uncomfortable *institutional* environment (inadequate staffing, unrealistic workloads, and poor morale) is more difficult—but a critical first step if staff development specialists are to accomplish their missions and goals and contribute positively to those in the institution.

The appendices also provide useful information that otherwise may not be easily accessible to readers.

My favorite parts of the entire book, however, were the stories that ended each chapter. The situations described in these vignettes are realistic and familiar. The stories clearly illustrate the concepts presented in the chapters. More importantly, they are a celebration of staff development "best practices." They were a joy to read.

This book is targeted toward individuals currently in staff development practice or contemplating entering this specialty area. The contributors have done a monumental job—not only in reflecting current staff development practice, but also in leading it into the next century. At once reflective and energizing, this book is a must-read.

Belinda E. Puetz, PhD, RN
Founder and Administrator
National Nursing Staff Development Organization
Editor-in-Chief
Journal of Nursing Staff Development
Pensacola, Florida

Preface

Staff development is many things to many people. To some, it is a program. To others, it is a process. To yet others, it is a product. This book attempts to make some sense of the various approaches to staff development that occur in health care settings. I have recently begun to refer to this work as *clinical staff development*. With this term, I am attempting to capture the nature and essence of programs, processes, and the product of staff development, competence. I believe that the product of staff development is and should be competence. Thus, the continued focus of this book is competence assessment and development programs and processes that are designed to produce that elusive state of competence.

Though the term *competence* continues to be defined in a variety of ways, this book, as a second edition, focuses on competence more as the most prominent theme of staff development as it has evolved since 1990 when the formal work on the first edition began. Those familiar with the first edition will note a shift in this text.

The shift is toward staff development programs and processes designed to assess and contribute to the development of competence among clinical care providers. Clinical care providers are those health care professionals who provide direct services to patients and have direct contact with patients. Patients may be very sick people in hospitals, people in need of some long-term therapy such as rehabilitation in ambulatory settings, or people investing in their health through participation in screening and surveillance programs like those found in most ambulatory care settings. Other patients who receive care may be in extended care facilities and receive care from clinical care providers like nurses and certified nursing assistants, as well as therapists from many specialties, such as physical therapy, occupational therapy, recreation therapy, music therapy, and others. The awkward term *unlicensed assistive personnel* also describes some care providers in these settings. Though nurses continue to be the largest group of health care providers—at more than 2 million—adding other kinds of health care providers increases that number to more than 10 million.

This shift toward describing staff development programs and processes that provide competence assessment and development as being a service to the patient is a deliberate one. It recognizes and centers on the purpose of staff development: to provide competent providers of clinical care to patients. Defining the *purpose* of staff development in this way creates a shared vision of the possibilities. Some may view this as a shift away from what nurses need and do; I see it as including nursing staff development as an extension of a nursing caring model that has been integral to staff development traditions of the past century. Indeed, principles from one of the first publications about nursing staff development still apply today.

To illustrate that shift, this second edition is organized differently. The first edition used a problem-solving approach (also known as the nursing process) to describe what nurses do to help nurses and other care providers to maintain and develop competence primarily in hospital settings. This edition moves toward what nurses and others may do to produce competent clinical care providers in a variety of settings. The text is organized into four sections:

- staff development practice (Chapters 1–4)
- competence assessment (Chapters 5–8)
- competence development (Chapters 9–12)
- staff development operation and administration (Chapters 13–15)

The reader interested in staff development as a practice discipline will find the first and fourth sections of value, as they cover theory, models, outcomes, management and leadership issues, and development of the field. The reader new to the field of staff development—for example the physical therapist or clinical specialist newly assigned to an aspect of staff development—will find the second and third sections more useful for getting started. These two sections focus more on the how-to aspects of staff development.

A new feature in this edition is the story. At the end of each chapter, an individual who has experienced providing a staff development program or process was asked to write a first-person account. The purpose of each account is to shed further light on the everyday practice of staff development and communicate its richness. As a field of practice, staff development is full of texture.

Karen J. Kelly-Thomas, PhD, RN,C, CNAA

Introduction to the Second Edition

The first edition of this book was written to help new and experienced specialists learn how to "do" staff development. After spending 15 years in this field of practice and learning much from my colleagues, I wanted to give something back. I wanted to help other nurses who found themselves in this role, either by design or by default, to consider a variety of strategies for developing themselves in their role.

During the past 5 years, many of you have come forward to thank me and offer suggestions for this edition. Great changes are occurring and will continue. Our roles in our respective agencies are also changing. Restructuring, reengineering, retooling, and revisioning are but a few of the frequently heard re-do words today. We are all involved with these *r* words. This book is about those experiences and what has worked and what hasn't. It provides some of the best practices to help novice staff development nurses learn their work and to help experienced nurses consider new approaches.

The book also expands these principles to cover clinical care providers. Our experience and traditions have served us well, and many of us have had the opportunity to provide staff development services to a broader audience. This text is focused on the provision of staff development programs and services to nurses, therapists, technicians, and care support staff. Within a framework of clinical care, these roles are selected to address the common care providers in health care today. Individuals in these roles have unique and common needs for competence assessment and development. Common needs are addressed across roles. Unique needs of different care providers are also addressed in this edition. Though the principles are the same across various target audiences, performance expectations of the care provider have changed. Common among all is the need to learn new skills and new ways of thinking, and new ways of working together. Collaborating with individuals in new roles, while new technical and critical thinking skills are being learned and developed, is a collective need. Team learning as new technologies emerge for improved patient care is another need. Central to this edition is the distinctive character of the caring community created in the clinical settings of patient care.

This edition has been reorganized to focus on the two essential components of a staff development program: competence assessment and competence development. In the previous edition, I proposed a model that included a third component, competence maintenance. This component is included in the competence assessment component.

The text also includes new models and structures to help specialists develop relevant programs for clinical staff. The term *clinical staff* is used interchangeably with the term *clinical care providers* to describe that delivery of services role in health care systems today that has a direct patient care aspect.

Acknowledgments

There are many in my life that I would like to acknowledge. And since the first edition of this book, much has happened in my world, and I'm sure yours, too. Despite the complex but alive world we live in, we sometimes get to take a moment and give thanks for simple things. Carpe diem! Here's my simple thanks to people who have been important to me during the past 5 years or so.

To Nancy Diekelmann, who gave me gentle good counsel during my visit to the Heideggerian Institute at the University of Wisconsin and gave me confidence to inquire in a way that was good and right for me and my nursing heart. Thank you.

To Dorothy del Bueno, who continues as my rabbi and my model for clear, crisp, and entertaining writing. Thank you.

To Mary Silva, who gave me the gift of her scholarship. Thank you.

To my cancer care team, Kathy Alley, Carolyn Hendricks, Harriet Handler, Terri Leonarczyk, Nancy Endler, and Barbara Summers, thank you for helping me through all the therapies, and for helping me keep my breasts beautiful for me and my man. Thanks!

To Lisa Marshall, whose patience and kindness as an editor during the past 2 years are just what I needed to keep writing. Sincere thanks.

To Lorry Schoenly, who agreed to write another chapter on a topic important to me. Thanks again.

To Diana Murk Russell, who helps me bring beauty to my Deep Creek gardens. Thanks, girl!

To Belinda Puetz, who gave me the gift of her friendship. Thank you.

To my mother, who always guides me gently toward my spiritual self. Thanks, Mom.

And of course, to my man Mike. AKA, my Legal Officer in Charge of Validation and Energy Renewal and my friend. I love you and thank you for being there for me during the past 12 years of our lives together.

Contributors

Lorraine C. K. Anderson, MEd, RN is an organizational learning consultant for the University of Minnesota Health System. She has been consulting, writing, and helping health care professionals learn for over 15 years. Ms. Anderson has been a leader in the development, implementation, and evaluation of the competency process across the organization. She facilitates educational opportunities and practical techniques for staff to develop and improve competency. She has published and presented across the nation on topics including creative teaching strategies, competency assessment, and oncology nursing.

Julia W. Aucoin, DNS, RN,C has led the education department in several hospitals and presented staff development topics to national audiences. Certified in continuing education and staff development, she has taught the review course for the certification exam (CE/SD) and studied the effects of this certification on participation in continuing nursing education. She is currently teaching at North Carolina Central University and performs consultation for providers of continuing education. A charter member of the National Nursing Staff Development Organization, she has served as a member of the board and chaired task forces.

Freddica L. Brubaker, MSN, RN, CCRN, CEN is the Clinical Resource Nurse for the Emergency Department at Howard University Hospital in Washington, DC. She has 22 years of experience working in urban hospitals in emergency departments, critical care units, and in staff development. As an educator, she has developed, implemented, and taught courses targeted toward emergency department and critical care nurses. She was instrumental in developing a 6-month Critical Care Internship Program for newly licensed RNs. Ms. Brubaker received her BS in Nursing from the University of Miami in Coral Gables, Florida; her MS in Nursing Administration from George Mason University in Fairfax, Virginia; and is certified in emergency and critical care nursing. Ms. Brubaker has published in the areas of hemodynamic monitoring and arterial blood gas interpretation.

Barbara Brunt, MA, RN,C has worked in various staff development roles (educator, coordinator, director) for the past 19 years. She has functioned in centralized and combination staff development structures, as well as a hospital-wide education program. She is certified in Nursing Continuing Education and Staff Development, as well as medical–surgical nursing. Ms. Brunt has presented many programs locally and nationally, and has written numerous articles related to staff development topics. She was a section editor for *Core Curriculum for Nursing Staff Development* and wrote a chapter in that same publication. As a charter member of the National Nursing Staff Development Organization, she is currently serving as treasurer.

Bette Case, PhD, RN,C, an independent consultant, assists health care organizations and professional schools to achieve their goals by using innovative educational approaches. She frequently presents continuing education offerings and publishes on a variety of professional development topics. She also edits a critical thinking column in *Dimensions in Critical Care Nursing* and serves on the editorial board of the *Journal of Continuing Education in Nursing.* During her 30 years in health care and nursing, Dr. Case has focused on education for all levels of students and practitioners of nursing, and has directed nursing in critical care and emergency services settings. Immediately before beginning her own consulting practice, she directed staff education for the 3,500 employees of Michael Reese Hospital and Medical Center in Chicago. Dr. Case earned her BSN from Syracuse University and her MSN and PhD in educational psychology from Loyola University in Chicago. She is Membership Chairperson for the National Nursing Staff Development Organization.

Barbara J. Daley, PhD, RN is currently an assistant professor of adult and continuing education at the University of Wisconsin-Milwaukee. After working as a staff nurse, head nurse, and clinical nurse specialist, she entered the education arena as a staff development instructor in an acute care facility. She then served as a director of education in acute care, a coordinator of continuing nursing education in a community college that serves a three-county rural area, and as the director of continuing nursing education in an urban university setting.

Kathleen J. Fischer, MA, RN,C, CNA is currently the Director of Educational Services for Nursing at the University of Michigan Health System. She has presented nationally on topics related to health care, administration, and education. She has co-authored the ANA standards for the profession, and two books on performance improvement in staff development and continuing education, in addition to other publications. She is actively involved in professional organizations including the National Nursing Staff Development Organization (Executive Board), Sigma Theta Tau (Regional Board), and the Michigan Nurses Association.

Donna Gloe, EdD, RN,C, CCRN currently holds several positions, as the Knowledge Information Module Manager in Quality Resources at St. John's Health System, Education Director for the Dermatology Nurses Association, and as an adjunct faculty member at Southwest Baptist University. She has been involved in staff development and quality issues in nursing for seven years. She serves on the editorial board for the *Journal of Continuing Education in Nursing, Heart and Lung,* and *Dermatology Nursing.* Dr. Gloe also serves on the Test Development Committee and Board for Certification of Nursing Staff Development and Continuing Education at the American Nursing Credentialing Center.

Mitzi T. Grey, MEd, RN,C is President of Grey and Co., Inc. in Mocksville, NC, a private consulting firm specializing in contract education and consultation to health care systems. She has been an educator in four hospitals and is currently an adjunct faculty member with the University of North Carolina in Greensboro, NC, and Quality Manager at Davie County Hospital. She is certified in continuing education and staff development and serves as national faculty for the National Nursing Staff Development Organization Certification Review Course. She has published in the areas of competence assessment and quality management.

Susan B. Jeska, EdD, MBA, RN is Director of Organizational Learning for Fairview Hospital and Healthcare Services in Minneapolis, Minnesota. Dr. Jeska has over 20 years of experience in a variety of practice, education, and management roles at the University of Minnesota Hospital and Clinic and the Fairview Health System; for the past 11 years, she has had a leadership role in education administration. Dr. Jeska holds a baccalaureate degree in nursing, a master's degree in business administration, and a doctorate in educational leadership. She has given over 40 national presentations and seminars and has several publications on leadership and staff development practice to her credit. Dr. Jeska is adjunct faculty at the University of Minnesota, serves on the editorial board of the *Journal of Nursing Staff Development,* and has her own consulting and teaching business.

Rebecca Katz, MA, RN,C has over 30 years of progressive experience in staff, management, and education positions.

Currently she is the Senior Director of Learning and Education for Mount Carmel Health System, Columbus, Ohio, where she is responsible for the integration of the education departments of three separate hospitals. In addition, she is developing a strategy for matrix management of all educational resources within the new system.

She has led multiple teams in competency preparation during regulatory team preparation, as well as redesigned performance management systems to reflect the philosophy of competency as a building block in the performance process.

Karen Kelly-Thomas, PhD, RN,C, CNAA is an experienced nurse administrator and staff development specialist. She has 26 years of experience in nursing, many of which have been focused on administering developmental programs and projects in multiple settings. She owns and operates a private consultation practice, Kelly Thomas Associates. She recently served as Administrative Director at Suburban Hospital, Bethesda, MD, where she was responsible for the Clinical Education, Research, and Development Department and Oncology Services. Presently, Karen is the Director of Practice and Research, Association of Women's Health, Obstetric, and Neonatal Nurses in Washington, DC. In her private consultation practice, Dr. Kelly's clients range from 90-bed rural hospitals to 1500-bed complex teaching health care systems, as well as health care associations.

Karen has a diploma from Holy Name Hospital in Teaneck, NJ, a BSN from Regents College, Albany NY, and an MS in adult education from Virginia Tech. She recently completed her doctorate in nursing and health care administration at George Mason University in Fairfax, Virginia. Her research is focused on expert practice and the nature of intuition among staff development experts.

Dr. Kelly presents regularly to national and international groups. Her presentations primarily focus on competence assessment systems, organization development, quality management, and strategic thinking. Karen has published more than a dozen articles and chapters in books. Her book *Nursing Staff Development: Current Competence, Future Focus* was selected as a 1992 Book of the Year by the *American Journal of Nursing.* She is certified in nursing administration, advanced and nursing continuing education, and staff development. Karen also is a founding member of the National Nursing Staff Development Organization and served as the NNSDO 1992–94 president. Karen received the Belinda Puetz Excellence in Nursing Staff Development award from her colleagues in 1994—a cherished testimonial.

Karen loves what she does and does what she loves!

David J. Massello, BA is the founding partner and President of the Business Performance Institute. Before founding this forum, Mr. Massello served as President and Chief Operating Officer of Doctors Hospital in Ohio. He also has served as the Senior Vice President, Chief

Financial Officer, and was Vice President of Human Resources for 8 years. He has 26 years of experience in the health care field, with a background in finance, expert behavior, and operations.

He has had extensive training in the team management and storyboard practices of Walt Disney and in research in human factors, models of expert behavior, and the role and impact of leaders in organizations.

Mr. Massello is a Certified Practitioner in neuro-linguistic programming.

The Business Performance Institute and Mr. Massello offer a specialized "in the trenches" consulting strategy and teach leaders from CEOs to nurses and physicians with their Creating Great Leaders™ Education Program. Mr. Massello has conducted seminars for hospitals and universities, and consulted with clinical professionals in nursing and radiology on a variety of topics such as Advanced Leaders Skills, NLP techniques, and Strategic Thinking Patterns of Success.

Donna Miller, MEd, RN,C, CCRN has over 20 years experience in nursing as an RN, and also as a CLPN. She has held several educational positions in schools of nursing, radiology, and acute care, with a clinical specialty of critical care. In her role as an educator, she has been responsible for orientation, in-service, and continuing education of critical care staff. Ms. Miller has published and presented on a variety of critical care and staff development topics. She is a member of the Executive Board of the National Nursing Staff Development Organization.

Denise M. Petras, MA, RNC is Associate Director of Patient Care Services Education at the University of Pittsburgh Medical Center, Shadyside, Pennsylvania. She has 17 years of experience in nursing education and staff development and patient/community education. In addition to published articles, Ms. Petras has developed videotapes on negotiated care and the role and responsibilities of nurses. She is certified in Nursing Continuing Education and Staff Development through the American Nurses Credentialing Center. Ms. Petras received a BSN from Carlow College, Pittsburgh; an MA in Adult/Community Education from Indiana University of Pennsylvania; and an MSN as Community Health Nursing Specialist from LaRoche College in Pittsburgh. Ms. Petras is currently serving as Vice Chair/Program Chair of the Staff Development Network of Western Pennsylvania.

Linda Ristow Puetz, BSN, BA, RN is Education Coordinator for Children's Mercy Hospital in Kansas City, Missouri. In this role, she serves as the education consultant/facilitator for seven critical care units, the trauma and code blue programs, nursing research, patient rights, organizational ethics, and human resources. She is also Chair of the multidisciplinary Information Systems and Media Support Team, and a member of multiple organizational development projects and activities. Prior to this, Ms. Puetz had 15 years of clinical experience as a staff nurse and charge nurse in neonatal and pediatric critical care units, and 1 year of adult ICU/CCU experience in Missouri, Illinois, Wisconsin, and Kansas. She obtained a BA in biology from the University of Kansas in 1973 and her BS in nursing from the St. Louis University Accelerated Nursing Program in 1974.

Lorry Schoenly, DNSc, RN,C is Director of Education for the National Association of Orthopaedic Nurses, a professional nursing association with over 8000 members dedicated to advancing education, research, and nursing practice in musculoskeletal healthcare. Lorry has spent more than a decade in staff development, holding positions as Staff Development Educator,

Director of Education, and Assistant Vice President for Education and Development in the acute care setting. She received her Doctorate in Nursing Science in 1997 from Widener University, Chester, Pennsylvania. Certified in Nursing Staff Development and Continuing Education through the American Nurses Association since 1992, she is a charter member of the National Nursing Staff Development Organization and has held the position of Research Chair as well as Informatics Committee member. Dr. Schoenly speaks and has published widely in the areas of staff development, continuing education, and nursing informatics.

Suzanne K. Sikma, PhD, RN is currently Assistant Professor in the Nursing Program at the University of Washington-Bothell. She has over 20 years of experience in staff development and administration in health care. She has held roles as staff nurse, unit manager, staff development instructor and director, clinical director, and consultant in a wide range of clinical settings including critical care, acute care, long-term care, and community health nursing. Her research interests include developing caring organizations and health care programs and organizational evaluation.

Dori Taylor Sullivan, PhD, RN,C, CNA is Assistant Vice Chancellor for Quality and Performance Improvement at the University of Connecticut Health Center in Farmington, Connecticut. She completed her BS and MS in nursing at the University of Connecticut School of Nursing. Her doctoral degree is in the area of educational psychology/evaluation research and measurement. Known as an entertaining speaker who enthusiastically brings theory alive and assists others in the application of new insights to practical real-life situations, Ms. Taylor Sullivan is a frequently invited presenter at a variety of regional and national conferences, and she has published numerous articles and book chapters.

Janice A. Ward, MSN, RN,C, is Director of Education at Puetz & Associates, Inc., an association management company in Pensacola, FL. Formerly Director of Central Staff Development at Indiana University Medical Center in Indianapolis, Indiana, Janice was responsible for orientation, continuing education, and the development of staff in the Department of Nursing and Patient Care Services. She collaborated with the clinical nurse specialists and educators for nursing and other health care professionals to plan and provide a staff development program.

Janice has worked with adult learners in a school of nursing, a community-based hospital, and a university medical center. She has also practiced as a family nurse practitioner in a community health center and with a physician in private practice. Her experience has been extensive both as a director and as an instructor.

Janice was also active in creating the National Nursing Staff Development Organization. She was a member of the steering committee and has been secretary of the organization. Within Indiana she is a charter member of the Indiana Nursing Staff Development Organization.

Francie Wolgin, MSN, RN, CNA is Director, Operations Support and Practice Development at St. Joseph Mercy Hospital in Ann Arbor, MI, and President, National Nursing Staff Development Organization. Her department is responsible for the training and development of all patient care associates, including the orientation and ongoing competency assessment of nurses, and the Patient Care Assistant and Patient Care Technician training programs. Ms. Wolgin also serves as an adjunct faculty member at the University of Michigan

School of Nursing. Previous positions she has held include Director of Nursing Practice Development and Clinical Associate, School of Nursing, Duke University Medical Center, as well as several management, staff development, and administrative positions at the University of Cincinnati Hospital and a College of Nursing & Health faculty appointment. Ms. Wolgin serves on the *Journal of Nursing Staff Development* editorial board and is the Deputy Editor for *Perspectives on Research*. She has published books and many articles and contributes to books on staff development, competency, and advanced nursing assistants.

Donna K. Wright, MS, RN is currently working for Creative Healthcare Management as a staff development specialist and consultant. She works with health care organizations to help them establish cost-effective, quality education and competency programs. She has had many years of experience in staff development and education. She has worked for the University of Minnesota Hospital and Clinic, the American Diabetes Association, and the Minnesota Association for Public Teaching Hospitals. She is also an adjunct faculty member at the University of Minnesota School of Nursing.

Contents

Staff Development: Growth in Practice

KAREN J. KELLY-THOMAS

The trend is crystal clear: great changes in the health care environment have brought about great changes in the structure, process, and delivery of staff development services, and these changes will continue. Clinicians who dedicate their time to staff development, at both novice and expert levels, must change the design and delivery of these services to make their critical contribution to patient care.

All roles in health care are changing; few can say with certainty that they are performing the same tasks they were a few years ago. Re-engineering, restructuring, retooling, and revisioning are but a few of the frequently heard re-do words today. We are all involved with these R words. However, our traditions have served us well and will continue to do so in our continuous pursuit of improved staff development services. Chapter 1 discusses some of those traditions and shows how they can serve as an anchor for growth in our practice. This chapter describes some of the many changes confronting new and experienced staff development specialists and presents new and relevant trend data. Using change as the organizing framework, our changing environment, needs, systems, and settings are examined. In addition, the chapter explores the continued evolution of staff development as theory-based practice. The historical survey of staff development in this chapter also serves as a backdrop to the changes in the field. We must understand this history to evaluate the extension of this practice and these principles to all clinical care providers.

Growth in practice is also evidenced by practitioners in the field of staff development. Expert clinicians and educators continue to be drawn toward the field, rewarded by the knowledge that specialists can make a difference in patient care. Self-development is a prerequisite, so the novice-to-expert skill-acquisition model is again included in this edition, to guide the development of new and experienced clinical staff development specialists.

Finally, a new mental model is proposed to provide a backdrop for the rest of this text. This model provides a mental image to guide novice staff development specialists as they learn about this work. For experienced specialists, it will provide an intuitive understanding of our growing practice and an opportunity to consider how our ideas have been blended to create that practice.

CHANGING ENVIRONMENTS

Profound changes are occurring in the environments where staff development services are provided, and these changes will continue to occur. Such environments include all settings where health care is provided (e.g., the traditional hospital, new single-purpose ambulatory care settings, the home, long-term care settings, subacute care settings, and other settings where patients receive health care services from clinicians). The providers

1

of that care are considered the target audience for staff development services, and the health care agency or setting is the consumer of staff development services. The purpose of staff development services is competence assessment and development, quality, and excellence in patient care. The patient remains at the core of health care environments. In some settings, the patient may be called the client or consumer, but this text will use the term *patient* to describe the person who is the focus of health care services.

The patient is provided health care services by clinical staff who use thinking, technical, and interactive skills to provide care and who work to design an environment in which the best outcome for the patient may be achieved. Management of that environment by clinicians and other administrators has transformed the face of health care. The imperative to re-engineer nursing and health care is essential as this era of reformation continues (Blancett & Flarey, 1995).

Technology will continue to drive health care advances, and health care providers will continue to be challenged to focus on patient needs. To support healthy outcomes, clinicians must serve as advocates for patients, who can easily become lost in complex health care environments. Indeed, clinicians are constantly confronted with technology that can threaten the healing and well-being of patients entrapped in the high-tech health care settings of today. Maintaining day and night light cycles and stimulating certain senses for healing (*e.g.*, with music and sound) are some of the measures used by clinicians to create an environment of care that will stimulate healing.

Cost, access, and quality are the three major factors generating the most change in health care. One change generated is the migration of patients to settings considered more efficient. Such migration is driven by various factors, including a common goal of most providers and recipients: to reduce costs. Cost control and resource management remain at the core of the health care industry. National health care spending increased by 6.4% in 1994, to $949.4 billion from $892.3 billion in 1993. Although this is the smallest rise seen in the past 20 years, the share of the gross domestic product grew to 13.7% in 1994, up from 8% in 1975 (Prospective Payment Assessment Commission, 1996).

With costs approaching 15% of the gross national product and expenditures at the trillion dollar mark, it makes sense that so many have a stake in reducing and controlling costs. Managed care calls for the provision of the least amount of service in the least expensive place to an informed consumer. This is a remarkably different approach from earlier care models, which included competition for the most patients who needed or wanted the most advanced technology in everyday care. The cost of that care was paid by indemnified plans or government entitlement programs. This type of health care delivery system is rare in today's cost-conscious and constrained environment.

Public policy and the market are also (some say finally) driving efforts to control runaway costs. In 1995, more than 56 million Americans were enrolled in HMO plans, up from 11 million in 1982. Medicare continues to be a major contributor to the federal budget deficit, with spending more than $169 million, a 5.3% increase over the past two decades. Of great concern is the continued insolvency of the Medicare trust fund, with predictions that it will be bankrupt by 2002. With 76 million baby boomers set to retire in 2011, the solutions to this crisis will be draconian (Lamm, 1996).

The site of care delivery is also undergoing significant shifts. For example, the National Center for Health Statistics (1996) extracted data from 118,000 medical records from 494 hospitals and ambulatory care centers and found that 28.3 million surgical and nonsurgical procedures were performed in 1994 during 18.8 million visits. Although 16 million (85%) of the ambulatory surgery visits occurred in hospitals, an increasing number (15%, or 2.9 million) occurred in freestanding centers. The four procedures performed more than 1 million times on ambulatory patients include extraction of lens, endoscopy of the large intestine, insertion of prosthetic lens, and endoscopy of the small intestine. These shifts call for changes in the way staff development services are designed and delivered to the clinicians involved in this care. New care delivery designs, such as subacute facilities or units, also call for new staff development services for care providers.

Unfortunately, as the full effect of changes has been observed, not all patients or providers have been served well. Patients are learning more about what they can expect before, during, and after their health care system experiences based on their health care plan (or lack of it). Care providers are learning through everyday experience how to deliver care in new settings outside of the traditional hospital setting. As the scramble to reduce costs continues, the environment of health care is changing to be one with a greater emphasis on costs and benefits to more stakeholders—such as third-party payors, federal and state government, and taxpayers—than just patients. Never before has the process of staff development, in which care providers are helped to solve everyday problems and develop new competencies, been so important. However, in some environments staff development is considered to be an extra—something expendable or too costly. Patients continue to suffer as a result.

Health care workers are also affected by the shift to new settings in which new technologies and skills are used. Some of these skills did not exist just a decade ago. Advanced technology that reduces costs (*e.g.*, cholecystotomy using laser surgery) changes postoperative patient needs, the requisite clinical skills of care providers, and the setting where that care is delivered. Advancing technology will continue to change the environments where health care is delivered and the competence required of care providers.

Access to health care is the second major factor creating change in the health care environment. Of 267 million Americans, more than 35% remain uninsured or underinsured. Immigration and homelessness also affect patients' access to consistent health care that helps them stay healthy. Access issues—where and how health care is provided in the United States—continue to be important. As nurses and others expand their practice as primary health care providers, access issues can be addressed in innovative programs. New skills are required of advanced practice nurses and others in settings administered as community health models.

Shifts in the place that patients seek care are also driven by income. For example, unlike the patient with a high income, a patient with a low income is likely to seek primary care in a hospital outpatient department rather than in a physician's office (NCHS, 1996). Health care systems are accommodating these trends by creating new service delivery strategies, with primary care provided by nurse practitioners, physician's assistants, and others in settings other than emergency departments. This shift in provider and place of care also calls for new thinking about the design and delivery of staff development services.

Quality is the third major factor that has created change in health care. Total quality management and the use of continuous quality improvement strategies underpin many changes in the health care environment. Changing the look, feel, and name of labor and delivery rooms to "birthing inns" grew out of efforts to improve the birth experience for all involved. By using the results of research, monitoring quality, and making an effort to retain volume, health care systems responded to customer demands to change the manner in which care was provided to women and families during birth. The environment was significantly changed to accommodate this improved approach using limited interventions and supportive care.

Changes in where nurses practice and how they deliver services create a different environment of care than that experienced in the past by patients and care providers. Although the 1995 national sample of RNs showed that 60% of the employed RNs work in hospitals, more nurses are realizing the potential of nursing practice in new settings and are seeking new opportunities. Of concern to staff development specialists, however, is the finding from the survey that 50% of RNs in management positions still are not prepared at the baccalaureate level; this represents no change since 1992. These nurses need significant staff development services and also need assistance to return to educational programs and acquire the academic credentials needed for these roles.

In March 1996, there were almost 2.6 million RNs in the United States, of which 2.1 million are employed in nursing (HRSA, 1997). With the U.S. Census Bureau reporting a population of 266,920,753 in March 1997, this represents the highest nurse-to-population ratio in the world—that is, one nurse for every 127 Americans. The reallocation and redeployment of clinicians has created role and job crises for many nurses. Staff development services are frequently required for these redeployments. The continuing disruption in the nursing profession will primarily be caused by closure of hospitals (Lamm, 1996).

Another shift in the design of staff development services will be driven by the nature of hospitalized patients and the care they require. Of the 1.26 million RNs working in hospitals, 40% work in critical care settings. Changes in care delivery patterns will call for more advanced practice nurses and allied health care providers in new settings, another emerging role for staff development specialists. Educational programs are changing to meet the demand for advanced practice nurses in a variety of specialties. The Pew Health Professions Commission estimated that double the present number of 25,000 nurse practitioners will be needed (Finocchio et al., 1995). Advanced practice nurses, regardless of their chosen setting, bring a whole new set of competence assessment and development needs to be addressed through staff development programs.

Other clinical disciplines have also evolved. Advancing technology has created new breeds of health care providers. For example, radiation oncology has created positions for therapists, technicians, and radiation care nurses that were unknown two decades ago. High-tech advances have created a group of highly skilled health care providers with sophisticated technical competence. These new care providers interact with patients in significant ways that call for clinical judgment as well as technical expertise. Although not all may focus on the whole patient as nurses do, most readily acknowledge the importance of seeing the patient as a human being with needs specific to their particular specialty of care. Regardless of their specific role, they also recognize the need to maintain and develop their individual and collective competence for continued quality improvement of care.

CHANGING NEEDS

Experience and traditions have served us well, and many of us have had the opportunity to provide staff development services to a broader audience. This text is focused on how staff development specialists provide programs and services to nurses, therapists, technicians, and support staff.

Within a framework of clinical care, these roles are selected to address the development of providers in health care today. Persons in these roles have both unique and common needs for competence assessment and development. Common needs are addressed across roles, and some unique needs of different care providers are also addressed. Although the principles are the same across various target audiences, performance expectations of the care provider have changed. However, all must learn new skills, new ways of thinking, and new ways of working together. All must learn to collaborate with persons in these updated roles with their new technical and critical thinking skills. Team learning as new technologies emerge for improved patient care is another need. Central to this text is the distinctive character of the caring community created in the clinical settings of patient care.

Patients

The patient is the focus of care in clinical staff development. Health care services are provided to patients through competent care providers. Patients' needs have also changed. New environments may require that patients be helped to find their way to the service setting; in other instances, patients may need to help care providers find their way to them. This concept is not new, but changes in technology and the organization of services add complexity to simple tasks. Patients may see themselves as having certain roles or certain relationships. These aspects are considered in the development of clinical care providers.

Nurses

Some staff development needs of nurses have changed significantly in the past 5 years, and others have remained the same. Some needs are shared by other clinical care providers. The competence assessment and development needs of nurses will always be driven by the skills their patients require. These performance skills include:

- Thinking skills
- Technical skills
- Interpersonal skills.

These performance skills may not seem different from those required in other clinical care disciplines. However, what makes nurses' skills unique is the focus on the whole patient during diagnosis and treatment. As in other clinical disciplines, nurses use standards of care to define the scope of practice and provide guidelines for continued development. The term "superordinate standards of care" has been used when defining the term "standard of care." She noted that nurses organize their care and perform many tasks for patients related to the patients' needs for skin care, hydration and nutrition, elimination, psychological and sociologic care, pain management, and education.

Even Florence Nightingale referred to areas of nursing practice to organize her *Notes on Nursing: What It Is, and What It Is Not*, originally published in 1859. Although she cautioned that her notes were not intended to serve as rules or standards, Nightingale believed her thoughts might give hints to women who have personal charge of the health of others. Despite her caveats, Nightingale's chapters were organized around 13 aspects of nursing practice, most of which continue today in some form. They were:

- Ventilation and warming
- Health of houses
- Petty management
- Noise
- Variety
- Taking food
- What food?
- Bed and bedding
- Light
- Cleanliness of rooms and walls
- Personal cleanliness
- Chattering hopes and advice
- Observations of the sick.

Nightingale's thoughts continue to influence modern nursing and often serve as the basis for nursing's scientific knowledge base. Competence in these areas is the ability to use the body of related nursing science during the daily practice of nursing. Organizations and groups of nurses may focus on specialized aspects of these standards. For example, Wound, Ostomy, and Continence Nurses is a group that focuses on the development and promulgation of skin care standards of nursing practice. The ssional performance of these standards is monitored by the professionals in the association and the nurses who practice them. Through the staff development activities of competence assessment, these standards are used to provide a framework for the development of comprehensive staff development programs.

Other needs of nurses have changed due to technology and advances in science. Genetic research and the massive knowledge being generated by the Human Genome Project have created entirely new roles for nurses in health education, teaching, and counseling.

The changing roles and needs of nurses are even evident in the symbols of nursing. As Margretta Styles (1992) wrote:

> In recent decades we have searched for a new identity and a new significance for nursing through a succession of symbols. The starched, pristine, maidenly uniform and cap were abandoned for the lab coat or blue jeans or business suit. The modest bandage scissors tucked in the pocket were visually exchanged for the bold stethoscope dangling conveniently (and conspicuously) around the neck. The lamp was replaced, generations later, by telemetry. The chart, for some, gave way to the clipboard, which in turn has yielded to the computer. In our self-portrayal the hospital has receded as the community and the college campus loomed larger. None of these modern physical symbols belongs to nursing alone.
>
> And words. "High tech/high touch," as we describe ourselves, expresses not only the breadth and demands of practice but an internal tension within each of us and within the body of nursing. . .
>
> Our symbols of the late 20th century are not a mirage. They rightfully and accurately reflect changes in nursing and changes in nurses. (p. 73)

Clinical Care Providers

The term "clinical care providers" is used here to mean persons and groups other than nurses who provide direct clinical care to patients and share a patient-focused approach to the organization and delivery of their services (*e.g.*, physical therapists, occupational therapists, mental health counselors and therapists, and others). Some persons are already part of a defined professional group; others are technicians and may or may not be part of a group of similar technical care providers. For example, technicians who provide care to patients within the clinical context of testing or assisting with diagnostic procedures, such as those who work in freestanding gastroenterology centers, are an example of high-tech technicians. Technicians in hospital-based cardiac catheterization laboratories who also provide angioplasty services are another example.

Many new configurations of patient care services in traditional and innovative settings are creating new types of clinical care providers. The term "unlicensed assistive personnel" is commonly used to refer to persons who provide care to patients under the direction, supervision, and training of nurses (ANA, 1994). Although this term is clumsy, it is an attempt to describe and categorize the clinical care providers who assist nurses in technical tasks. The problem with this—and any—categorization is consensus development about what these persons can and cannot do in various settings. The difference in these roles, when compared with nursing roles, is the unknown element of clinical judgment.

The needs of administrative assistants and support personnel also change as their roles change. New office technology and new means of communication, documentation, and information dissemination all contribute to a different set of skills for persons in patient support roles. Competence assessment for many of these persons often follows the development of a new skill just acquired for a task to be performed tomorrow. Further, the person doing the assessing may have just learned the new skill, with no opportunity to gain experience with the skill due to rapid change. This situation is an aspect of all competence assessment and development programs.

The judgment or thinking aspect of any role is the most difficult to grasp, because judgments are always made within a certain context. That context or situation involving the patient can never be predicted because of the myriad of unknown variables that are part of any patient care situation. Assessment of thinking or clinical judgment competence remains one the most difficult areas. Later chapters in this text illustrate this further and propose creative models and structures to help staff development specialists with this task.

CHANGING SYSTEMS

As mentioned previously, the settings where patient care is delivered, and the persons providing that care, have changed significantly in the past 5 years and will continue to change.

For instance, administrators in tertiary care settings must figure out how to provide enough routine care to pay for the highly sophisticated and technical care often required in unusual cases. Referrals to these settings are made now because they are the regional (and sometimes only) center at which a certain level or kind of care can be received. For example, a level 1 trauma center delivers a very different service than a level 3 center. Competence assessment and development needs of care providers in these different settings vary, despite the focus on trauma. Although some efforts to standardize competence across various settings have been successful due to standardized courses such as advanced cardiac life support and advanced trauma life support, the limitations of these types of programs are evident: competence varies, based on everyday experience with course content, which may or may not be relevant to the patients commonly served in these settings.

University-affiliated and academically based medical centers with a primary focus on research have a different set of changes to deal with, such as the shift in funds for medical education and training from entitlement programs such as Medicare. Greater competition for limited resources through grant programs also has changed the nature of patient care delivered in academic medical centers. Managed care and an emphasis on primary care received at local levels for most health care problems have also changed referral patterns and outreach efforts.

A return to the notion of community care has also changed systems. The idea of taking care to the patient is certainly not a new one to nursing, but the kind of care nurses and other care providers can take to patients in a variety of communities has changed. Providing high-tech home care for technology-dependent patients has changed the kinds of skills required of these providers, including how they use the resources available to them in the home or field. For instance, care providers in communities have organized care for small groups of infants infected with the AIDS virus who were abandoned at birth. Care providers who work in community settings bring a new set of competence assessment and development needs due to the unique nature of their work and the goals of care.

Systems of care have also changed due to health insurance or the lack of it. The American public is no longer willing to pay through indemnity plans for care received by those less able to pay for their health care. Due to the cost of insurance, many employers are no longer willing to pay the full amount of premiums, so deals are negotiated with insurance companies based on the number of covered persons in a group. Actuarial data about vulnerable populations now serve to raise the potential cost of insurance to employers. The larger the number of healthy persons in a group, the more negotiating power the employer has and the more attractive the employer is to the insurer.

Arrangements and affiliations with other care providers who were considered competition yesterday is common. As mergers and other enterprising arrangements are made to provide care to healthy persons and vulnerable populations, new roles for care providers will continue to emerge. Their competence will need to be assessed and developed to meet the quality expectations of patients and care providers alike.

CHANGING SETTINGS

Competence assessment and development programs are no longer considered solely hospital-based. The tradition of health care provided by nurses in many settings will continue to serve as a legacy for the future. Whom those providers care for in the various settings will also continue to change. The notion of performing certain patient care tasks in a single place has clearly changed, as has who performs those tasks, under what supervision, and in what context.

Nurses and others have moved solidly into the primary care role. Nurses now work with advanced practice nurses to deliver primary care to adults, families, children, women, and other groups. Nurses also work directly with families to assess family caretakers of patients at risk, such as the elderly or those on ventilators or other life-support technology at home.

Other care providers work in partnership with these nurses, bringing their unique therapeutic role or technical tasks to improve patients' health and quality of life. Specialists who provide competence assessment and development services for providers of patient care are well served if they reconsider the whole notion of where care is delivered, by whom, and for what purpose. Advanced technology and cost will continue to complicate this issue.

Some places of service delivery to patients will remain the same; such places include acute care hospitals, ambulatory care settings, extended care facilities, rehabilitation settings, subacute care facilities, homes, hospice programs and sites, and primary care groups. New settings specializing in selected aspects of care as well as new configurations for primary care will also emerge.

Redefining the terms in health care—that is, who does what for whom and at what cost—will continue to be the main challenge for all health care providers and recipients. The common goal—the right care at the right time in the right place by the right provider at the least cost—will be the challenge for staff development specialists. The assessment and development of competence of providers in myriad settings for various patient groups must always be associated with these services to ensure quality care for patients.

FROM NURSING IN-SERVICE TO THEORY-BASED PRACTICE

The tradition of nursing staff development has been a long and rich one, and, as with all things that are growing and evolving, new traditions will continue to form. Some of these traditions provide a solid foundation for the evolution of this field of practice. Is it a field of nursing practice? It all depends on the context of practice. If the practice of the field is limited to nurses providing staff development services for nurses and nursing personnel, it can be viewed as nursing staff development for the purposes of focus, mission, and program outcomes.

The four common roles nurses assume in practice are:

- Clinician
- Educator
- Administrator
- Researcher.

The staff development specialist who is a nurse is functioning in the educator role.

This text is based on everyday practice, and this viewpoint is reflected in the writing and experience of the contributors. What began in my mind as a field of specialized nursing practice has changed. Daily experience taught me that staff development services can be provided by nurses and other care providers who value a patient-centered approach.

This is not a new notion. What is new is the concerted attempt to arrange a collaborative working relationship among persons who share a patient care philosophy that includes the shared goal of competent provision of care. The principles of staff development, as they have been developed within the tradition and view of nursing, can be expanded to be inclusive, rather than exclusive. This text attempts to demonstrate a movement toward inclusivity; thus, one chapter and two stories were contributed by persons who are not nurses.

As the practice of staff development evolves, so too will the experience and titles of its specialists. The nature of the field—that is, a focus on revealing the competence of clinical care providers for assessment and development—will remain the same. Who does it and where it happens will grow.

We have learned about the nature and developing character of this and any specialized field of practice. Without the acknowledgment of this evolutionary and developmental state, the field will not continue to emerge as a viable and necessary component of nursing practice in health care organizations.

In 1996, organizations budgeted $59.8 billion for the continuing formal training of their employees, $13.4 billion more than in 1990. Almost 60 million employees were represented in this report by 150,000 U.S. organizations. Health service industry trainers reported an average total budget of $259,000 (Training Industry Report, 1996). A portion of this is dedicated to the continuing development of clinical care providers such as nurses, therapists, and technicians. Specialists in the field of clinical staff development are responsible for using these resources judiciously in programs designed to assess and develop the competence of staff members, as defined in job and performance expectations of the organization.

Because more than 72% of the dollars go toward the salaries of staff development specialists and support personnel, the practices and procedures used by these specialists are the most significant feature of this work. The manner in which each staff development specialist goes about this task varies. However, over time, consistent practices have emerged that have been successful.

Grounded theory tells us that we can look to our past as well as to current practice to define our future. A rich tradition exists within staff development, and this tradition will be used to define our present practice and form our future.

Traditions

Hospitals and other health care agencies have organized opportunities for nurses to develop their expertise since the time of Nightingale. Her often-quoted statement "Let us never consider ourselves finished nurses" set the stage for the expectation of continued development as a professional practice standard. In 1928, Pfefferkorn discussed issues related to improvement of the nurse in service. Hospitals assigned "in-service education" responsibilities to senior nurses and organized orientations and classes for the nurse "in service." Thus, the term "in-service education" was used for many years to describe this work.

Few papers and books were written to help nurses learn how to provide staff development. Nurses in hospital-based schools of nursing often served in the dual capacity of teaching student and graduate nurses. It was unusual for a nurse to be assigned solely to the continuing development of nurses in service. In the early 1960s, the role began to emerge as nursing became more complex. Senior nurses, sometimes those who could no longer manage the strenuous duties associated with direct care, were assigned to a role called in-service education. Few resources were available to help these nurses with this assignment. Staff development nurses had to rely on their own innate ability to identify the learning needs of nurses and to define methods to meet those needs. These experienced nurses used a problem-solving approach, intrinsic to the nursing process, as a framework to help organize this work. Learning needs were assessed; educational activities were planned, implemented, and evaluated; and practice was re-assessed for improvement and continued learning needs.

Paralleling the development of organized in-service education programs for nurses by nurses, some hospitals and health care agencies organized hospital-wide or comprehensive education programs to develop all staff in all roles using various approaches. These organizing frameworks included human resource development, adult education, and performance instructional technology approaches. Some of these programs and departments were planned, implemented, and administered by nurses; some were developed by others with education, personnel, or health care backgrounds.

Many nurses were assigned or "promoted" to staff development positions because of their good clinical skills. However, there were few support systems and limited coursework to help in this transition from a clinical to management position. In 1974, Tobin, Yoder-Wise, and Hull made a significant contribution to the field with their textbook *The Process of Nursing Staff Development: Components for Change*. This text and the later 1979 edition defined the field of practice until the early 1980s.

The ANA, through the work of the Council of Professional Nursing Education and Development, continues the tradition of publication and promulgation of standards for staff development begun in 1976 with the pamphlet *Guidelines for Nursing Staff Development* (ANA, 1976). Their 1994 publication *Standards for Nursing Professional Development: Continuing Education and Staff Development* is used by nurses and others in this field of practice as a reference to help organize and deliver staff development services.

Professional associations such as the American Physical Therapy Association and the American Respiratory Therapy Association continue to develop and promulgate standards and guidelines that define competence for their clinical care providers; these serve as curricula for many organizations' staff development programs. Specialty clinical nursing organizations such as the Association of Women's Health, Obstetric and Neonatal Nurses, the American Association of Critical Care Nurses, the Oncology Nursing Society, and the Association of Operating Room Nurses also develop and promote standards and guidelines that describe competencies for nurses who practice these specialties.

Regulatory bodies recognize the need for an organized staff development program. In 1978, the Joint Commission on Accreditation of Hospitals, as it was then known, required that a position be established for overseeing and coordinating staff development activities such as orientation and in-service education. Although a dedicated position is no longer required, the leaders of health care organizations are held accountable for providing an organized and systematic staff development program to assess and develop competence. Most facilities with staffs greater than 100 assign someone to the role of staff development on at least a part-time basis. Many health departments responsible for licensing health care organizations also review staff development activities to determine if organizations are meeting selected standards and criteria.

Many nurses have raised superb questions and issues to help staff development specialists consider how best to achieve their goals within their specific work settings. For example, O'Connor (1986) defined the following issues that must be addressed by nursing staff development specialists:

1. Who is responsible for staff development? And who benefits?
2. How can participation in staff development activities be promoted?
3. What should be the content of staff development?
4. How can adult learning principles be applied to the design of staff development offerings?
5. How can the educator ensure that staff development offerings are relevant, with applicability to the professional lives of participants?
6. What are the best teaching strategies for staff development?
7. What measures should be used to demonstrate the effectiveness of the staff development program?
8. How can the staff development program most efficiently use limited resources?
9. How can quality in staff development programming be ensured?
10. Does staff development make a difference?

These questions provide a sound basis for the design of a clinical staff development program. The answers to some of these questions are still emerging; others have definitive responses, to be discussed later in this text.

Bille (1982), using a systems approach to nursing staff development, wrote that staff development is an integral component of every organization, and expanded the list of components advocated by Tobin et al. Bille further argued that staff development is only one component of the total organization and does not exist in a vacuum, nor can it solve all the ills of the organization. In looking at staff development within the organization, Bille advocated using a systems approach that looks at all parts and structures in an organization and the way they relate to organizational goals or outcomes. He defined three basic components of staff development, using a classic systems approach to job performance:

- Inputs: entry staff behavior, level of education, and prior experience
- Throughputs: orientation, policies, procedures, and managerial direction
- Outputs: the final staff behavior and quality patient care.

This approach to portraying how nursing staff development fits into the larger scheme of organizational behavior and development also serves as a sound basis to assist the staff development specialist with program planning and design. Recent concerns with outcomes measurement have created an opportunity for staff development specialists to return to a systems approach to define anticipated outputs or outcomes for measurement.

In the past, staff development specialists often turned to other fields such as adult education, human resources development, instructional technology, and organization development for help in designing staff development programs. These activities were practical and rational, but they required neophyte staff development nurses and clinicians to adapt this information to the unique setting of clinical staff development in the health care organization.

Staff development nurses sought out staff development nurses in other organizations and created formal and informal networks to help each other learn and adapt to this emerging role. As more nurses began to identify with the staff development role, the need to develop this field of practice became increasingly recognized. Professional groups of care providers formed special-interest groups or networks for those who provided training, education, and other staff development services.

The 1980s brought several significant contributions to the development of the field, including:

● Publication of several texts specific to nursing staff development
● Publication of the *Journal of Nursing Staff Development*
● Recognition of the specialty by the addition of the words "staff development" to the ANA's Council on Continuing Education and Staff Development
● Formation of the National Nursing Staff Development Organization.

Nurses now seek out positions in staff development and look for graduate programs to help them prepare for this role. Indeed, several of the first tasks of the newly formed National Nursing Staff Development Organization were to:

● Identify graduate programs that included curricula that would enhance the practice skills of the staff development specialist
● Explore the feasibility of a certification process for staff development specialists
● Provide continuing education and networking opportunities for nurses engaged in this field.

Experienced practitioners in this field generally agree that a graduate degree is appropriate for this field of practice, but few graduate programs exist to prepare clinicians specifically for this role as an educator and manager. Despite this, nurses and other clinical care providers have sought the requisite coursework and knowledge to help them meet the challenges of this changing and evolving role. Indeed, since it first offered a certification examination that recognized the practice in 1992, the ANA has certified 2078 nurses as generalists in nursing continuing education and staff development. Further, the ANA and the National Nursing Staff Development Organization have formed a task force to examine the notion of staff development as an advanced practice field.

Recent Experiences

As a field of health care practice, staff development is dynamic, diverse, and developing. The commitment of nurses and other clinical care providers to helping people become independent and cope with their health is the essence of a clinical practice. The continuing development of nurses and other clinicians as they attempt to achieve the right level of involvement with a patient is the specific assignment of the clinical staff development specialist. To attenuate that assignment with responsibilities to many departments is to weaken the effectiveness of the specialist. Conversely, it is appropriate to assign nurses and other clinicians to the staff development responsibilities of departments with a clinical focus.

Collaboration across disciplines to plan a comprehensive staff development program is required for the efficient and effective use of scarce resources. For example, it makes no sense to assess competence related to universal precautions using many different knowledge tests, because the principles are the same. What requires assessment is the application of these principles in the clinical settings by all care providers. The savvy staff development specialist organizes this form of competence assessment activity efficiently to meet myriad regulatory and quality monitoring needs. Data gathered through competence assessment activities are used both to demonstrate compliance and to create continued competence development activities. This is the dynamic nature of clinical staff development.

Any organization's approach to the development of its human resources should include clearly communicated expectations by the administration about the role of staff development professionals and the scope of responsibilities assigned to them. In this regard, the recruitment and retention of knowledgeable workers, such as clinical staff development specialists, should include the recognition that some clinicians choose to fulfill their career aspirations through a staff development role.

The staffing of health care organizations will continue to challenge administrators. How many clinical staff development specialists are needed? Is there a ratio of specialists to the number of patients served or the clinical care providers needing development? When clinical staff development providers are organized to provide services across several settings in the same system, what efficiencies are gained? What is the right mix of staffing for this level of complexity? Some anecdotal information exists and is examined at convention and conference presentations and in the literature, but the search for answers to these questions continues. What is known is that with the myriad talents and creativity of nurses and health care professionals available to the health care industry, all should be able to find fulfillment and satisfaction in the many roles needed to continue to improve patient care services.

To be most effective and able to influence the improvement of patient care, clinical staff development departments or programs should be organized within a clinical patient care department. The leader of the department should hold an advanced degree in nursing, adult education, or a health care-related field. The leader should answer directly to the top executive over most or all of the clinical operations. In large organizations, the leader of the staff development department should be in a line position and should hold equal title and rank to the operational leaders of the various divisions within other clinical departments. Only within such a structure can the staff development leader have access to key information and participate in making essential clinical practice decisions. This information is vital if a staff development program is to be responsive to the changing practice expectations of the organization's clinical leaders.

A successful practice model for clinical staff development is the consultative approach. Ulschak and SnowAntle (1990a) believe this approach improves costs and services and fosters collaboration and cooperation. Assuming that an organization is willing to forego traditional "turf" issues, this model is a powerful organizational development tactic that can enhance effectiveness. With more than 8 million health care workers and 2 million nurses, the competence of all workers can be enhanced through improved collaboration and cooperation skills.

Also of note is the role of staff development within career development and promotion programs. Often called clinical ladder programs, staff development specialists are expected to participate in the design, implementation, and administration of these programs. Although many clinical ladder programs as we knew them in the 1980s are being revised or dismantled, the role and activities of staff development specialists enhance these programs. Clinical ladder programs have used the staff development process to enhance career options for professional nurses. They often use skill acquisition and recognition strategies to reward and engage nurses in their continuing development. Staff development specialists should be intimately involved with career development and promotion programs. New approaches are needed to expand clinical advancement programs in the changing health care environment; a detailed discussion of these programs can be found on pp. 311–313.

Specialists in clinical staff development have gained perspective and continue to define the body of knowledge, the best practices, and the way of knowing about the field. Sovie

(1983) described three stages of professional career development in nursing that have applicability to clinical staff development:

- Professional identification, in which persons become oriented toward the field
- Professional maturation, in which the potential for development and expansion of competencies is recognized
- Professional mastery, in which the potential is realized.

At present, many staff development specialists are in the stage of professional maturation. As the field of nursing staff development continues to be defined by practitioners and others, nurses will readily recognize the essential contribution of staff development activities to the professional development of individual nurses and nursing as a whole.

The issue of staff development as a noun, verb, or adjective is of concern as the field attempts to define itself. Specifically, the misuse of the term "in-service education" causes confusion. Phrases such as "in-servicing of staff" and "in-serviced clinicians" are bewildering. Clear, concise, and accepted use of terms is essential to the field, and the appropriate use of these terms by staff development specialists is a hallmark of professional practice.

Abruzzese (1996) made a significant contribution to nursing staff development with her textbook that featured strategies for success. She provided strategies to help staff development educators excel in the crucial aspects of their teaching and learning activities, and experts in nursing staff development from various settings provided practical guidelines for novice and experienced staff development educators in the areas of foundation, management, process, and professional issues.

Alspach (1995) wrote a textbook expanding the process of nursing staff development within an adult education framework, as well as a text (1996) about competence assessment. Several other titles on staff development have been published by National Nursing Staff Development Organization.

Swansburg (1994) used a human resource development and administrative approach to staff development. A key element in all of these newer developments in the field is that they apply strategies and methods to more than just nurses and nursing personnel; all acknowledge that structures and personnel in staff development are changing and expanding to include others.

The contributions of these authors and specialists are significant and have helped to develop this practice discipline. As with most emerging disciplines, various theories, frameworks, and concepts are blended to create some semblance of organization in the field. Those mentioned above and others will continue to help clinicians define the uniqueness of clinical staff development within a framework of common themes. Understanding of clinical staff development will grow as it is practiced.

Theories in Use

This new understanding of staff development of clinical care providers continues to blend concepts from other theories. In some clinical staff development programs, a theory serves as an organizing framework; in others, selected concepts from the following theories and frameworks serve as the basis.

The theories and beliefs that underlie the clinical staff development model include:

- Change
- Systems
- Roles
- Competency-based education
- Adult learning

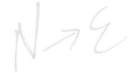

- Adult development
- Human resources development
- Organization development
- Interaction
- Contingency
- Quality management.

Like any new model, this one requires testing and validation. It is hoped that this offering may also provide incentive and opportunity for the processes required by an evolving discipline. Chapter 3 expands these thoughts and addresses progress in staff development research and evaluation.

The issues of who we are and what we do have been answered. Although continued research is needed to refine these definitions and models, the outcome of staff development activities is what counts. Hence, the emphasis in this text is on competence as the outcome of organized clinical staff development programs.

Patients continue to speak out about what is important to them. For everyday health problems, they want a primary provider who is approachable, affable, convenient, and competent. Although managed care programs attempt to direct patients toward the use of primary providers as gatekeepers, Americans continue to demand a choice and want to continue to see the same provider, often their previously established one.

The 35 million uninsured Americans are also saying something when they use emergency rooms for their primary health care. New systems have been and will continue to be developed to care for vulnerable populations. Use of these systems will be driven by cost and the availability of various providers. Never before has there been such an opportunity for developing efficient and effective collaborative care arrangements. Nurses and other health care professionals are moving into the arena of primary care in innovative ways as the system continues to be re-engineered.

CRAFTING STAFF DEVELOPMENT PRACTICE

Many of the trends predicted by Naisbett and Aburdene (1990) in *Megatrends 2000* have been realized. They include:

- A global economic boom in the 1990s
- Renaissance of the arts
- Emergence of free-market socialism
- Global lifestyles and cultural nationalism
- Privatization of the welfare state
- Rise of the Pacific Rim
- Women in leadership
- The age of biology
- Religious revival of third millennium
- Triumph of the individual.

These trends are relevant to clinical staff development specialists, who are interested in societal change and how populations of patients affect and are affected by these trends. Recent welfare reforms will create changes in health care access, cost, and quality. Change-oriented leadership and women in leadership roles create different challenges and opportunities for patients and providers. Ensuring competence in new areas of technology and decision making will require the participation of staff development specialists.

New leadership methods will require people to learn to coach and inspire others and gain patients' commitment to participate in their health care. As Naisbett and Aburdene wrote, "the dominant principle of the organization has shifted, from management in order to control an enterprise to leadership in order to bring out the best in people and to respond quickly to change" (p. 218). Patients are also responding to that change with new empowerment, new thinking skills, and new health care problems to manage.

Women will have an important role in all future initiatives because they have reached a critical mass in virtually all professions. Nursing's tradition of helping people and its experience in coping with stress and illness will play a significant role in helping the health care system celebrate the human spirit, and nursing staff development programs will play a clear role for the future. This role will focus on helping nurses realize and achieve new levels of caring using both technology and the human spirit to guide the healing and coping processes.

Trends in health care education were analyzed by Ulschak and SnowAntle (1990b). Their key issues included:

- Shortage of providers
- Financial stability
- Management and supervisory training
- Flexibility and creativity
- Effective use of resources
- Retention
- Service orientation
- Aging population
- Need for return on investment for education
- Increased acuity of patient conditions
- Uninsured and indigent patients
- Total organizational development
- Technological advancements
- Continued rapid change.

They set out five requirements for planners:

1. To plan for a future where there will be a shortage of health care professionals in hospitals as they migrate to other service settings
2. To plan for ongoing turbulence
3. To approach education as a business, with a clear mission and objectives that will make a difference in the life of the organization
4. To share key trends with top administrators and explore ways education can assist with development
5. To attend to personal needs to avoid burnout and manage work to maintain optimal energy.

Ulschak in 1988 advocated adopting new thoughts about the process of change. He used a metaphor from a martial-arts exercise: to take as a given that staff development will be knocked off center, and thus to maintain as a goal the ability to recenter as quickly as possible. He argued that staff development specialists have been knocked off balance by the changes in health care delivery brought about by changes in health care financing. He advised them to keep the ongoing goal of learning to refocus and recenter, with the expectation of being knocked off balance on an ongoing basis. This advice still has merit in today's continuously changing environments.

Role shifts as organizations change to respond to new imperatives are inevitable. The successful clinical staff development specialist will seek new roles and make transitions to new expectations.

Despite the need to advance to new roles in response to organizational change, there is a need for a consistent title for persons who serve in a staff development specialist capacity. Titles of nurses and others engaged in staff development practice abound. Some samples are:

- Staff development specialist
- Staff development coordinator
- Education specialist
- Instructor
- Nurse educator
- Clinical educator.

One title must be chosen to communicate the role and services of staff development. The advantages of one title are:

- A common bond among specialists
- Identification of the role by consumers
- Clearer expectations of the role
- Common understanding of services provided by the role
- Opportunity to change perceptions about staff development by upgrading titles, qualifications, and services.

Disadvantages of using many titles include the inability of nurses and others to understand and use the resources available to them because of role confusion. If a title sounds powerless and ill defined, the organization may fail to appreciate the contribution the clinician makes; this could lead to cuts in these services.

Staff development personnel, with the assistance of their leader, must define and communicate the services, expectations, and limitations of the role. This is essential to the success of any staff development effort.

The preferred title of the clinical staff development role is specialist, and we will use it throughout this text. This term imparts authority, mastery, expertise, and an expected level of professionalism. Specialists are dedicated to a particular branch of study and practice. The distinguishing mark of the staff development specialist is the commitment to the continued professional development of clinical care providers, using strategies, tools, and skills unique to the field. The specialist also assumes the responsibility to continue to transform and refine the role and the field through systematic inquiry. The title "specialist" communicates to consumers these essential components and characteristics. With an understanding of the specialized nature of the field, more clinical care providers will benefit from the distinctive skills of the staff development specialist.

Clinical staff development specialists with licensure or certification in clinical disciplines should consider including those designations on their name tags, badges, and signs, displayed prominently for patients to see. These designations may include, among many others, RN, RPT (registered physical therapist), OTR (occupational therapist registered), LCSW (licensed clinical social worker), RRT (registered respiratory therapist).

The transition to new titles often provides an opportunity for staff development specialists to clarify and communicate new roles that are responsive to the changing organization. Professional clinicians of today have increasing autonomy, and the need to support them in their need for continued development is evident. Having a person specifically dedicated to clinical patient care and its development through competent care providers will make a vital contribution to patient care.

CLINICAL STAFF DEVELOPMENT TODAY

Some accepted definitions of nursing staff development can be expanded to include other clinical areas. The ANA (1994) defined staff development as including both formal and informal learning opportunities to help persons perform competently in fulfillment of role expectations within a specific agency. Resources both within and outside the agency would be used in this process.

We propose a new definition, given the current emphasis on efficiency, quality, and effectiveness:

> Clinical staff development is the systematic organization of prescribed assessment and development activities to provide data about the competence status and outcomes of health care providers in a designated health care setting to achieve shared patient care and quality goals.

Key concepts in this definition include the role of clinical staff development in the achievement of organizational goals. All staff development activities must be linked in some way to organizational goals. Other key concepts include the activities of assessing and developing clinical competencies. Activities must be related to knowledge, and skills related to performance expectations. To relate staff development activities to performance expectations requires the assessment of competence to plan for the continued development of staff. The goal and outcome of all staff development activity is competence—hence the emphasis on the assessment and development of competence.

Earlier, maintenance activities were suggested for some nursing skills and knowledge, but present thought excludes maintenance activities per se, including them in either assessment or development. For example, it was previously thought that a certain skill level in topics such as CPR, fire safety, patient safety, employee safety, universal precautions, and blood-borne pathogens standards requiring common knowledge needed to be maintained. This is still true, but now the requisite level of knowledge or skills is routinely assessed. Development of new knowledge and skills related to these and other topics is required as new science and technology becomes available. Changing health care needs, changing technologies, changing clinical practice patterns, and changing expectations will also dictate the form that competence assessment and development activities will take in comprehensive staff development programs. Figure 1 illustrates a conceptual model of this staff development program.

This definition of clinical staff development is grounded in education and the needs of organizations for continued response to changing health care technologies and health care needs of communities and patients. In addition, the future will also require staff development specialists to help nurses and other clinical care providers make increasingly sophisticated judgments about which patients receive what kind of care, under what circumstances, and with what expected outcomes.

The evolution of clinical staff development will depend on the continued development of the persons dedicated to this role. Clinical staff development specialists are frequently advanced or placed in these roles based on their strong clinical skills and a desire to teach. It is up to each specialist to seek education and self-development in this field. Initiative in this area is a characteristic of successful clinical staff development specialists.

Some nurses and other clinicians specifically seek roles in this specialized field of practice. Any clinician entering this field should recognize the need to accumulate new experiences and learning in areas different from clinical practice. A development model for the new clinical staff development specialist is discussed in Chapter 3, in which the Dreyfus (1986) model of skill acquisition is used as a framework to help the novice

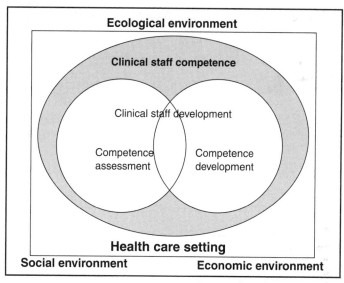

FIGURE 1-1. Clinical staff development model. (Copyright Karen Kelly-Thomas, 1997.)

clinical staff development specialist learn about and understand the characteristics of expertise development.

THE FUTURE OF CLINICAL STAFF DEVELOPMENT

There are six major priorities for the future of staff development programs in health care organizations.

The first goal is to agree on the name of this kind of practice. We suggest clinical staff development, but other titles will continue to emerge, such as performance improvement, research and development, and professional development. Efforts to reach consensus about a name for this important work in health care should continue. Otherwise, consumers and patients will continue to be confused about the services that staff development provides toward quality patient care outcomes.

Second, the role of the clinical staff development specialist should be communicated. Regardless of their title, clinicians providing staff development are responsible for defining their role and communicating it to the organization. Similar but distinct roles must also be differentiated. The role of clinical specialist is a complementary one to staff development, but it is not the same. Balancing the clinical component of the staff development specialist role with the expectation of managing a case load of patients in some way is an expectation. The clinical competence of the staff development specialist must also be defined and developed. This balance can be defined through assigned areas of responsibility and a clear expectation in job descriptions and performance standards regarding the percentage of time spent in clinical practice and the scope of that clinical practice.

The third goal is continued definition of the field, what it includes and what it does not. Tobin et al. (1979) defined the components of the field as orientation, in-service education, continuing education, leadership development, skills training, and incidental learning. Others have added components such as competency assessment, clinical affiliations, patient education, career counseling, and health and wellness education. Central to any staff development program is the assessment and development of clinical staff competence. The resources that are necessary to achieve defined outcomes must also continue to be examined. The planning and design features of staff development are the same as for any learning activity, regardless of the adjectives used to define the education. A mechanism for a rational and reasonable accreditation process of the staff development program is needed.

Fourth, staff development programs should be organized to meet the future needs of patients in our ever-changing health care system. Puetz's 1989 editorial about a report by the American Society for Training and Development is still relevant today. This report discussed 13 essential skills for the workplace. The seven directly relevant to clinical staff development are:

- Knowing how to learn
- Listening
- Speaking
- Creative thinking
- Problem solving
- Organizational effectiveness
- Leadership.

Integrating these basic skills into clinical staff development programs will help prepare clinical care providers for the continuous challenges of providing care in a constrained health care economy with rapid knowledge obsolescence. Staff development specialists must serve as catalysts for acquiring these and other skills.

The fifth goal is to work hard to build bridges to all clinical disciplines, with a shared vision and focus on patient care. Mutual goals and contributions to patient care should be acknowledged and shared or common skills identified. This work is enhanced in health care delivery systems that have adopted new strategies that re-engineer care, reform corporate and organizational systems, and return to a mission of care that has patient needs as the core. Working on teams, which are the fundamental re-engineering work unit, the clinical staff development specialist creates new opportunities to assess and develop competence of care providers. Deciding what competencies are performed by whom in what context generate the core of staff development programs in restructured and innovative systems.

Finally, serious research should be conducted about the outcome of staff development activities. This evaluation component is essential for any program designed to produce change in behavior and performance. Formulas, strategies, and approaches are needed to strengthen the case for the value and actual return on investment. If the outcome of a quality clinical staff development program is competent care providers who consistently deliver quality patient care, how can we demonstrate this? What measurement should be used? What mixture of clinical staff development specialists produce the best outcomes? And what specific staff development strategies produce the best outcome at the least cost? These questions and many others related to outcomes must be answered to confirm the belief that staff development makes a difference in patient care. Chapters 4 and 8 explore this goal further.

The future depends on the evolving competencies of today's staff development specialists. Challenge and opportunity will help this work.

New Mental Model

The momentous changes discussed in this chapter have created a new "mental model": many clinicians joined in a collaborative effort to assess and develop the competence of care providers for the purpose of continuously improving care. These clinicians will continue to contribute to the development of many nurses, joined by therapists and technicians, with a mutual interest and focus on the quality of clinical practice and outcome of the care provided.

A new clinical staff development model is shown in Figure 1. Although the model will continue to evolve with use and change, it represents what staff development in health care organizations is all about today. Viewed within systems thinking concepts (Senge et al., 1994), two new definitions are proposed:

1. A *competence assessment system* is a management tool that samples an array of competencies that are meaningful to the organization using a variety of strategies to provide data about the overall capacity of the clinical staff to provide quality patient care.
2. A *competence development system* is an organized program planned to cultivate, enhance, and produce competent providers of health care services capable of improving personal job performance and quality care outcomes.

These concepts and the new model are discussed further in Chapters 2 and 3.

A final word for both the novice and experienced staff development specialist is warranted within the context of this change. Waldrop (1992) elegantly presented compelling reasons for continued evolution. He described the work at the Santa Fe Institute, a "think tank" observing common patterns across theory development in diverse disciplines such as biology, mathematics, artificial intelligence, and economics. The scientists there propose complexity theory as one way to understand changing systems. Today's systems are complex, capable of undergoing spontaneous self-organization, and adaptive. The unique feature is their seemingly innate ability to bring order and chaos into a distinct kind of balance, called the "edge of chaos." This is a place where components never quite lock into place, nor do they spin off into turbulence; rather, system components achieve a new but temporary sense of balance on the edge of chaos. Complexity theory helps explain the need for change to survive. These systems—biological, economic, intelligence, health care, and others—have demonstrated the maxim of change or die.

Summary

This chapter examined the growth and history of nursing staff development as a specialized field of practice. The potential for expansion of this nursing practice field was explored, and conclusions about the inclusion of other clinical care providers were drawn. Change served as the organizing framework to survey the environment, needs, systems, and settings. The history and tradition of nursing staff development were used to provide strength to the proposal of including others in staff development activities for the common goal of quality patient care. With an focus on patient care and what patients want, a model for developing skills in clinical staff development using the novice-to-expert skill-acquisition model was suggested. A new mental model with an emphasis on two primary staff development activities, assessment and development, was proposed as an archetype to generate competent nurses and clinical care providers.

Staff Development: Growth in Practice, or How I Learned to Stop Worrying!

JANICE A. WARD

As I read this chapter, several words and themes became apparent—change, environment, technology, patients, nurses, and staff development. Reflecting on these words, I realize how they have shaped and will continue to shape the practice of staff development.

First, staff development. Whether it is nursing staff development, human resources development, education and development, it is in every organization and a part of everyone's job. It may be an orientation program, an in-service on a new piece of equipment, a secretary explaining the complexities of a word processing program, an interdisciplinary continuing education program, or a consultation on how to develop an educational program. It is seen everyday, in many places. It has always been there, sometimes not named, but present nonetheless. It will continue to be present, even if it is not titled staff development. We must have the vision and the courage to continue to bring staff development to the forefront and remind ourselves, and those we work with, of its importance to the organization and ultimately to those for whom the organization provides care.

Patients and nurses are words used every day by each one of us. Patients are the indirect recipients of our work in staff development, and we cannot lose sight of this fact. The programs and services that staff development provides do affect patient care. What we have not done is to provide proof of that link. We often say that we know and just feel that what we do affects patient care, but we cannot provide concrete data for ourselves and others. This continues to be a major challenge, and we must begin to provide this information. This data will validate what we have known all along, that staff development does make a difference.

There are many "customers" in today's organization. Our future will be more secure as we provide services and programs to more and varied clients, both inside and outside the organization. We must think beyond the walls of our offices and buildings and not let our geographic location limit our practice.

For most of us, nurses are our primary clients and nursing is our own basic educational background. Nurses are still providing care, but in settings different from what many of us were accustomed to. As nursing is changing, so is staff development. What is difficult for many nurses to accept—delegation of patient care, new roles and responsibilities—is also difficult for staff development personnel. Often we must help nursing staff with the changes before we have come to terms with them ourselves. We are often caught in a conflict between our job and our philosophical and educational background. As when caring for patients, however, we must place our own concerns second and proceed to help the nursing staff.

However, we cannot neglect ourselves, or our practice will begin to suffer. We must begin to support each other with these conflicts. Support from peers, if only as a sounding board, is needed as we continue to provide staff development.

Technology was instrumental in the formation of the staff development role. Often expert clinical practitioners were asked to present information (in-services) to others on the use of new equipment or the development of new skills—for instance, the interpretation of arrhythmias. Today new technology and the acquisition of new skills continue to influence our practice. However, the challenges are now how to use technology to teach or evaluate the knowledge and skills of nurses, technicians, managers, and indirect caregivers and how to use technology in our own practice. Video conferencing, the Internet, satellite feeds, and videotapes are only a few examples of how technology will expand staff development outside the walls of the organization.

The environment in which most of us practice staff development has changed as health care and in turn nursing have changed. Staff development can be practiced in acute settings and long-term care, ambulatory and home care, rehabilitation and subacute care, a physician's office, and a school of nursing—indeed, any setting where patients and families receive health care or where health care professionals work or are educated. The arenas for the practice of staff development are limited only by our imagination. As health care changes, so will staff development. We must be proactive in identifying where and when we will practice.

Change cannot be ignored or wished away. It has always been present and will continue to influence us. We cannot, as nurses and as staff development professionals, return to the "good old days." We must to face the change and the problems it brings; we must turn these problems into opportunities. We cannot be in control of everything that happens to us, but we can be in control of how we respond. For us and staff development to survive and flourish, we must strive to develop new work philosophies and habits. Pritchett (1994) advised us to adopt the following ground rules:

- Become a quick-change artist.
- Commit fully to your job.
- Speed up.
- Accept ambiguity and uncertainty.
- Behave like you're in business for yourself.
- Stay in school.
- Hold yourself accountable for outcomes.
- Add value.
- See yourself as a service center.
- Manage your own morale.
- Practice *kaizen* (quality improvement).
- Be a fixer, not a finger-pointer.
- Alter your expectations.

Acquiring these habits and making the resulting changes in our basic philosophy are not easily or quickly accomplished but are necessary if staff development is to continue.

REFERENCES

Abruzzese, R. S. (1996). *Nursing staff development: Strategies for success.* St. Louis: Mosby.

Alspach, J. G. (1995). *The educational process in nursing staff development.* St. Louis: Mosby.

Alspach, J. G. (1996). *Designing competency assessment programs: Handbook for nursing and health-related professions.* Pensacola, FL: National Nursing Staff Development Organization.

American Nurses Association. (1976). *Guidelines for nursing staff development.* Kansas City: Author.

American Nurses Association. (1994). *Standards for nursing professional development: Continuing education and development.* Washington, DC: Author.

Bille, D. A. (1982). *Staff development: A systems approach.* Thorofare, NJ: Slack.

Blancett, S. S., & Flarey, D. L. (1995). *Reengineering nursing and health care: The handbook for organizational transformation.* Gaithersburg, MD: Aspen.

Dreyfus, H. L., & Dreyfus, S. E. (1986). *Mind over machine.* New York: Macmillan.

Finocchio, L. J., Dower, C. M., McMahon, R., Gragola, C. M., & the Taskforce on Health Care Workforce Regulation. *Reforming health care workforce regulation: Policy considerations for the 21st century.* San Francisco: Per Health Professions Commission, December 1995.

Health Resources and Services Administration. *National sample survey of registered nurses, March 1996.* Rockville, MD: US Department of Health and Human Services, Bureau of Health Professions, Division of Nursing, 1997.

Lamm, R. D. (1996). The coming dislocation in the health professions. *Healthcare Forum Journal,* Jan/Feb, 58–62.

Naisbett, J., & Aburdene, P. (1990). *Megatrends 2000: Ten new directions for the 1990s.* New York: Morrow.

National Center for Health Statistics. *Health, United States, 1995.* Hyattsville, MD: Public Health Service, Table 75 (p. 188), 1996.

Nightingale, F. (1859/1946). *Notes on nursing: What it is, and what it is not.* Philadelphia: Edward Stern & Co.

O'Connor, A. B. (1986). *Nursing staff development and continuing education.* Boston: Little, Brown.

Pfefferkorn, B. (1928). Improvement of the nurse in service: An historical review. *American Journal of Nursing, 28,* 700.

Pritchett, P. (1994). *The employee handbook of new work habits for a radically changing world: 13 ground rules for job success in the information age.* Dallas: Pritchett & Associates, Inc.

Prospective Payment Assessment Commission. *Medicare and the American health care system: Report to Congress, June 1996.* Washington, DC: Author.

Puetz, B. (1989). Preparing tomorrow's workers today [editorial]. *Journal of Nursing Staff Development, 5*(5), 209.

Senge, P. M., Roberts, C., Ross, R. B., Smith, B. J., & Kleiner, A. (1994). *The fifth discipline fieldbook.* New York: Doubleday.

Sovie, M. (1983). Fostering professional nursing careers in hospitals: The role of nursing staff development (Part 2). *Nurse Educator, 8*(1), 15–18.

Styles, M. M. (1992). Nightingale: The enduring symbol. In F. Nightingale, (Ed.), *Notes on Nursing: What it is, and what it is not.* (commemorative ed., pp. 72–75). Philadelphia: Lippincott.

Swansburg, R. C. (1994). *Nursing staff development.* Boston: Jones & Bartlett.

Tobin, H. M., Yoder Wise, P. S., & Hull, P. K. (1979). *The process of nursing staff development: Components for change* (2nd ed.). St. Louis: Mosby.

Training Industry Report (1996). *Training, 33*(10), 37–79.

Ulschak, F. L., & SnowAntle, S. M. (1990a). *Consultation skills for health care professionals.* San Francisco: Jossey-Bass.

Ulschak, F. L., & SnowAntle, S. (1990b). A glance at the future: A Delphi study of trends affecting health care education. *Journal of Healthcare Education and Training, 5*(1), 3–6.

Ulschak, F. L. (1988). *Creating the future of health care education.* Chicago: American Hospital Association.

United States Census Bureau (March 21, 1997). *POPClock Projection.* http://www.census.gov/cgi-bin/popclock

Waldrop, M. M. (1992). *Complexity: The emerging science at the edge of order and chaos.* New York: Simon & Schuster.

BIBLIOGRAPHY

Benner, P. (1984). *From novice to expert: Excellence and power in clinical nursing practice.* Menlo Park, California: Addison-Wesley.

Brunt, B. A. (1988). Continuing education and megatrends. *Journal of Nursing Staff Development, 4*(4), 174–178.

2

Structure and Process: New Models of Nursing and Clinical Staff Development

BARBARA BRUNT

Staff development departments provide a variety of services and functions in a very diverse array of settings. This chapter describes the role of belief systems, philosophy, vision, mission, and goals in determining the best structure for staff development. Educational structures and organizational structures are differentiated, with examples of each type of structure given. Examples of integrative activities, roles, and credentials of educators and administrators are also discussed. Processes of staff development include program planning and service delivery mechanisms. However, regardless of the structure and processes of staff development, the focus must be on outcomes, so ways to define, measure, and report outcomes are included.

BELIEF SYSTEMS

Belief systems must be analyzed before we can examine the structure and processes of staff development. Some of the basic beliefs of the ANA (1994) relating to continued professional development, which includes staff development, are:

- Professional development needs of nurses are influenced by many factors. Some of these include accountability for one's own practice, knowledgeable consumers, changing health care delivery systems, advances in nursing practice, and technological advances, as well as political, socioeconomic, and legislative factors that influence nursing and health care.
- Lifelong learning is essential to maintain and increase competence in nursing practice.
- Many educational options are needed to meet the diverse needs of the nursing population.
- Ongoing evaluation of structure, process, and outcomes is essential to maintain and enhance the quality and cost-effectiveness of health care.
- The practice of nursing continuing education and staff development is guided by principles of ethics.

Competence

O'Brien (1995) emphasized the role of competence and stated that the development of able, proficient, and self-renewing human resources affects the success of every system and process within the organization. Staff development merges personal fulfillment with organizational purposes for comprehensive organizational development. It is the development through educational processes of all employees of the organization to their highest level of competence in all dimensions of the organization (p. 149).

Kelly (1992) introduced a model of competence development as a framework for basic beliefs related to clinical and nursing staff development. She defined staff development as:

> A field of nursing practice that describes the organized program and process assigned the responsibility for assessing, maintaining, and developing nurses' competence, as defined by the employing agency, most often using learning activities such as orientation, in-service education, continuing education, leadership development, and skills training, and most often occurring within health care organizations and agencies. (p. 31)

Figure 1-1 in Chapter 1 shows a new schematic of nursing staff development that incorporates the idea of competence within a health care organization developed further by Kelly (1998). The primary processes were defined by Kelly (1992) as:

ASSESSING COMPETENCE   Processes and programs designed to measure and evaluate the competence of nurses in relation to expected performance standards

DEVELOPING COMPETENCE   Processes and programs designed to cultivate, generate, and extend the competence of nurses related to expectations and performance standards new to the person or new to the organization (p. 31).

The new model removes "maintaining competence" as an element and assumes that those processes and programs are included within competence assessment and competence development. The notion of maintenance is too static in today's dynamic health care environment. Assessment programs and processes yield data about current competence.

Philosophy

Factors influencing staff development must be considered when developing or revising a philosophy statement. In 1994 the ANA developed a model for nursing professional development that displays the factors influencing nurses' professional development (Fig. 2-1). These factors are not limited to nurses but also apply to the professional development

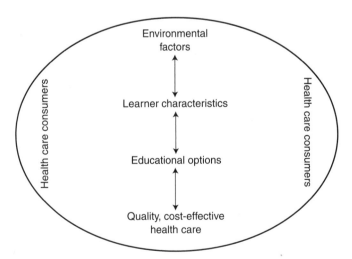

FIGURE 2-1.   Professional development of nurses and clinicians.

of other personnel. Some environmental factors are changing client demographics and cultural backgrounds, changing health care delivery systems, the growing body of knowledge, mandated requirements, health care consumers, organizational needs, and professional development goals. Characteristics of learners include their learning style, education, experience, cultural background, and motivation. Educational options include both formal means (*e.g.*, academics, continuing education, staff development, and research) and the informal means of consultation, professional reading, and other self-directed activities. All of these factors relate directly or indirectly to the competence of health care providers providing services to the health care consumer, which contributes to quality, cost-effective health care for all members of society.

The philosophy statement should reflect the beliefs and value of educational services and should:

- Be grounded in organizational beliefs and norms
- Address the value of knowledge as a strategic resource
- Address the need for lifelong learning
- Address globally the manner in which services and products are provided
- Provide guidance for practice, including decision making, in accomplishing education services (American Society for Health Care Education and Training [ASHET], 1994, pp. 1–2).

Svenson and Rinderer (1992) liken the philosophy statement to a creed. It can hang on the wall to remind everyone of the department's principles when it is time to make tough decisions. Questions that should be considered when developing a philosophy statement could include:

1. Why is the organization interested in staff development?
2. What do we expect staff development to accomplish?
3. What are staff development's limitations?
4. What responsibility is expected of each employee?
5. What responsibility does the organization assume?
6. What is generally expected of supervisors and managers?
7. What is expected of the staff development department?
8. Is staff development an investment or an expense?
9. Do we eagerly embrace the value of continual learning and improvement or learn only when we can prove it is necessary? (pp. 137–139)

Cody (1996) defined philosophy as:

a statement of the values and beliefs that direct an organization in its attempt to achieve a purpose. An organization's philosophy explains the reason procedures and tasks are carried out in the way that they are. A philosophy serves as a directive to the way a purpose is achieved. (p. 45)

A philosophy articulates the beliefs and values that direct all the work of the staff development department. It is a guide not only to the mission and values of the institution, but to the profession of nursing. It also is a guide to the establishment of the department's purpose, goals, and objectives, as well as setting the grounds for the conceptual framework and the basis for the staff development curriculum.

According to Cody (1996), a philosophy should be:

- Unique and descriptive of the values of the setting
- Simple, clear, and meaningful to the reader
- Applicable and pragmatic

- A basis for structure, direction, and action
- Nonrestrictive
- A shared vision of employees and managers
- Practiced as it is stated.

The staff development philosophy must also be consistent with the organizational and nursing department philosophies. Wolgin (1992) pointed out that it is important to recognize the constant state of flux of the health care environment. The astute staff development specialist acknowledges that philosophies are ever-evolving and change as the organization changes. Turnover in administration or significant changes in health care delivery or reimbursement systems may cause a philosophy to be modified to accommodate new variables. The movement within health care organizations toward restructuring has created an opportunity to redefine nursing staff development to include other clinical care providers, such as unlicensed assistive personnel and respiratory or physical therapists. All these providers are assisting nurses in the delivery of quality patient care. It is important to include these concepts in the philosophy in organizations that are choosing a clinical staff development model. Display 2-1 gives an example of a philosophy statement of an educational department in a large urban two-hospital system.

Peters (1987) emphasized the importance of developing a philosophy that enables everyone to understand clearly what the organization is trying to achieve. He suggested that the philosophy be:

specific enough to act as a tie-breaker (*e.g.*, quality is more important than volume) and general enough to leave room for the taking of bold initiatives in today's ever-changing environment. (p. 398)

Vision

Many staff development books discuss philosophy, mission, and goals, but few address the role of vision in this process. Developing a strategic vision and goals is thinking about the big things. Vision is "a story that you make up to describe the future (the big things), and the goals are a short list of things that must be done if today's vision is to become tomorrow's reality (the small things). Both are important if you want to get there" (Svenson & Rinderer, 1992, p. 153).

A partial list of items that should be included in a vision statement include:

- A brief overview of today's training system
- Training support for important business goals
- Training as an instrument of change
- The kinds and quantities of training to be provided
- Important training systems to be used
- Strengthening parts of the training system
- Organization and administration of training
- Governance of training
- Present and future comparison charts
- The costs and benefits of training (Svenson & Rinderer, 1992, p. 156).

Mission

Ulshak (1988) described a mission statement as a written statement that reflects the department's core values. It defines the direction and target for the department and provides a guideline that allows educators to go about the business of education. He stated

DISPLAY 2-1

Summa Health System Department of Education Philosophy

The Summa Health System Department of Education functions on the following principles:

- Adults are self-directed.
- Teaching-learning is a continuous, dynamic, and interactive process between the learner and the educator.
- Learning is a positive change in behavior.
- Learning takes place in an atmosphere of mutual respect and helpfulness.
- The adult learner brings various learning styles and experiences to the educational process.

We Believe the Learner is Responsible for:
- Identifying and achieving own educational needs.
- Participating in organizational needs assessments.
- Attending and actively participating in educational programs/activities.
- Maintaining own competence.
- Enhancing own career.
- Integrating continuous learning into personal and professional life.
- Evaluating the effectiveness of educational activities.
- Evaluating the effectiveness of own learning.

We Believe the Educator is Responsible for:
- Analyzing needs.
- Developing systems to facilitate educational goals/endeavors.
- Developing core education/curriculum and training roles.
- Designing curricula.
- Developing a variety of training methods and techniques.
- Developing educational materials.
- Creating educational opportunities for customer/learner.
- Delivering and coordinating instruction.
- Providing the most effective, efficient, cost-effective methods and techniques.
- Encouraging application of interpersonal and critical thinking skills.
- Developing collaborative education/learning plans/methods with customers/colleagues.
- Evaluating outcomes and education systems.

We Believe That Leadership is Responsible for:
- Working with the education department in an atmosphere of cooperation and collaboration to achieve organizational and educational goals.
- Knowing what skills and knowledge are required for high-level performance within their teams.
- Developing collaborative education/learning plans/methods with customer/colleagues and work group/team.
- Facilitating employee access to training (educational systems).
- Evaluating effectiveness of educational activities.
- Participating in evaluation of team and individual competency of performance regarding skills and interpersonal relationships.

that "until there is agreement about purpose, a department has no direction, no tool to measure progress, no real reason to be motivated, and no clear focus for its energy" (p. 39).

In ASHET's *Standards for Health Care Education and Training* (1994), the mission statement defines a direction for education and essential functions to be accomplished. This statement should relate what education does for the organization; focus attention on actual needs of the organization, as derived from corporate and professional information sources; and change as the needs and priorities of the organization change.

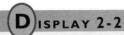

DISPLAY 2-2

Department of Education Mission

The Summa Health System Education Department supports the mission, values, and goals of Summa Health System through the appropriate use of collaborative educational systems to meet current and future customer needs.

The Mission will be accomplished by:

1. Providing job skills and specific education/curricula that assist employees to become members of a competent, motivated, flexible work force.
2. Using knowledge and techniques from the behavioral sciences to increase organizational effectiveness by integrating individual and organizational goals.
3. Supporting and providing community education projects and activities on health care issues in collaboration with other providers.

Rodriguez et al. (1996) outlined the steps required to develop a mission statement:

1. Identify your customers.
2. Identify the major roles that the department will take.
3. Identify the role of the learner.
4. Identify the relation between cost and quality.
5. Identify the department's responsibility to meet strategic directives.

Quality care should be included in a mission statement. Alspach (1995) noted that a health care agency's mission statement typically includes statements related to provision of the highest quality of health care for the community served, and provision of quality services by competent professionals who provide state-of-the-art health care services. Display 2-2 shows a sample mission statement of an educational department in a large urban two-hospital system.

O'Brien (1995) stated that the staff development department's mission statement gives clear direction to planning, implementation, and evaluation. The purpose should be operational rather than idealistic; it should describe the contingencies to be satisfied and what the department is and should be.

Consistency among the various levels of the organization or within several training units is critical. In a large organization, an important reason for developing the mission statement is to reveal role conflicts or gaps between the various training units (Svenson & Rinderer, 1992). Important areas of overlap or gaps can be identified by laying all the mission statements for the training units next to each other on a table. The mission statements for the organization, nursing and patient care services, and the staff development department should be consistent and should demonstrate how one mission statement builds on the others, based on their focal point of interest.

Goals

Goals are statements of broad direction or general intent (ASHET, 1994). The goals of a nursing staff development program are broad statements of what the program is intended to accomplish. These goals are derived from and are consistent with the mission and philosophy statements of the program but are more specific and concrete than either of these (Alspach, 1995). Goals serve as a basis for developing more detailed outcomes for each component of the staff development program. Because the primary mission of staff development is to provide educational programs and services that assist nursing staff to gain, maintain, and improve competence in patient care, goals related to each of these responsibilities need to be specified. This could include such areas as orientation, in-service, continuing education, and career development. Cody (1996) divided these components into:

- Staff development objectives and strategies for action
- Curriculum building
- Designation and allocation of resources
- Priorities for action
- Organizational structure (p. 54).

Goals address both the desired outcomes of specific educational efforts and the processes to be used to achieve these outcomes. Thus, one goal for a staff development department might be to increase the self-directed learning activities of staff nurses (an outcome goal); another might be to establish and maintain a technically sophisticated and comprehensive learning resource center to support self-directed learning (a process goal).

Practical Application

The practical application of the philosophy, vision, mission, and goals is the development of a strategic plan. A strategic plan provides education with a focus and should include (ASHET, 1994):

- Mission
- Assessment of educational services' strengths and weaknesses
- Assessment of organizational strengths and weaknesses
- Identification of educational services' goals and objectives
- Identification of the gap between what is and what needs to be
- Action steps to move toward what needs to be
- Contingency planning (p. 5).

This plan should be reviewed and updated annually. Other items that should be part of the strategic planning process, as identified by Cody (1996), include viewing the future, assessing the present and past, formulating strategies, ranking critical strategies, review and approval, and evaluation and control. Strategic planning gives the staff development unit a process by which to examine the elements of the organization and to develop plans to guide the organization through change.

The practical application of an organization's belief system will lead to the development of a "world-class learning system," as outlined by Svenson and Rinderer (1992). The following are characteristics of such a system:

1. Cultural values that support full competence development and lifelong learning
2. Strong executive leadership and participation
3. Participation across all levels of the organization
4. A learning system driven by business performance goals and competency-based
5. Tight linkages between training departments and the users of their services
6. Resources matched to needs and objectives
7. Competent training staffs that include a balanced mix of expertise
8. A balanced array of strategies
9. Strong administrative coordination of education and training
10. Internal education and training resources leveraged through appropriate use of outside resources (pp. 16, 18–20).

The process of articulating beliefs into philosophy, vision, and mission statements prepares the staff development professional to act in a proactive manner in harmony with the larger system. These documents should be living documents, regularly reviewed to reflect the setting, nursing practice, and patient care. These concepts become the framework for the curriculum and operations of the staff development unit and more importantly the basis for experimentation and innovation necessary to keep up with a rapidly changing world (Cody, 1996).

STRUCTURES

Settings

The ANA (1990) defined nursing staff development as:

> a process consisting of orientation, in-service education, and continuing education for the purpose of promoting the development of personnel within any employment setting, consistent with the goals and responsibilities of the employer. (p. 3)

Hitchings (1996) identified the following factors influencing the organization of staff development activities:

- Philosophy and mission of the organization
- Organization of the nursing department
- Scope of staff development roles and responsibilities
- Educational preparation of the staff development director and educators
- Educational preparation of nursing service executives, managers, and staff nurses
- Availability and use of clinical nurse specialists
- Diversification of patient care services
- Physical layout of the hospital
- Financial status of the institution (p. 88).

Alspach (1995) differentiated between the educational and organizational structure of nursing staff development. The educational structure describes how nursing staff development fits into the overall scheme of professional nursing education. The organizational structure describes how the staff development program is situated within the overall organization of the health care facility. Both of these structures are addressed in the section on models.

The architect's maxim "form follows function" applies to the design of organizations. The organizational structure is form; what it is supposed to accomplish is function. The structural design should be driven by the strategic vision and goals and by the quantitative plans developed for the amounts of work to be performed and the resources to be organized to accomplish the work (Svenson & Rinderer, 1992). These authors suggested the following guidelines for developing a viable organizational structure:

1. Create a position for a high-level training officer.
2. Make the training department large enough to support the specialized expertise needed to fulfill its responsibilities.
3. Centralize curriculum architecture and common instructional materials development.
4. Establish one organizational unit to provide leadership in the areas of instructional methodology, technology, and procedures.
5. Do not try to mix instructional design and training materials development and instruction in the same job.

It may be difficult for a small department or a typical staff development structure to achieve some of these guidelines. Departments must determine what guidelines are appropriate based on their organizational setup.

There are many different models outlining how staff development departments are organized. Two categories will be used to describe staff development models; one will address models that determine how the educational function fits into the overall educational structure, and the other will describe how the education department is organized within that structure.

MODELS OF EDUCATIONAL STRUCTURE

Models that describe how education fits into the overall organization include institution-wide, nursing-based, product- or service line-based, matrix, or consortium-based.

Institution-wide departments centralize all educational operations, including patient education, in a single department that is on a level with other departments within the organization. Staffing of the department is usually multidisciplinary, although all members share expertise in education. Nursing staff development educators report to the director of education, who may or may not be a nurse, and have neither line nor staff positions in the nursing division. Institution-wide education departments act as a service center to meet all the educational needs of the organization (O'Connor, 1986).

The relation of a hospital-wide education department to nursing services varies. Nursing-based staff development departments typically report to a nursing administrator and focus on the educational needs of nursing service personnel. With different types of personnel becoming part of the nursing department (*e.g.*, unlicensed assistive personnel, multidisciplinary therapists), staff development specialists usually are involved in education for other groups in addition to nurses.

Product or service line organizations identify services that they want to provide, and then all categories of employees contributing to that service become part of that group. For example, the psychiatric services might include nursing, social services, and admitting. Thus, the manager of the department would oversee a variety of disciplines working on the same services (Sheridan, 1996). Educators functioning within that service would also provide education for the diverse group within that service line.

Consortiums provide another way to organize education. Cooperation to provide staff development activities can be carried out not only between colleges and hospitals, but also among two or more hospitals. Cooperative ventures can be related to almost any aspect of staff development activities, including orientation, in-service, and continuing education (Hitchings, 1996). Advantages of this approach, as outlined by O'Brien (1995), include being able to provide more and better programs at a lower cost. Collaboration and shared planning are essential. Planning is needed to reach agreement about the nature of the shared service, the physical facilities and financial resources needed, and the methodology for delivering the education. Examples of success with this approach have been noted in the literature (Lyon, 1988; Stetler et al., 1983).

MODELS OF ORGANIZATIONAL STRUCTURE

Models that describe how staff development functions are operationalized include the decentralized model, the centralized model, and a combination of the two. Table 2-1 outlines the advantages and disadvantages of these three operational models.

Decentralized models may locate the responsibility for nursing staff development at the level of the nursing department, at some subdivision of that department, or at the unit level. One form of a decentralized structure involves placing the responsibility for nursing staff development within a central nursing administration. A second form may have some nurse educators assigned to a centralized nursing staff development program

TABLE 2-1

ADVANTAGES AND DISADVANTAGES OF STAFF DEVELOPMENT STRUCTURES

	Advantages	Disadvantages
Centralized	Coordination of resources	Centralized decision making
	Uniformity in implementing standards	Unresponsive to unit needs
	Coordination of regulatory and agency-required programming	Lack of coordination between general and unit programs
	Comprehensive and collaborative orientation activities	Lack of identity with specific areas
	Consistent education content and teaching methods	Dissatisfaction of educators with role
	More efficient use of educators	Possible reduced autonomy
	Support services readily available	Potential loss of clinical skills of educators
Decentralized	Educational needs more easily identified	Coordination may be ineffective or inefficient
	Increased opportunity for feedback and application	Duplication of education and efforts of personnel
	Increased educational leadership and involvement in departments	Inconsistent education and teaching methods
	Programming implemented in a timely manner	Lack of support services
	More flexibility in educational programming	Inadequate or inconsistent recordkeeping
	Educators seen as clinical experts	Educators may be used for service
Combination	Identification of individual unit needs	Cost of maintaining both designs may increase staffing
	Timely response to both centralized and decentralized education	Educators may lose sight of overall staff development goals
	Use of clinical experts for unit-based programming	
	Increased flexibility	
	Availability of support services	
	Coordination to reduce duplication and inappropriate use of resources	
	Collegial support for all educators	

and others to various clinical divisions within the nursing services department. The most extreme form of decentralization places all responsibilities for nursing staff development on individual nursing units, where unit-based educators who are specialists in their clinical area are assigned these functions (Alspach, 1995). Decentralized models often flatten the organizational hierarchy. The success or failure of decentralization often depends of the ability of the designated person and the amount of involvement educators have in delivering nursing care. Because of the limited staff available to provide a unit's patient care or because of budget constraints that require staff development educators to perform dual responsibilities, educators have sometimes been required to serve as direct caregivers. The key element in successfully assigning educators who are also required to give patient care hours is a trusting relationship between the educators and unit managers (Hitchings, 1996).

In centralized models, all staff development activities are performed by a central staff. Staff development specialists report to a director, who assigns all programs and tasks. Communication often flows through the nursing or human resources administrator to the director to the specialists. The staff development department is responsible for the entire process of assessing needs, planning programs, implementing them, and evaluating outcomes. This approach is considered by many nurse leaders to be the most economical and effective for meeting quotas and standards (Wolgin, 1992). If the centralized structure is within a human resources department, it may represent one small part of a much larger department that is responsible for very diverse functions, such as recruitment and retention, personnel policies, job descriptions, employee benefits, leadership development, patient or community development, and community relations (Alspach, 1995). If the staff development program is placed within a hospital-wide education program, the focus will probably be more on education than personnel issues, but nurses will be only one of many categories of health care workers whose learning needs must be met.

Staff development specialists may be organized by either function or patient services. Functional areas could include (Hitchings, 1996):

- Orientation
- Product-related issues and in-service classes
- Regulatory agency and organizational requirements
- Hospital-wide continuing education programs
- Unit-based continuing education programs
- Management development.

Patient service areas could include medical-surgical, critical care, obstetrics, behavioral health, outpatient services, and home health. Each service area may have one or more educators assigned to it.

The combination approach uses portions of both the centralized and decentralized structures to try to maximize their advantages and minimize their disadvantages. Educators provide centralized instruction that addresses learning needs common to many members of the nursing staff, but they are often assigned to specific areas to address these areas' unique needs. In some settings, certain instructors may be assigned to the centralized functions while other instructors cover decentralized areas.

Cummings and McCaskey (1992) outlined how the combined model was successfully implemented in a 540-bed research facility. Four centralized educators reported to a director of professional development, who was responsible for generalized learning needs and universal nursing department orientation. Eight decentralized educators reported directly to the nursing administrator of their clinical area and were responsible for addressing specialized learning needs and coordinating the specialty orientation for their clinical areas. The decentralized educators had no formal line relationship with the centralized nursing educators, but there was a formal communication system within the educator role group, which included both centralized and decentralized educators. This group met twice a month for communication, collaboration, professional networking, peer support, and project work. All educators met the same qualifications, except for clinical specialty. The four basic elements of the job descriptions for both groups were:

1. Assess, plan, and implement educational programs designed to meet the varied and specific learning needs of a wide range of professional nursing staff practicing in a complex biomedical research environment.
2. Develop and use methods, measurements, and tools to evaluate achievement of learning goals, effectiveness of curricula content, teaching strategies, and quality assurance.
3. Provide educational and clinical consultation to unit, service, and departmental professional staff in the areas of program development, professional development, and educational practice issues.
4. Assist in the application of research findings and facilitate and/or conduct research with an educational or clinical focus (p. 23).

There is no one best way to structure the nursing staff development function within an organization. The specific institution must find the structure that works most effectively in that setting. Clarity in lines of communication, collaboration, authority, and responsibility are more important than the precise positioning of the nursing staff development unit in the facility (Alspach, 1995).

FRAMEWORK

Regardless of the organizational structure or model, staff development usually refers to learning activities designed to facilitate the clinical staff's job-related performance. Staff development has three dimensions: orientation, in-service, and continuing education (ANA, 1994). Orientation socializes new clinical staff members, introducing them to the organizational culture and philosophy, goals, policies, role expectations, and other factors necessary to function in a specific work setting. Orientation typically occurs at the beginning of employment and any time there are changes in roles and responsibilities. In-service education helps clinical personnel acquire, maintain, or increase their competence in fulfilling assigned responsibilities. Examples could include instruction about a new piece of equipment or a briefing on changes in policy and procedure. Continuing education, on the other hand, refers to learning experiences designed to enrich the clinician's contributions to quality health care and professional career goals. Continuing education includes programs and independent studies that meet specified criteria for contact hours.

There is often confusion between continuing education and inservice (Table 2-2). In Chapter 1, Kelly-Thomas proposed two dimensions—competence assessment and competence development—that would encompass all the dimensions of staff development.

A framework for role and responsibilities in staff development, identified by the ANA (1992), is shown in Figure 2-2. This framework is conceptually based in nursing knowledge of the factors and relationships required to understand, predict, and affect environment. By engaging in the educational process, clinical staff members learn to maintain and increase their competence to practice in a constantly changing health care environment. Staff development interventions, which promote lifelong learning, are based on and influenced by changing client demographics, changing delivery systems, increasing knowledge, and changing learner characteristics. An increasing focus on individual, organizational, and patient outcomes also influences the provision of educational interventions.

Phelps (1990) described a framework for providing structure and direction to a staff development department. Educators monitored the impact of educational programs on the profession, the community, and the market in which the institution functions. The

TABLE 2-2

COMPARISON OF CONTINUING EDUCATION AND IN-SERVICE

	Continuing Education	In-Service
Definitions	Professional experiences designed to enrich the nurse's contribution to health care	Activities intended to help nurses acquire, maintain, or increase the level of competence in fulfilling assigned responsibilities specific to the expectations of the employer
Examples	Programs, independent studies	New equipment; changes in policy and procedures; updates on patient care or staff issues or concerns
Time Frame	Must be at least 50 minutes or 1 contact hour. Contact hours based on amount of time spent on content (not breaks, lunch, welcome, exhibits).	Anywhere from 5–10 minutes to several hours; usually less than 50 minutes
Target Audience & Need	Must be identified and included on application form	Must be identified; may be determined by administrator or educator
Planning Committee	Must include 2 RNs; one of whom is a BSN. Must include LPN if LPNs will be attending.	Determined by institution; may be sales representative or assigned to educator
Faculty	Education and professional qualifications included on application	Selected by institution or educator based on knowledge in that area
Objectives	Must be identified and included on written evaluation by participants	May be verbally stated; may or may not be evaluated by participants
Publicity	Materials must indicate number of contact hours and approval statements.	Usually flyer or memo
Evaluation	Specific items must be included on a written evaluation given to each participant.	Return demo, verbal feedback, exercises, or other means
Recordkeeping	Application form, attendance sheets, summary of evaluations, and other paperwork must be kept secure for 6 years.	Usually attendance sheets kept on file; other records determined by institution or regulatory agency
Requirements for Relicensure	Varies by state	No requirements

Developed by Barbara Brunt, 1995.

development of problem-solving skills for care of patients who were increasingly ill, the ability to make ethical decisions in the high-technology environment, and cost-effectiveness were essential to the development of a successful program. The pinnacle of this model (Fig. 2-3) is peak performance. This was based on Garfield's (1986) definition of peak performers as people who possess "the ability to achieve impressive and satisfying

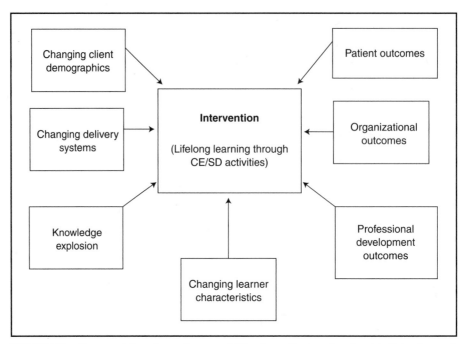

FIGURE 2-2. Framework for roles and responsibilities in continuing education/staff development.

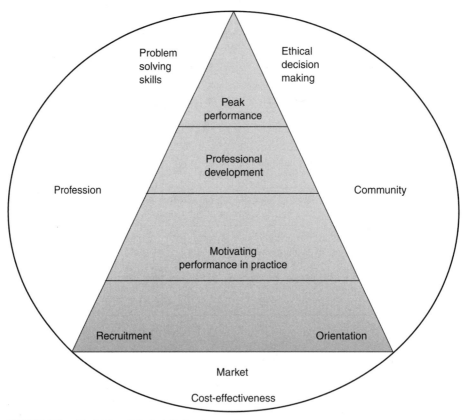

FIGURE 2-3. Model for clinical staff development.

results in their careers on a consistent basis" (p. 16). The education department developed a clinical staff of peak performers through recruitment and retention activities, educational offerings designed to motivate performance in practice, and programs that supported professional development. A staff development department using this framework could have a major influence on health care in the community it serves.

Integration

Integration of staff development activities can be facilitated by developing close working relationships with other departments or agencies to coordinate services and programs. Relationships between institutions and schools of nursing can offer unique and creative opportunities for staff development. Shared or joint appointments can be successful in providing additional resources for developing staff. In a joint appointment, faculty from a local or affiliated college or university and hospital personnel have responsibilities at both the academic institution and the health care agency. This can promote collegial working relationships and helps both parties become more aware of the trends and realities in the other setting. Theory-based practice is reinforced within the hospital setting by academic personnel, and educational resources are communicated and shared, preventing duplication and creating cost-effectiveness.

Frequently cited opportunities for affiliation between service setting and academic nursing institutions, as described by Malia and Propst (1995), include:

1. Theory development in the field of nursing staff development
2. Research affiliations that enable faculty to have access to hospital staff and patients (with informed consent and in appropriate hospital policy), and that enable staff to obtain the support of experienced nurse researchers
3. Joint appointments to maximize the experience and skill of faculty and nursing service staff
4. Curriculum design that merges the needs of the academic institution and those of the service institution
5. Opportunities for practicing nursing staff development specialists to contribute to the development of graduate programs in nursing staff development (p. 109).

School affiliations are often developed through requests by local schools and universities for clinical placement for students. Staff development personnel frequently are involved in developing the contract and coordinate the clinical experiences for these students. An important element that should be included in any contract is the responsibility of the institution to ensure patient safety. Often provisions for joint meetings with the institution for planning purposes or participation in curriculum design are included. Limits on the number of students permitted on each unit and coordination with other clinical experiences for employees of the organization also must be considered.

The role of clinical nurse specialists within the institution may provide opportunities for collaboration. They may function as a clinical expert, a staff educator, or both. Boyer (1986) described the collaboration and cooperation between the clinical nurse specialist ("the expert in clinical knowledge and skill") and the staff development educator ("the expert in educational process") as a means to provide "ongoing cost-effective programs to insure nursing excellence" (p. 23).

Increasing number of unlicensed assistive personnel are being incorporated into institutions, and this provides opportunities for the staff development department to integrate educational activities for these workers into the overall staff development program. Radcliffe (1995) described the regulatory influences, instructional strategies, continuing education, quality improvement, and competence needs of these workers. She outlined the following activities as providing a solid framework for assistive personnel:

1. Examine programs in place to meet Joint Commission on Accreditation of Healthcare Organizations criteria as a baseline that will provide guidelines and data for further curriculum development.
2. Develop an awareness that most activities for RNs also have implications for assistive personnel. Maintain communication and instruction for new information related to equipment, quality improvement, and practice changes.
3. Explore the role of the assistive worker in the current delivery system for educational support to perform job responsibilities, ensure competence, and address problems.
4. Seek involvement in the development of new or changed nursing service delivery.
5. Serve as a role model for problem solving, change, and recognizing diversity in the workplace (p. 193).

Recent reports and recommendations from the Institute of Medicine (Wunderlick et al., 1996), the Pew Health Commission (1995), and the Pew Task Force on Health Care Workforce Regulation (1995) have implications for the education of personnel, as well as the practice of nursing. These ultimately affect the staff development specialist and provide opportunities for education of staff and integration of educational activities to ensure and document quality-of-care initiatives. Staff development educators can set an example by doing the following and encouraging others to do likewise. Specific strategies identified by Brunt (1996) included:

1. Become visible and take every opportunity to educate our consumers on the value of nursing.
2. Keep informed about current initiatives and how they could affect nursing; share with others this information.
3. Keep informed about current legislative initiatives, both in your state and nationally. The Pew Task Force members are working with governors and legislators to implement proposed regulatory changes that would reduce the power of nursing boards relating to competence, delegation, and unlicensed personnel.
4. Set up networks of information or other coalitions to ensure that you stay informed.
5. Take every opportunity to look at and evaluate care provided by unlicensed assistive personnel. The Institute of Medicine could find little empirical evidence that hospital quality of care was being harmed by workforce restructuring and was "shocked" by the lack of current data showing the status of hospital quality of care (pp. 2–3).

Roles

The ANA has outlined various roles for staff development specialists across all settings: educator, manager, consultant, and researcher (ANA, 1992). As educators, staff development specialists provide an appropriate climate for learning and facilitate the adult learning process, which is outlined later in this chapter. As managers, they manage the educational experience and support the administrative functions related to their role. As consultants, they help integrate new learning into the practice environment or serve as a resource for the professional growth and development of other personnel. As researchers, they integrate relevant research into staff development and nursing practice. Extensive information on each of these roles can be found in *Core Curriculum for Nursing Staff Development* (Avillion, 1995).

The role of staff development personnel as internal consultants and change agents is also outlined in the *Standards for Health Care Education and Training* (ASHET, 1994). Educators cross organizational boundaries to facilitate change. This includes active involvement in organizational activities, committees, task forces, and projects. It requires coaching and mentoring skills, as well as knowledge and skill in data collection, performance analysis, problem solving, communication, team building, and change theory.

Staff development personnel also need to foster career development. They are in an ideal position to participate in the design, implementation, and administration of programs to enhance career development or promotion. Sovie (1983) described the role of staff development in fostering professional nursing careers in hospitals. This model, which can easily be adapted to various settings and personnel, outlined three phases of a nurse's development:

1. Professional identification, in which the nurse becomes oriented to the career
2. Professional maturation, in which the potential for development and expansion of competencies is recognized
3. Professional mastery, in which the potential for self-actualization is reached.

Staffing

Both the ANA (Appendix A) (1994) and ASHET (1994) have standards relating to staffing of the education department. ASHET's standard states, "Education services are delivered by a sufficient number of competent individuals who are able to implement an organized schedule of educational programs, services, and activities to meet the organizational needs" (p. 4). ANA's standard states, "Qualified administrative, educational, and support personnel are responsible for achieving the goals of the provider unit" (p. 8).

CREDENTIALS

Credentials of both the administrator and staff members are outlined in the ANA's *Standards for Nursing Professional Development: Continuing Education and Staff Development* (Appendix A) (1994):

> The administrator of the provider unit has a baccalaureate or higher degree in nursing, and a graduate degree in nursing or a related field. The administrator demonstrates managerial and educational knowledge and skills. . . .
>
> Each member of the educational staff has a baccalaureate or higher degree in nursing and has demonstrated relevant educational, content, and clinical expertise in addition to interest and ability in providing education to adult learners. A graduate degree in nursing or a related field is preferred. (p. 8)

This is consistent with actual practice, as shown in a survey by Blocker (1992). Forty-eight responses were received from health care facilities in 30 states, representing all geographical regions of the United States. Thirty-two (66%) of the administrators had master's degrees; seven (15%) had a Ph.D. One administrator had an ADN, three had a BSN, and five did not respond. A similar trend toward master's-level preparation for the teaching staff was also seen. A total of 160 (36%) of the 448 educators that responded had a BSN; 187 (42%) had an MSN. Only 39 persons (9%) had an associate degree or diploma in nursing.

The number, titles, and responsibilities of staff development educators are as varied as the organizations where they work. The scope of services to be provided is the main criterion for determining how many positions are needed, the organizational design, and role functions. When institutions downsize, frequently it is the education department that loses staff members or is forced to cut back on services. This is why is it critical to tie in with the organizational goals and be able to document the outcomes of our educational endeavors. Survival in today's environment is directly related to the perception and value seen by the administration of the education department and services.

SKILLS AND EXPERIENCE

Staff development educators meet the educational needs of personnel and the mission and goals of the employment setting to enhance health care delivery. They use adult learning principles in the planning, implementation, and evaluation of activities. Their responsibilities, as outlined by ANA (1992), include:

- Managing overall program activities, including human and monetary resources as appropriate
- Providing relevant education to nurses to help keep them informed about current knowledge and practice
- Fostering a positive attitude about the benefits of lifelong learning
- Providing faculty with written guidelines regarding the development and implementation of educational activities
- Maintaining and enhancing clinical and educational competence
- Planning programs to increase the breadth and depth of the knowledge base of nurses
- Determining the need for, the type, and the extent of supervision in educational practice
- Applying adult education principles to the overall program framework
- Implementing learning needs assessments
- Evaluating the effects of educational activities
- Documenting the outcomes of educational endeavors
- Helping nurses deal with professional and workplace issues, such as patient acuity and the delegation of tasks to others
- Responding to the mission and goals of the institution, agency, or organization (pp. 9–10).

Shinn (1994) identified several competencies needed by staff development personnel in this era of health care reform:

1. Increasing one's knowledge is critical, especially in such areas as the institution's goals, priorities, and strengths and weaknesses, the cultural diversity of the staff and patients, the education and training needs of all staff, and technology. Staff development specialists also need to be aware of their own abilities.
2. Business acumen is important; this includes increased accountability for the outcome of training, skill at marketing services, and the ability to forge community partnerships.
3. Specialists must also be able to tolerate uncertainty. Today's environment is constantly changing, and the educator must be able to tolerate and thrive on chaos.
4. Staff development educators must take an active role in the political arena by arming themselves with facts and educating others.

The essential qualifications of the educator, as outlined by Lankford and Budzinski-Braunscheidel (1995), included scholarship, interpersonal relationship skills, teaching ability, creativity, business skills, and change agent skills.

CONTINUED DEVELOPMENT

Educators should be responsible for their own continued development, in addition to the development of others. Educators exercise autonomy and freedom within their scope of practice. As stated in the ANA's social policy statement (1995), this autonomy and freedom is based on their commitment to self-regulation and accountability for practice. One form of self-regulation is the accountability to develop and maintain knowledge and skills through formal and continuing education. Nurses also regulate themselves through peer review of their practice. Peer evaluation fosters the refinement of knowledge, skills, and clinical decision-making processes at all levels and in all areas of clinical practice. The *Standards for Nursing Professional Development* (Appendix A) (ANA, 1994) also address the need for both the administrator and educational staff to develop, maintain, and enhance their educational skills and expertise through self-evaluation and ongoing professional development.

PROCESSES

The processes of clinical and nursing staff development include both program planning and service delivery. Program planning includes the assessment, planning, implementation, and evaluation of individual sessions and the overall program. Service delivery includes identifying strategies, defining the target audience, and getting and using resources.

Program Planning

Standards for program planning are listed under the heading of "Educational Design" in the ANA standards (1994) and "Educational Process" in ASHET's *Standards for Health Care Education and Training* (1994). Both address the assessment, planning, implementation, and evaluation of programs. In staff development, the recipient is the nursing community within the organization, or the community itself. The ultimate client is the patient or consumer, who benefits from the knowledge and competence of the nursing staff.

ASSESSMENT

Assessment is the continuous process of data collection, analysis and synthesis, and diagnosis. The specifics depend on each institution's situation, philosophy, and needs. Learners must be included in the identification of their learning needs. Various strategies can be used to assess learning needs. While identifying needs, educators must be aware of the cultural differences that may exist in both patients and staff members. The ANA's *Roles and Responsibilities for Nursing Continuing Education and Staff Development Across All Settings* (1992) stressed the importance of safeguarding learners' rights while assessing learning needs.

PLANNING

Programs should be planned to increase the breadth and depth of the knowledge base of nursing personnel. The American Nurses Credentialing Center has set out criteria that must be met to give continuing education credit for educational programs or independent studies. The design should include documentation of a needs assessment, description of the target audience, educational objectives, content outline, teaching methods, evaluation strategies, and designation of appropriate physical facilities and resources. Promotional materials should accurately describe the content to be presented, the faculty members' qualifications, and the benefits of attending. Learning experiences should be organized to help participants understand the relation between theory and real-life situations. All content should be based on current information.

IMPLEMENTATION

Instructional technology should be geared to the learning outcomes to be achieved. Handout materials should have a clearly defined purpose and should be used to enhance the learning outcome. In the implementation process, educators assume a facilitator role rather than one of a lecturer or teacher. They must be aware of the characteristics of the learner and use a variety of teaching strategies, instructional techniques, and audiovisual materials to promote learning.

Flewellyn and Gosnell (1985, 1987) stressed the need for considering cost-effectiveness, practice efficacy, and preferred learning method, especially in relation to orientation programs for new nursing employees. They compared competency-based and traditional orientation programs in six hospitals over a 4-month period. Although the study findings did not show one method of orientation to be superior, it did show that the initial cost of competency-based orientation programs exceeded that of traditional programs. However, the long-term costs and benefits of competency-based programs are not known, and more and more emphasis is being placed on assessing and validating the competence of staff members.

EVALUATION

Both individual programs and the entire staff development program need to be evaluated, and methods for both will be described. Evaluation should be an integral, ongoing, and systematic process of all educational services. All educational programs should be evaluated, using a variety of methods that allow participants to evaluate the educational activity. Educators should then use the data to modify the content, delivery, or materials used. This design should include a mechanism for feedback to the learner when appropriate, and presenters should receive feedback for their component of the educational activity (ANA, 1994). Many methods can be used to evaluate individual educational programs: quizzes or tests, return demonstrations, satisfaction surveys after the session, verbal or written self-evaluation, and peer evaluation. Evaluation of outcomes of educational activities is discussed later in this chapter.

Chu and Chu (1991) discussed the power of feedback in helping staff nurses learn and grow. Hefferin et al. (1987) discussed trends in the evaluation of nursing in-service education programs, noting that evaluation is a simple concept but a complex process:

> For institutionally based educational efforts, to be both successful and cost-effective, their starting point must be the needs of nursing personnel related to their practice in that institution, and their end point must be the policies, procedures, and standards of practice that demand accountability for the utilization of newly acquired knowledge. (p. 40)

Many models have been developed to provide mechanisms for comprehensive staff development evaluation. Tiessen (1987) described a model that combined concepts from other models to provide a thorough approach to evaluation to demonstrate staff development's role in sharing accountability with nursing services for improved patient care. Set within a systems framework, three circles depicted the three components of staff development: orientation, in-service, and continuing education. For each of these components, five areas of evaluation were included: system assessment, program planning, program implementation, program improvement, and program certification. The outputs were the changes in knowledge, attitudes, and behavior that occurred within the employee as a result of participating in the educational program.

Fennel and Pollard (1995) described four types of evaluation and various methods of performing evaluations. Guidelines for developing data collection instruments, constructing written tests, and analyzing evaluation data are also included in their chapter in *Core Curriculum for Nursing Staff Development*. Mann Woith (1995) also wrote a helpful chapter on program evaluation in this same publication.

Quality improvement activities are also part of the overall evaluation process; they are addressed in Chapters 11 and 13.

Service Delivery

According to Wolgin (1992), staff development specialists provide services through a variety of mechanisms, including:

- Direct provision of services
- Coordination
- Collaboration
- Consultation
- Support.

Ulshak (1988) identified some strategies that provide a foundation for creative adjustments to the constant changes that education departments face:

- Know the decision makers.
- Know the mission of education.
- Develop control mechanisms for monitoring the work of the education department.
- Redefine the role of the educator.
- Examine revenue generation.
- Implement marketing efforts.
- Get close to the heartbeat of the organization.
- Promote a common language (pp. 151–153).

Strategies used to deliver services are based on the target audience and the resources available. Staff development educators often must juggle numerous programs and activities to meet the demands of multiple customers. Wolgin (1992) suggested cross-indexing delivery strategies. For example, with orientation the target audience is new nursing personnel, and the service delivery mechanism is primarily the direct provision of services. However, the staff development educator also must coordinate selected portions of the orientation with guest lecturers and must also collaborate with nurse managers to ensure that the orientation program is meeting their needs. This process can be used for other programs, such as in-services and continuing education.

Often requests for programs exceed the financial and time constraints of staff development personnel. Some requests may be handled through consultation and support rather than direct provision of services, coordination, or collaboration. Frequently, lack of compliance with institutional policies and procedures may been seen as an educational problem when it is actually a clinical one. In these cases, the staff development specialist may provide consultation or suggestions on how to deal with the issue. Not every problem can be solved with education.

An additional factor that must be included when assessing and using resources is the amount of time it takes to prepare or coordinate the program. Assessment data relating to learning needs may or may not be available. If data have been collected, then the staff development specialist may immediately use that information to begin planning activities.

The amount of time needed for preparation depends on the educator's familiarity with the content and his or her experience, the length of the program, the logistical preparations required (*e.g.*, dates, rooms, speakers, advertising materials, handouts), and the immediacy of the need.

OUTCOMES

In staff development work, both assessment and documentation of outcomes are critical. Henry (1989) analyzed evaluation research in staff development and concluded:

> It is apparent from this analysis that in our present environment of escalating health care costs, increased patient acuity, and a shortage of nurses, evaluation studies focusing on patient outcomes must assume a higher priority. (p. 138)

This section will include information on defining, measuring, and reporting outcomes.

Defining Outcomes

Outcomes can be defined in a variety of ways. Outcome evaluation can examine the achievement of learning outcomes, such as changes in knowledge, changes in clinical performance, and changes in patient care outcomes. Changes in knowledge can be assessed through a pretest and posttest format; this is very common in staff development. Changes in clinical performance are more difficult to identify and measure. One way of defining clinical outcomes is to tie into existing quality management activities. Quality monitoring has the advantage of providing information on both the magnitude and the persistence of performance improvement and can also address its impact on the general quality of care or patient satisfaction (Norgan, 1995). Performance problems identified by quality improvement activities can help identify and define desired outcomes.

It is much easier to identify and define changes in patient care outcomes than to measure these changes, or to infer that the patient care outcomes were directly related to the educational activity. Titler and Reiter (1994) stressed the importance of selecting and defining outcome domains that can be used by multiple disciplines involved in health care delivery. They suggested using some measure of functional status and patient satisfaction, which provide a common denominator to make comparisons across diverse populations. However, there must be consensus in deciding what domain of outcomes will be measured and how they will be defined.

Measuring Outcomes

Cervero (1985) described a model that emphasized the impact or outcome of an educational program. The measurement of the effectiveness of continuing professional education was conceptualized as behavior change. His model focused on four sets of variables affecting whether a continuing education program produced behavior change:

1. Characteristics of the program
2. Characteristics of the learner
3. Characteristics of the behavior change. A behavior change was most likely to occur if the proposed change was better than the idea it superseded; was compatible with needs, past experiences, and values; was simple to implement;

was amenable to being implemented on a trial basis; and had results visible to others.

4. Characteristics of the social system. Those shown to be positively related to adoption include system norms that were positive toward adoption, close communication among the members of the system, and the extent to which the social system's legitimizers were involved in the decision-making process related to the desired behavior change.

Another consideration to include in measuring outcomes is the period of time within which performance change will occur after a program. Norgan (1995) suggested that the interval required for application of learning can be predicted by examining the setting in which the newly acquired behavior is to be applied and answering specific questions about the behavior (p. 138):

- Is application of the newly learned behavior under the control of the individual learner?
- Does the behavior require the support or cooperation of others?
- Is the behavior complex, requiring further reinforcement before development of mastery?
- Is the general environment of the clinical setting conducive to rapid acquisition of new practices?
- Does the change in behavior require attitude change as well?

Measuring outcomes is important not only from the learner's behavior change and patient outcome standpoint, but also from the standpoint of the effectiveness of the overall staff development program. Waterstradt and Phillips (1990) discussed the use of a productivity tool to identify how a staff development department meets the needs of the institution. Use of this productivity tool provides an efficiency outcome measure for staff development. The education department can use productivity statistics to justify its existence. The value-based productivity tool they described provided an objective method of assessing the worth of classes offered and also a mechanism for generating statistics to quantify the value of the education department to the institution.

Reporting Outcomes

Educational records, which include evidence of competence, can be used to assess and evaluate employee performance for performance reviews and promotions, to meet regulatory requirements, to monitor risk management, and to serve as a form of protection in liability issues (ASHET, 1994). Evaluation techniques that specifically measure learning outcomes should be used; where appropriate, participants should receive a follow-up evaluation to determine change in skills, knowledge, or attitudes in work performance.

The ANA (1994) *Standards for Nursing Professional Development: Continuing Education and Staff Development* (Appendix A) (ANA, 1994) stated that mechanisms should be in place for systematic, easy retrieval of data on educational activities and participants. However, these records are confidential and should be available to authorized persons only. Periodic reports should be made to appropriate organizational or agency representatives to document and evaluate progress toward attainment of provider unit and organizational goals.

Care should be taken to ensure the participant's rights to confidentiality when reporting individual data. There may be times, especially with performance concerns in the clinical area, when the staff development educator must communicate a person's difficulty with certain skills or performance standards to the unit manager or preceptor. Care should be taken to do this on a need-to-know basis with only those persons directly involved. Inappropriate comments made about a person's lack of skill or expertise can alter co-workers' perceptions and make it more difficult for a new person to be accepted as a member of the team.

Reporting of aggregate data is also essential to documenting educational and patient care outcomes. Often quality management data are reported by unit or institution rather than by person. Results of educational activities should be communicated to staff members through appropriate departmental and organization channels. Educational systems, processes, and outcomes should be revised based on these results.

Competent providers can show that participants in educational programs actually learn something new, that they use the new skills on the job, that these skills benefit the patient, and that the whole effort is conducted in the most reasonable, cost-effective manner possible. In other words, educators must be able to determine what is learned and also to justify the cost of the learning effort. Educators can contribute to the improvement in quality of services by helping improve the performance of employees.

SUMMARY

This chapter presented factors that influence the structure and processes of staff development, with the framework of competence assessment and development used as the basis for any decisions relating to structure, processes, or outcomes. Belief systems, including philosophy statements, vision, mission, and goals, were described. Structures of staff development were delineated in terms of settings, integration, roles, and staffing.

Description of the settings for nursing staff development included factors influencing the organization of staff development activities, as well as models for educational and organizational structure. Integration activities included relationships with schools or agencies, the role of clinical nurse specialists, development of assistive personnel, case management activities, and the impact of recent national reports relating to health care workforce and staffing issues. Roles of the staff development specialist and staffing issues were also addressed.

The processes of staff development include program planning and service delivery. Discussion of assessment, planning, implementation, and evaluation activities were included in program planning. The section on service delivery mechanisms described strategies, methods to define the target audience, and resources needed.

Outcomes were identified as an important component of staff development practice today. Ways of defining, measuring, and reporting outcomes were discussed. Considerations in the reporting of individual and aggregate data were delineated. Competent staff development providers can be a powerful force in the institution by helping identify and quantify the impact of education on quality of care and patient outcomes.

A New Model of Clinical Staff Development

KATHLEEN J. FISCHER

At the University of Michigan Health System, we were presented with the opportunity to provide educational services differently. Historically, nursing had a three-tiered staff education system. Each patient care unit had a nurse responsible for unit-based education. Each clinical area had a master's-prepared nurse educator, called an educational nurse specialist, who was responsible for the education within the clinical area. In addition, there was a centralized education department, educational services for nursing; this department was responsible for educational activities across clinical areas. With these resources, there were extensive educational activities offered to staff and some redundancy of services.

As the clinical areas re-evaluated their financial and human resources, the patient care units decreased the amount of time the unit educators had available to provide unit-based staff education. Some patient care units decided to have a few nurses assume roles that a single nurse educator had done in the past. By decreasing the patient care unit educator's time, the need for additional unit support became apparent. In addition to the unit changes, the clinical area educators and the central educators became a single unit. The blending of these two groups of educators provided an opportunity to change significantly how staff education is done and perceived within the organization.

The redesign of the department of nursing staff education was a collaborative effort of the educational staff. The model was developed to be flexible and evolving. The following themes were considered critical operational goals in our new model:

- Enhance responsiveness to customer and organizational needs
- Provide educational services and support for performance development along programmatic lines
- Be responsive to the current system and inclusive of the continuum of care
- Forge stronger linkages between the clinical area and the staff education department
- Enhance integration of the educational nurse specialists into clinical area activities, including working with directors, managers, educators, and staff
- Provide a fluid and flexible structure and work activities to meet the immediate and long-term needs of clinical areas and nursing service.

The new nursing education performance development model is a blend of linking educational nurse specialists in an expanded role of performance development specialists with the central educational activity teams. Figure 2-4 reflects the interrelationship of the two components.

The paradigm shift from an educator with educational expertise to an educator with performance development responsibilities has been a major change, not only for the educator but also for the nursing staff.

The purpose of the educational nurse specialists with education and performance development responsibilities is to support the continuous improvement of nursing staff in providing quality health care to their patients. This is accomplished as the educational nurse specialist:

- Supports the achievement of:
  - Outcomes of clinical programs
  - Unit and area goals
- Collaborates with patient care units to:
  - Identify performance gaps
  - Determine the causes of performance gaps
  - Measure the impact of learning and nonlearning actions that are taken to change performance
  - Proactively identify performance implications for future goals and needs
- Assists groups to identify issues and develop solutions for themselves
- Is visible in the designated areas
- Establishes self as a resource for the staff
- Is knowledgeable of workload and the culture of the patient care units

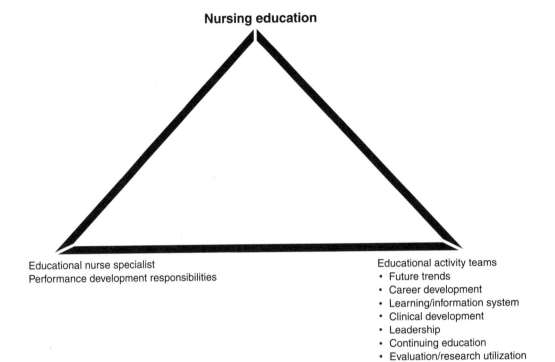

Nursing education

Educational nurse specialist
Performance development responsibilities

Educational activity teams
- Future trends
- Career development
- Learning/information system
- Clinical development
- Leadership
- Continuing education
- Evaluation/research utilization
- Formal communications
- Medicus monitoring

FIGURE 2-4. (*Above*) Nursing educational performance development model. University of Michigan Health System. (Used with permission.)

	Old Model of Development	**New Model of Development**
Environment	Education	Continuous learning environment
Focus/Outcome	Education only	Education and performance development including education, systems and processes, and structure
Customers	Unit educators	Whole unit, including director, managers, educators, and all levels of nursing staff (RN, UAP, and so forth)
Communication	Clinical educator groups	Manager and educator meetings, patient care unit meetings
Provider of Services	Single provider of services	Multiple providers of services: liaisons to areas and central teams
Performance	Isolated skill building/information transfer	Learning in context of the work environment; behavior- and outcome-driven
Skills	Primary skills Educational design Process facilitation	Expanded skills Team building, group dynamics Change, work redesign, and so forth

- Develops a link to each unit's education and leadership committees
- Participates in clinical area management meetings or communications
- Responds to staff needs in an efficient and effective manner
- Links education department activities with the unit or area
- Works to avoid duplication of activities.

It is too early to determine the outcome of changing to an education performance development model, but verbal feedback from the nursing directors, managers, educators, and staff has been very positive. Educational nurse specialists are more visible to their respective units and are contributing members to their groups. Specialists are included in the developmental stages of a wide variety of projects that help the unit operate more efficiently and effectively. They have demonstrated that they can assist in increasing staff's knowledge and skills, enhancing process and structure, and reducing barriers to getting patient care accomplished.

Will changing the role of the educator to a performance development specialist make a difference in patient care over time? As we begin to measure our outcomes, time will tell.

REFERENCES

Alspach, J. G. (1995). *The educational process in nursing staff development.* St. Louis: Mosby.

American Nurses Association. (1990). *Standards for nursing staff development.* Kansas City, MO: American Nurses Publishing.

American Nurses Association. (1992). *Roles and responsibilities for nursing continuing education and staff development across all settings.* Washington DC: American Nurses Publishing.

American Nurses Association. (1994). *Standards for nursing professional development: Continuing education and staff development.* Washington DC: American Nurses Publishing.

American Nurses Association. (1995). *Nursing's social policy statement.* Washington DC: American Nurses Publishing.

American Society for Health Care Education and Training. (1994). *Standards for health care education and training.* Chicago: American Hospital Association.

Avillion, A. E. (Ed.). (1995). *Core curriculum for nursing staff development.* Pensacola, FL: National Nursing Staff Development Organization.

Blocker, V. T. (1992). Organizational models and staff preparation: A survey of staff development departments. *Journal of Continuing Education in Nursing, 23*(6), 259–262.

Boyer, V. M. (1986). The clinical nurse specialist: An underdeveloped staff development resource. *Journal of Nursing Staff Development, 2*(1), 23–27.

Brunt, B. (1996). The changing workforce. *The Pacemaker, 37*(4), 1–3.

Cervero, R. M. (1985). Continuing professional education and behavioral change: A model for research and evaluation. *Journal of Continuing Education in Nursing, 16*(3), 85–88.

Chu, L. K., & Chu, G. S. F. (1991). Feedback and efficiency: A staff development model. *Nursing Management, 22*(2), 28–31.

Cody, B. (1996). Guiding principles: Vision, values, mission, and goals of staff development. In Abruzzese, R. S. *Nursing staff development: Strategies for success,* pp. 44–62. St. Louis: Mosby.

Cummings, C., & McCaskey, R. (1992). A model combining centralized and decentralized staff development. *Journal of Nursing Staff Development, 8*(1), 22–25.

Fennel, V. M., & Pollard, M. (1995). Evaluation. In Avillion, A. *Core curriculum for nursing staff development,* pp. 89–104. Pensacola, FL: National Nursing Staff Development Organization.

Flewellyn, B. J., & Gosnell, D. J. (1985). Comparison of two approaches to hospital orientation for practice efficacy and preferred learning methods of registered nurses. *Journal of Continuing Education in Nursing, 16*(5), 147–152.

Flewellyn, B. J., & Gosnell, D. J. (1987). Comparing two methods of hospital orientation for cost effectiveness. *Journal of Nursing Staff Development, 3*(1), 3–8.

Garfield, C. (1986). *Peak performers: The new heroes of American business.* New York: William Morrow.

Hefferin, E. A., Arndt, C., & Kleinknecht, M. K. (1987). Trends in the evaluation of nursing inservice education programs. *Journal of Nursing Staff Development*, 3(1), 28–40.

Henry, S. B. (1989). Evaluation in staff development education. In Holzemer, W. L. *Review of Research in Nursing Education, Volume II*, pp. 129–153. New York: National League for Nursing.

Hitchings, K. S. (1996). Organization of staff development activities. In Abruzzese, R. S. *Nursing staff development: Strategies for success*, pp. 83–108. St Louis: Mosby.

Kelly, K. J. (1992). *Nursing staff development: Current competence, future focus.* Philadelphia: J. B. Lippincott.

Kelly, K. (1996). *Nursing staff development: Our practice, ourselves.* Paper presented at the National Nursing Staff Development Organization Conference, Boston.

Lankford, B. P., & Budzinski-Braunscheidel, M. M. (1995). Role of the educator in staff development. In Avillion, A. *Core curriculum for nursing staff development*, pp. 235–250. Pensacola, FL: National Nursing Staff Development Organization.

Lyon, J. C. (1988). Shared staff development in the service setting: A model for success. *Journal of Continuing Education in Nursing*, 19(6), 248–251.

Malia, F. M., & Propst, J. (1995). Issues and trends. In Avillion, A. *Core curriculum for nursing staff development*, pp. 105–114. Pensacola, FL: National Nursing Staff Development Organization.

Mann Woith, W. L. (1995). Program evaluation. In Avillion, A. *Core curriculum for nursing staff development*, pp. 171–180. Pensacola, FL: National Nursing Staff Development Organization.

Norgan, G. H. (1995). Evaluation methods in human resource development. In Swansburg, R. C., & Swansburg, L. C. *Nursing staff development: A component of human resource development*, pp. 129–148. Boston: Jones & Bartlett.

O'Brien, W. M. (1995). Designing a staff development department. In Swansburg, R. C., & Swansburg, L. C. *Nursing staff development: A component of human resource development*, pp. 149–205. Boston: Jones & Bartlett.

O'Connor, A. B. (1986). *Nursing staff development and continuing education.* Boston: Little, Brown & Co.

Peters, T. (1987) *Thriving on chaos.* New York: Alfred A. Knopf.

Pew Health Professions Commission. (1995). *Critical challenges: Revitalizing the health professions for the 21st century.* San Francisco: UCSF Center for the Health Professions.

Pew Health Professions Commission Taskforce on Health Care Workforce Regulation. (1995). *Reforming health care workforce regulation: Policy considerations for the 21st century.* San Francisco: UCSF Center for the Health Professions.

Phelps, R. L. (1990). A working model for nursing staff development. *Journal of Nursing Staff Development*, 6(3), 126–130.

Radcliffe, K. (1995). Nursing assistive personnel in acute care: Framework for staff development. *Journal of Nursing Staff Development*, 11(4), 189–194.

Rodriguez, L., Patton, C., Steismeyer, J. K., & Teikmanis, M. L. (Eds.). (1996). *Manual of Staff Development.* St. Louis: Mosby.

Sheridan, D. R. (1996). The organization of staff development. In Rodriguez, L., Patton, C., Steismeyer, J. K., & Teikmanis, M. L. (Eds.). *Manual of Staff Development*, pp. 13–18. St. Louis: Mosby.

Shinn, L. J. (1994). Health care reform: Implications for competencies in staff development and continuing education. *Journal of Nursing Staff Development*, 10(3), 164–166.

Sovie, M. D. (1983). Fostering professional nursing careers in hospitals: The role of staff development, part II. *Journal of Nursing Administration*, 13(1), 30–33.

Stetler, C. B., McGrath, S. P., Everson, S., Foster, S. B., & Holloran, S. D. (1983). A staff education consortium: One model for collaboration. *Journal of Nursing Administration*, 13(10), 23–28.

Svenson, R. A., & Rinderer, M. J. (1992). *The training and development strategic plan workbook.* Englewood Cliffs, NJ: Prentice-Hall.

Tiessen, J. B. (1987). Comprehensive staff development evaluation: The need to combine models. *Journal of Nursing Staff Development*, 3(1), 9–14.

Titler, M. G., & Reiter, R. C. (1994). Outcomes measurements in clinical practice. *MEDSURG Nursing*, 3(5), 395–398.

Ulshak, F. L. (1988). *Creating the future of health care education.* Chicago: American Hospital Publishing.

Waterstradt, C. R., & Phillips, T. L. (1990). A productivity system for a hospital education department. *Journal of Nursing Staff Development, 6*(3), 139–144.

Wolgin, F. J. (1992). Staff development in the nursing service organization: Modeling for success. In Kelly, K. *Nursing staff development: Current competence, future focus.* Philadelphia: J. B. Lippincott.

Wunderlick, G. S., Sloan, F. A., & Davis, C. K. (Eds.). (1996). *Nursing staff in hospital and nursing homes: Is it adequate?* Washington DC: National Academy Press.

3

The Nature of Staff Development Practice: Theories, Skill Acquisition, and Research

KAREN J. KELLY-THOMAS

Clinical staff development (CSD) as a field of practice has seen significant progress in the past two decades. Nurses and other health care providers who choose this specialty often bring to it a knowledge of theory development as it is used in patient care services and other disciplines. When these clinicians apply this knowledge to development, new understandings of CSD practice emerge.

This chapter is written to help new clinical staff development specialists (SDSs) understand the theoretical basis of this field. An updated model for CSD, proposed in Chapter 1 (see Figure 1-1), is expanded on. Skill acquisition is central to the practice of CSD and is discussed in detail. Finally, this chapter presents some research findings about nursing and clinical staff development. Our future promises to be rich in development and learning.

THE NATURE OF STAFF DEVELOPMENT PRACTICE: THEORIES

Epistemology is the study of what we know. Schultz and Meleis (1988) described nursing epistemology as the study of the origins of nursing knowledge, its structure and methods, the patterns of knowing of its members, and the criteria for validating its knowledge claims. These ideas can be applied to nursing staff development to help understand the field and continue to cultivate the practice.

Carper (1992) recently updated her classic work about fundamental patterns of knowing in nursing and wrote, "the body of knowledge that serves as the rationale for practice has patterns, forms and structure that serve as horizons of expectations and exemplify characteristic ways of thinking about phenomena" (p. 216). She listed four fundamental patterns of knowing in nursing practice: empirics (as science), aesthetics (as art), experience (as personal knowledge), and ethics (as moral knowledge). These patterns can be applied to any field of inquiry and practice, including CSD.

Tripp-Reimer et al. (1996) described the embedded structure and knowledge undergirding nursing interventions and described three dimensions of care that may also be applied to clinical care and CSD: intensity of care, complexity of care, and focus of care. The dimensional structure suggested by this analysis also supports practice arenas shared by care providers in delineating the dimensional structure of health care interventions and the need for continuous competence assessment and development. Knowledge development work in the health care disciplines continues to emerge and inform us of our commonalities and differences.

In this chapter, no single theory is purported to be better than any other. As this field of practice evolves, new theories will be proposed. Diverse views and the discussions that accompany those theories will strengthen the field of practice. New theories will probably blend concepts and constructs from a variety of sources.

Some Imperative Questions

Questions to guide inquiry about CSD are:

- What are the origins of clinical and nursing staff development knowledge?
- What is the structure of CSD, and what are the methods?
- What are the patterns of knowing used by SDSs?
- What criteria are or should be used to validate this knowledge as it emerges?

To begin this inquiry, it helps to recognize that there are many ways of knowing. Chinn and Kramer (1995), citing the early work of Carper and others, described patterns of knowing that help us understand how we formulate what we know about nursing:

- Empirics: the traditional scientific approach; reality is viewed as an objective phenomenon that can be reduced and verified by multiple observers
- Ethics: what ought to be done
- Personal knowledge: that which concerns inner experiences and becoming a whole, aware self
- Esthetics: the art of nursing—that is, the comprehension of meaning in a singular, particular, subjective expression including imagined possibilities.

In the field of adult development, Taylor and Marrienau (1995) cited various barriers that adult women learners experience as they attempt to develop their competence through adult alternative higher education programs. Because development is the aim of most education, and a greater proportion of health care providers are women, it makes sense to consider their findings about how women's experiences in developmental programs differ from men's. The use of these findings will differ in the distinct settings of health care. Development of voice was described by Belenky et al. (1986) and Kegan (1994). They proposed a model of psychosocial development of both men and women as constructive developmental models that can be used in CSD and health care settings.

Who Was Doing What Then

In the late 1950s, nurses used the classic scientific approach to develop scientific theory for nursing. This approach reduced broad problems to manageable questions from which hypotheses could be formed and tested, ultimately generating results and findings that would contribute to the search for truth about nursing. A time-honored approach, this conventional method contributed to nursing knowledge. At the same time, other health care disciplines and providers considered their truths, discovered new knowledge, and developed caring health care practices. It is not surprising that different members of health care teams argue about "who is in charge here" or "the best way." Questions such as, "If you're the patient advocate, am I the adversary?" were raised. New work teams formed and began to search for new truths in caring practices.

During the next two decades, the reductionist approach mentioned above did not satisfy nurses because it could not capture the fullness of knowing and the knowledge that emerges from each caring experience. The nursing experience with patients also generated knowledge about care, as did the experiences of other clinical care providers.

Carper's work describing patterns of knowing in nursing has expanded our knowledge. Benner (1984) collected the personal experiences of expert nurses and analyzed them to develop new knowledge about nursing, expanding our knowledge about the caring practices of nurses. The work of these nurse scientists and many others has left fertile ground for continued inquiry in CSD. Through continued inquiry, we will gain knowledge and the ability to explain the process, cost, and outcome of CSD. The effect on the health of whole communities that occurs as a result of CSD actions is of utmost interest.

To start a discussion about the evolution of a staff development theory, I must explain the influence of nursing as primary in my view of CSD. The health promotion, health maintenance, and health restoration framework recently published by the Women's Health Expert Panel of the American Academy of Nursing (AAN, 1997) is consistent with my view of nursing and health care. Responsibilities of providers and consumers are delineated within an ecological environment. These activities of health care providers, and the acknowledgment that these activities take place systematically in some form of environment, is also consistent with my views. The AAN model for women's health also illustrates our mutual responsibilities in various health care consumer and provider roles. This work contributes to my thinking about the possibilities for CSD.

After spending some time thinking about what CSD is, I have developed a new view of CSD that involves more potential for continuous improvement of patient care. Central to this proposal is the patient who needs competent care providers for health promotion, health maintenance, and health restoration.

The rich traditions of this field date back to 1928 (Pfefferkorn, 1928), to a time when it was called "in-service education." Nursing staff development specialists have always been concerned with improving the competence of nurses in the service or clinical setting, rather than nurses in "pre-service" education; hence, the earlier identification of the practice as in-service education was common. As nursing evolved and preparation of nurses moved to academic settings, the field of nursing staff development developed. Faculty members of hospital-based schools of nursing were no longer available to assist in the continuing development of nurses. However, nurses knew that continued learning was an integral part of their professional lives. In the late 1960s, nurses were identified in organizations and given the assignment of organizing learning activities to help nurses maintain their competency.

Tobin et al. (1979) were among the first to propose an organizing framework for nursing staff development. Their landmark book gave definition to the field of practice. CSD was described as a process that includes both formal and informal learning activities that relate to the employee's role expectations and that occur within or outside the profession. They identified three major components of CSD: orientation, in-service education, and continuing education.

Professional practice issues related to new skills, expanding responsibilities, and increasing autonomy have caused the role of CSD in organizations to change. The role of universities in the continuing education of nurses has also had an effect.

Many other authors (Abruzzese, 1996; Alspach, 1995; Bille, 1982; Coye, 1976; O'Connor, 1986) have also described nursing staff development, and the extensive writings of Malcolm Knowles (1988), considered the father of adult education, are recognized throughout the literature. Recently, more information about competence assessment in industry (Portwood, 1993; Dubois, 1993), education (Manecke & Wild, 1994), and health care (Alspach, 1996; Avillion, 1995; Bennett, 1990; Jeska & Fischer, 1996; Wright, 1997) has emerged in various forms. Other health care providers (Johnson, 1994) have also begun to examine the notion of staff development of clinicians. Teachers in primary, secondary, and higher education also engage in staff development activities for practice improvement, as do bankers and computer scientists (Nierenberg, 1996; Glover, 1994). Performance improvement and outcome measurement are other areas of interest to SDSs and are examined in detail in other chapters in this book. These contributions have helped SDSs understand and improve their work.

Knowledge of clinical and nursing staff development work is developing and new theories will emerge; some are proposed in subsequent chapters. These new theories will blend rich traditions and current methods into new models for staff development practice. Future knowledge regarding staff development will bring into harmony theories from a variety of sources, including those mentioned above.

Theoretical concepts used in CSD are drawn from a variety of disciplines, including:

- Adult learning
- Adult education
- Adult development of men and women
- Change theory
- Human resources development
- Performance and quality improvement
- Nursing and other health care disciplines
- Organizational development
- Outcome measurement
- Systems.

Staff development specialists are challenged to build theories specific to this field of practice. Theory development may seem like a daunting task. A simplistic but helpful way to think of theory is merely as a way of viewing the world. How one views the world is influenced by many factors; elements such as beliefs, values, culture, and experience all blend to formulate a personal view of the world. This personal view of the world can be considered a theory about how one should exist in the world.

Consider this line of thought for CSD practice. What is your view of staff development? What words would you use to begin to describe it? Think about how your background as a clinician has influenced this view. Consider the effect of your upbringing, values, and cultural practices on your staff development theory. These are the beginning questions that one asks and answers to develop a theory. The crucial factor is thinking, which is central to any theory development effort. Serious analytical thinking about the continuing evolution of nursing staff development knowledge is critical to the growth of the field. Eventually, staff development theory will have to answer questions related to the evaluation and criteria used to examine the worth of any theory.

Meleis (1997) described the development of the discipline of nursing as a "convolutionary" process, one that is a complex, twisting, winding form or design. She cited a pattern of progress in nursing's accomplishments, carefully critiquing what has been accomplished and what is yet to be accomplished. This eloquent analysis of the discipline of nursing can also be applied to clinical and nursing staff development. Consider the complex forms and structures of CSD programs in health care organizations. Think about the progress made during periods of plenty and the reduction of services during times of economic duress. Contemplate the accomplishments and contributions of staff development specialists to patient care. It becomes evident that CSD may follow a pattern of development similar to that of other disciplines.

As specialists continue to develop a world view of their practice, the field will evolve and at times will be revolutionized. Del Bueno's (1978, 1990a, 1990b, 1993, 1995) and

Del Bueno et al.'s (1987) continuing work with competence development and evaluation revolutionized the field in the late 1970s. Other authors have written about staff development in a variety of journals, from "how-to" articles to comprehensive program planning and evaluation models. This is the beginning work of a discipline. Continuing work will involve research to support many of the beliefs, theoretical frameworks, systems, and processes already in use.

Meleis (1997) proposed a strategy for theory development in nursing that can also be applied to staff development. This process includes stages that occur in theory development, but not necessarily in a particular order. The process begins in the practice situation with the observation of a phenomenon—an event, incident, or occurrence that attracts the observer. The next stage includes beginning efforts to define, describe, or delineate the phenomenon. In CSD, a common phenomenon is the acquisition of new knowledge and skills through planned learning activities. How does this competence development phenomenon occur? How does it compare to what happens in other learning activities, such as formal academic classes? Meleis suggested that another stage is the formation of analogies and labels, which communicate the interpretation of the phenomenon.

Somewhere in this theory development process, Meleis wrote, a concept emerges. Concepts are organized perceptions that have been labeled. As concept definitions emerge, propositions are advanced as tentative statements about the phenomenon under scrutiny. Explicit and implicit assumptions are analyzed throughout the process.

Key mental activities that must occur during all stages of theory development are questioning, reflecting, studying, appraising, thinking, writing, altering, and modifying. Meleis cited intuition as one of the most significant tools for theory development.

Clinicians and nurses who choose to engage in theory development for CSD will find the process challenging and rewarding. The experience of clinicians who specialize in staff development will be the primary source of theory development for this field.

The First Proposal

In 1992, I proposed an early definition in an effort to describe nursing staff development and contrast it to other education programs for nurses (Kelly, 1992):

> Staff development can be described as the organization of prescribed developmental activities that assist the organization in reaching defined goals through the assessment, maintenance, and development of nursing competencies. (p. 7)

I further described nursing staff development as a field of nursing practice that describes the organized program and process assigned the responsibility for assessing, maintaining, and developing nurses' competence, as defined by the employing agency, most often using learning activities such as orientation, in-service education, continuing education, leadership development, and skills training, and most often occurring within health care organizations and agencies that employ predominantly nurses. This definition drew on traditional definitions and experience and used a label that had been assigned to this work for years.

A schematic of nursing staff development that incorporates this proposal is shown in Figure 3-1. This diagram identifies the primary processes used in nursing staff development at that time:

- Assessing competence: processes and programs designed to measure and evaluate the competence of nurses in relation to expected performance standards
- Maintaining competence: processes and programs designed to conserve, preserve,

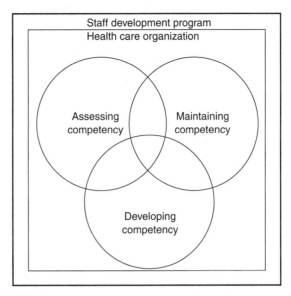

FIGURE 3-1. Nursing staff development in health care organizations. Kelly, K. J. (1992). *Nursing staff development: Current competence, future focus.* Philadelphia: Lippincott. Used with permission.

support, and sustain the competence of nurses in relation to organizational expectations

- Developing competence: processes and programs designed to cultivate, generate, and extend the competence of nurses related to expectations and performance standards new to the person or new to the organization.

Figure 3-1 shows these processes and programs as interrelated. In practice, programs may be designed to accomplish several processes. The schematic also places these processes against a program background, because the nursing staff development program may include processes or assignments not clearly associated with the above three processes. Many of these unknown processes are related to an organization's history and tradition. For example, does the organization place a research component within the staff development program? The organization often decides these elements.

Finally, Figure 3-1 shows the staff development program within the environmental boxes of the health care organization and health care systems. As the definition proposed, nursing staff development occurs within and is funded by health care organizations and agencies. This work was the beginning effort to illustrate nursing staff development as it existed in many organizations.

Although nursing staff development is not completely understood, certain concepts are emerging. For example, most CSD programs include standards and guidelines for organizational activities such as orientation, the use of preceptors, the management of new graduate nurses, and new product orientation. The satisfaction of nurses and subsequent retention of staff is a concept frequently integrated into staff development programs.

Another concept is the interrelated role of SDSs and clinical managers. The natural link of persons responsible for clinical care differentiates clinical staff development from other human resource development programs; the common understanding about direct patient care serves as a bond between the persons. The concept of linkages—the importance of linking program planning to organizational goals and priorities—is another concept that continues to surface. The concept of competence development through processes designed to assess, maintain, and develop the abilities of clinical care providers in practice continues to be a concept woven throughout CSD programs.

These concepts are intertwined throughout this text to provide a wealth of information about the experience of staff development to the new specialist and program manager. Minor discrepancies exist between some views and are evident in the models, systems, and advice provided in various chapters. You will notice these differences more as you begin to develop your own view of CSD. However, the primary pattern of staff development work that continues to emerge is this: CSD involves planning activities designed to assess and develop competence of health care workers in their employment settings for quality care.

A Second Proposal

Chapter 1, Figure 1-1 illustrates a new model of CSD. This version demonstrates a convergence of competence assessment and competence development activities within broader environments, such as the health care system, the social environment, the economic environment, and the ecological environment.

The intent of this updated model is to illustrate three changes from earlier thinking. The first is the consideration of the many environments that influence staff development work and the care of patients. The second is grounded in the fact that few staff development specialists can spend time helping clinicians maintain their competence. An SDS is responsible for and should be engaged in only two services: competence assessment and competence development. This second change is the recognition of the complex interaction of competence assessment and development activities with various systems that affect those activities. Third, the addition of a circle representing the "universe" of staff competence in a given organization is purposely represented as a larger universe than is possible for a clinical competence assessment and competence development program to be responsible for, or to even consider. There will always be more staff and competencies that cannot be assessed or measured by SDSs and CSD activities. The key is to identify, with others, the important few that should be assessed and developed. These concepts are discussed and applied more fully in Chapters 4 through 8.

The activities in the former model were previously considered maintenance issues and included "mandatory" topics, such as those topics thought to be required by one regulatory or accrediting body or another. However, experience has shown that clinicians are motivated to improve their practice by a variety of factors. Required training often did not reach the skill maintenance levels thought to be adequate, or outcomes expected to result from required training were not realized.

Despite unclear outcome expectations, programs were offered on a plethora of topics related to resuscitation (e.g., BLS, ACLS, PALS, ATLS), infection control, safety, and so forth. Although they were designed to improve care, many of these programs failed cost-benefit analysis. Lists abounded with names, titles, assignments, and job responsibilities organized in a variety of ways for a variety of federal, state, and local health department inspectors, consultants, and consumer groups.

Over a period of time, systematic competence assessment found that most care providers are willing to demonstrate their competence in a variety of ways using an array of strategies. Therefore, the new proposal updates or replaces concepts in the nursing staff development model with concepts applicable to CSD.

CSD in health care organizations may be organized as a program or a department. Is one structure better than another? Many approaches work; some do not. What works best? Are certain procedures and methods more efficient than others? As the field matures, these questions and many others need to be answered through systematic research and evaluation of staff development practices.

SKILL ACQUISITION IN CLINICAL STAFF DEVELOPMENT

As we acquire skill in the theoretical constructs that underlie a CSD program designed to assess and develop competence for quality patient care, we must also help others assess and develop skills relevant to their practice. The following section is written for the novice SDS unfamiliar with the Dreyfus (1986) skill acquisition model. Experienced SDSs may find this information useful as they design updated orientation programs for new specialists and other clinical staff.

These principles apply across many disciplines. The Dreyfus skill acquisition model is also known as "novice to expert" because Benner (1984) demonstrated congruence about the skillfulness of clinical nurses in daily practice and stages. The stages of novice, advanced beginner, competent, proficient, and expert are used here to parallel Benner's findings and to attempt to apply them to the skill development of clinical CSSs. Of course, every specialist brings a wealth of experience to the role, and this experience influences the acquisition of new skills required in new roles.

Simpson (1990) presented a skill acquisition plan that continues to be useful to today's SDS. Grounded in the Dreyfus model of skill acquisition and also using Benner's work, she suggested a progression to peak performance for the new staff development specialist, with characteristics and developmental activities for each level (Fig. 3-2). Sample programs are also proposed to challenge the SDS at various levels.

SDSs will find this useful in planning their own orientation, particularly in organizations where only one or two staff members are dedicated to this role. Large and complex

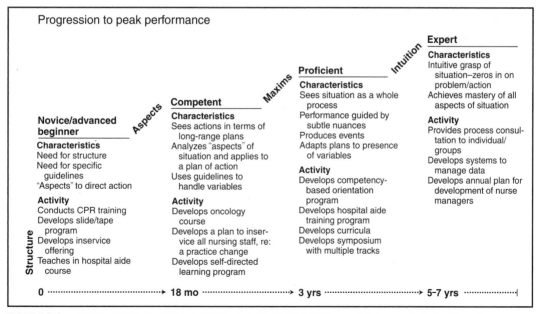

FIGURE 3-2. Staff development skill acquisition plan. Application of "Benner's Framework Novice-Expert" to development of the staff development specialist. Source: Mary Simpson, MSN, RN, Director of Nursing Staff Development, Ohio State University Hospital, Columbus, OH. Used with permission.

organizations also create staff development roles in various clinical departments that may or may not be linked to central departments, either formally nor informally. Astute SDSs who work in complex organizations will find ways to link to others performing similar work.

Getting Started as a Specialist

The novice SDS will want to gather information about the organization, its environment, expectations of others, and the status of the existing competence assessment and development activities and program. The specialist needs to know the:

- Organizational priorities
- Care imperatives
- Client or customer status
- Target audience
- Differences between "nice to know" and "need to know" competences of the staff groups the specialist is responsible for developing.

In small departments of one or a few, specialists may have to design their own orientation while simultaneously designing orientation plans for other new employees. Data from the skill acquisition model used here (Benner, 1984; Benner & Tanner, 1987) revealed that most clinical care providers need about a year to feel some confidence in their competence. New specialists should bear this in mind as they work on their own personal development program and programs for others.

A useful model to use for program design was illustrated by Holmes (1989) and is displayed in Chapter 10, Figure 10-1. Using classical program planning strategies, Holmes presented a step-by-step process. However, experienced specialists know that the linear appearance of the model is used only for illustration and does not necessarily reflect the order in which some of the planning activities occur.

NNSDO's (1994) critically acclaimed booklet *Getting Started in Nursing Staff Development* has served many novice specialists well during the first year of their practice.

Skill Acquisition

The following suggestions are derived from the knowledge gained from various applications of the Dreyfus model, as illustrated by Benner (1984), Benner et al. (1987, 1992), and others.

Novice SDSs usually have refined and well-developed clinical expertise. Although the novice SDS may have the capacity to see the whole picture of patients they were caring for in their clinical care provider role, the ability to see the whole picture of staff development and its potential in organizations is acquired during the first few years in practice. It takes about a year to feel as if everyday practice is manageable and less full of surprises. This is frustrating for highly skilled clinicians, who view themselves as quite competent. Some may return to the clinical settings in which they feel comfortable. Savvy staff development specialists, novices and otherwise, learn to balance clinical time with important staff development activities such as competence assessment.

Novices will also look for rules, guidelines, and resources to help guide their practice. Resources abound in many forms. New specialists may find it helpful to join local and national professional organizations, read journals, network, seek mentors, and engage in other personal development activities during this period of rapid growth and a steep learning curve.

The advanced beginner level seems to occur around the second year. Benner (1984) identified novices as student nurses and advanced beginners as new graduate nurses; this seems to apply to the staff development specialist role as well. During this developmental stage, the specialist will bend the rules or create new ones through innovative program offerings and responses to requests for various services. Some creativity is evident. Available resources are used and new ones are developed. Specialists begin to work more efficiently. Often, the specialist in this stage begins to develop confidence in his or her ability to influence practice and improve care.

The competent level was designated (Benner, 1984) as the stage in nursing practice development in which the nurse gets the whole picture, sets reasonable goals that can be accomplished, plans for the future, and develops flexibility. Staff development specialists often find themselves at this juncture in their development after about 2 or 3 years in practice. A certain level of comfort and an ability to predict outcomes based on past experiences are evident.

The proficient and expert levels are difficult to separate in this application and are treated as one level. After about 3 years of active engagement in the practice, some staff development specialists gain a significant understanding of the potential of competence assessment and development, its role in patient care, and the possibilities inherent in this work. Maxims are formulated and experience plays an important role. Politics and organizational decisions are readily understood and can often be predicted. Collaboration with a variety of other health care providers and managers is evident. The influence of these staff development specialists is often manifested in the numbers and kinds of change projects that the specialist is involved in or asked to lead. The expert staff development specialist welcomes these opportunities and creatively responds to them. Intuition, knowing what will and will not work, comes easily and naturally. The specialist can use political savvy to sell new ideas to stakeholders and care providers.

Kelly (1994) examined the nature of intuition among nursing staff development experts through extensive interviews about their experiences with intuition. Four themes emerged:

1. Struggling to find the knowing: forming and informing intuition
2. Informed knowing about the possibilities
3. Listening to the moment
4. Transforming the everyday nature of practice.

Intuition was defined as trusting the "whole-knowing" of the inner voice. The experts who participated in this dissertation research illuminated the phenomenon of intuitive knowing. They have made a rich contribution to understanding how staff development is practiced in health care organizations.

Specialists must continuously improve their staff development skills. Role development over time is a somewhat linear pattern. Some days, even expert staff development specialists identify new personal development needs to improve their practice and that of others. The knowledgeable specialist will recognize those moments as natural in the evolution of the role. Roles that do not change cease to exist; role development is continuous.

DEFINING ROLES IN THE FUTURE

The role of staff development within organizations will evolve as the roles of health care organizations and individual providers change. The continuing need to respond to change contributes strongly to the robustness of this field. Staff development specialists must acquire and use characteristics that will help them thrive.

Stream and Herrin (1990) studied successful staff development specialists and found three basic types:

- *The examiner*: Performs literature review to gather data; attempts to identify all available options and will keep researching and thinking to identify these; prefers to work alone; likes to deal with complex issues—the bigger the challenge, the better; questions fundamental assumptions, such as, "Why do we have to start orientation on Monday?"; is cautious
- *The collaborator*: Consistently consults colleagues; believes in group process; emphasizes role complementarity; enjoys and is good at mentoring; accepts the status quo to keep the peace; doesn't like to rock the boat
- *The specialist*: Reflects on own past experiences when making decisions; acts decisively and seizes opportunities; acts autonomously; appears self-confident in field of specialty; prefers hands-on management style—does it rather than delegates it.

Each of these clusters of characteristics has advantages and disadvantages. For example, the examiner knows the literature but may spend too much time analyzing; the collaborator has a strong network of colleagues but may be overly concerned about how others perceive him or her, which may interfere with appropriate decision making; and the specialist can make quick decisions, but these decisions may be premature.

Stream and Herrin (1990) found that successful staff development specialists are aware of their own characteristics as well as those of others and can comfortably draw on different behaviors as indicated. In other words, they can use the examiner approach to analysis in some situations and the quick decisiveness of the specialist in others.

These investigators also provided advice about enhancing each basic type. To enhance their skills, examiners should:

- Read more.
- Use formal problem-solving processes, such as force field analysis.
- Break down complex problems into workable units; develop PERT and GANT charts.
- Persevere in tasks.
- Train to be assertive.
- Ask why.

Collaborators should:

- Surround themselves with competence; hire people to complement their own limitations.
- Trust subordinates and allow them freedom.
- Reward good performance.
- Engage in mentoring relationships.
- Join organizations for networking.
- Learn to accept compliments.

Specialists should:

- Engage in positive "self-talk."
- Take an inventory of their own skills.
- Define their expertise and "turf."
- Publicize their skills.
- Trust their judgments.
- Think through worst-case scenarios—for instance, "What would be the worst thing that would happen if we tried this new strategy?"

These basic types have been validated with an instrument developed by the investigators and have proven to be useful to help staff development specialists learn about how they perform their work. Specialists can learn much through self-inventories and should use them to help understand how to position themselves and their work for success within the organization.

Role Development

Like the field of staff development itself, the role of the specialist is varied and poorly defined. Job descriptions and performance expectations help the specialist interpret organizational expectations for the role, but they rarely define the full range of competencies often expected of the specialist. The elementary reason for this may be simply the need for a role that is broadly and flexibly defined to allow the specialist the freedom to redefine the role in response to new and ongoing organizational initiatives.

This may be frustrating for specialists who prefer structure and a predictable work environment. Role definition efforts are worthwhile; if nothing else, the process causes the specialist to think through the most important components of the role as it is currently defined or implemented. The role of the SDS is complex, varied, and changing and includes many components.

Characteristics and Competencies

SDSs should examine the changes in health care system structures, processes, and outcomes to analyze how these elements will help them understand more about role expectations and what needs to be done to advance the competence assessment and development of clinical personnel for quality care.

The Delphi study conducted by the American Society of Training and Development is a helpful attempt to identify these many components and roles. It reviewed the trainer role throughout industries, and application can be made to the CSD role. McLagan (1989), in a review of this study, wrote, "There will clearly be great economic and personal value in being able to optimize the performance of individuals, teams and entire organizations" in the future (p. 51). She listed 11 key outputs by role:

1. Administrator
2. Evaluator
3. Human resources development manager
4. Human resources development materials developer
5. Individual career development adviser
6. Instructor or facilitator
7. Marketer
8. Needs analyst
9. Organization change agent
10. Program designer
11. Researcher.

She further listed four types of competencies:

1. Technical competencies: adult learning understanding, career development skill, competency-identification skill, computer competence, objectives preparation skill, performance observation skill, electronic systems skill, facilities skill, subject matter skill, and training and development understanding
2. Business competencies: business understanding, cost-benefit analysis skill,

> delegation skill, industry understanding, organization behavior understanding, organization development theories and techniques, and project and record management skills
>
> 3. Interpersonal competencies: skills related to coaching, feedback, group process, negotiation, presentations, questioning, relationship building, and writing
> 4. Intellectual competencies: data reduction skill, information search skill, intellectual versatility, model-building skill, observing skill, self-knowledge, and visioning skill.

Achieving these competencies may seem daunting and perhaps even impossible, but learning about these competencies is the beginning of acquiring the skills needed for the future. This study serves as a useful model to challenge staff development specialists in their continuing development and role definition. Careful consideration of these sample competencies will help specialists continue to evolve as sophisticated providers of staff development services.

The shifts in practice in health care, nursing, and staff development require shifts in practice patterns. These practice patterns can be explored and documented as an integral part of performance standards when a framework such as this is used to discover how SDSs spend their time at present and how they should spend their time in the future.

The most meaningful contribution the SDS can make to the competence of nurses is the ability to "learn how to learn." People learn in a variety of ways and have preferred learning styles. In pursuing new knowledge or skills, people seek experiences and engage in learning in ways that are personal and meaningful. People can be helped to think about how they think. Termed "metacognition" by cognitive scientists, the process of how people think can be expanded to how they go about acquiring new knowledge. If the staff development specialist can simply raise the awareness of learning as something that is done by people rather than to people, then progress can be made toward this goal.

Certification

An option open to the experienced staff development specialist to demonstrate competence is certification. Various organizations offer different certifications. Some specialists seek certification to become certified health education specialists. Nurses may seek certification as a staff development generalist from the American Nurses Credentialing Center (ANCC). In 1996, the ANCC reported that 111,164 nurses had been certified through its 16 specialties and 2,078 (2%) had successfully completed the staff development generalist certification examination. Others may seek other forms of certification from different accrediting or certifying agencies. Courses, programs, and study materials are available to help staff development specialists and educators pass required tests. The purpose of most of these certifications is to demonstrate competence in the field. The certification is often used as a hallmark of the person's commitment to quality practice.

A recent Delphi study by the ANA's Council for Professional Nursing Education and Development and the NNSDO (1997) about advanced practice in continuing education and staff development is also of interest to SDSs. Results of three Delphi rounds yielded six major areas of advanced practice competencies:

- Level of awareness
- Educational process repertoire
- Establishing relationships
- Interacting with the practice environment
- Contributions to the profession
- Individual characteristics.

Seventy-seven competencies were identified in the second Delphi round and rated by 727 participants, further yielding significant data about the competencies of advanced practice in staff development. Whether these identified competencies can be offered in some form of certification examination has yet to be determined; the task force recommended conveying this information to the ANCC for consideration. This study provides rich data about the perceptions of thousands of practicing staff development specialists.

STAFF DEVELOPMENT RESEARCH

The need to inquire about any field of practice is clear. If a group of persons who call themselves something want to add legitimacy to their discipline, they must provide a systematic collection of data to support their theories, ideas, and projected outcomes. Thus, the field of CSD, like any other, calls for inquiry, exploration, examination, and experimentation. Only through systematic scientific methods will our field, practice, and discipline grow. The following section provides examples of the interests that some experienced staff development specialists have pursued; it is not intended to be exhaustive.

NNSDO Research Committee

Some SDSs have formed a community of learning and inquiry. The NNSDO and other clinical specialty professional associations sponsor research committees or staff development special interest groups or councils. Members of these groups share a view of staff development—what it is and what it can be. Inquiry, theory testing, and continued examination of the best practices are required as this field evolves.

Each group sets goals and envisions a future. The NNSDO Research Committee in 1993 described itself as "a structure and process in which research activities, relationships, and accomplishments related to staff development advance the specialty practice and contribute to quality patient care." Activities of the committee were described as making regular contributions to the association newsletter, providing ongoing support for a Delphi study being conducted by a committee member as part of her doctoral studies, designing convention activities to highlight CSD research, and raising money to establish a small grants and scholarship program. The committee set nursing staff development outcomes as a inquiry focus and conducted an exhaustive literature search. Reviews were categorized into five areas:

- Reference and study focus
- Sample source and size
- Measurement used
- Types of outcomes found
- Strengths and limitations, and comments

A monograph with these findings is scheduled for distribution in 1999.

Results of the Schoenly (1994) Delphi study supported by NNSDO yielded the following research priorities and gave the organization direction and momentum. The following were the top three questions as ranked by a staff development panel after three rounds:

1. How can the benefit of staff development programs be measured as related to improved patient outcome and reduced health care costs?
2. Which staff competency measurements (*e.g.*, written examination, supervised skills, self-assessment, performance appraisal) are the best predictors of actual nursing competency?
3. Does competency-based education or orientation improve quality of care?

As a result of these findings and the literature review, the committee sponsored a colloquium at the 1996 convention to explore benchmarking, best practices, and outcomes. The participants in the colloquium agreed to provide data about their experiences with staff development outcomes. Data are being analyzed, and reports are imminent. Plans to extend the study are also underway.

In addition to these activities, the committee continue to promote the need for research-based practice among clinicians for clinical care and staff development specialists for competence assessment and development.

Research-Based Practice

The core of staff development work is the evidence available to support particular procedures, tasks, and other ministering provided to patients. For example, procedures such as CPR require a systematic response and a series of activities by a variety of clinicians and support staff to give the patient the best chance of recovery. The team should review each member's performance. This review can be arranged in a variety of configurations, including:

- Quality monitors
- Procedure evaluation by self-assessment using a checklist after the fact
- Procedure evaluation by checklist during the arrest by an observer
- Videotape review by an expert panel, with recommendations
- Discussion during routine team meetings
- Other strategies in which participating clinicians examine their practice.

Some inquiries are arranged in a controlled clinical trial design; others are less rigorous. Although the controlled clinical trial is considered the gold standard for certain inquiries, others do not require or cannot support an experimental design. Important data can be gained through a variety of systematic approaches to inquiry, examination, and exploration. The SDS brings real-world knowledge to any research design that is valuable to and valued by most organizations.

Other Relevant Studies

Recently, experienced staff development specialists have conducted systematic investigations to answer questions. For example, Aucoin (1997) conducted a study to identify reasons for staff development specialists' participation in continuing education programs and how that participation relates to certification. Surveying 600 staff development specialists using a "participation reasons" scale, Aucoin reported that specialists participated because they want to develop new professional knowledge and skills, keep abreast of new developments, and be more productive in their role.

We must begin to define specific and contributing staff development outcomes to continue to demonstrate our value and contribution to care of patients. To that end, the definitions and models proposed earlier in this chapter are presented for discussion and inquiry.

CSD research is also found in the literature of other fields. For example, a group of administrators and educators (McLaughlin et al., 1995) surveyed more than 200 hospital-based chief nurse executives to examine the number of hours and the related costs spent by staff in orientation and job retraining as part of their care delivery system changes. The number of hours spent in orientation or job retraining of nurses to prepare them to work with unlicensed assistive personnel were measured; the hourly cost was reported to be $33.66, with a total mean cost of $814.14 for 24 hours of training. These cost reports did not include on-the-job follow-up training.

Another study (Jelinas & Manthey, 1995) also investigated improvement of patient outcomes through systems change. Through structured telephone interviews, 13 executives provided important data about the impact of work redesign on the roles of hospital executives. This study was relevant to future staff development activities for many levels of hospital staff, including clinicians.

A great deal more could be written about the importance of research to staff development. Staff development specialists use research in their practice much the same as clinicians do, and staff development specialists must study their own practice to continued improvement and understanding. Models have demonstrated their usefulness, in practice and research, for understanding (McSweeney et al., 1997). Moving forward, with inquiring minds, is the only direction open to SDSs.

SUMMARY

This chapter examined the nature of CSD and presented several ideas that merged concepts from a variety of disciplines. A new definition and model of CSD was illustrated, with a rationale for its use. Advice for the novice staff development specialist was provided, and selected research issues and studies were included.

The purpose of this chapter was to give a flavor of an evolving field of practice that is dedicated to producing competent care providers. Future definitions of the field will better merge concepts from many theories: adult learning, adult development, performance improvement, outcome measurement, and the theories of change, systems, and organization development. This blending of knowledge from various sources will strengthen CSD practice and will make this knowledge relevant to the complex reality of staff development in health care organizations. It will also affirm the value of the diverse background, experience, academic preparation, and beliefs of staff development specialists.

The Education of an Educator

DONNA MILLER

My entry into the practice of staff development occurred quite unintentionally. I was working part-time in a coronary care unit while completing my BSN. A few months before graduation, the head nurse of that unit called me into her office. She was curious to know what career plans I had upon graduation. I told her I was uncertain about what direction in which to head, but that I loved to teach. Despite my love of teaching, I was very clear that I did not want a position within staff development. My impression of the staff development educator at that time was a nurse who provided in-service education on products. This short-sighted impression came from my observation of educators I had encountered in the past. The only time I saw the educators was for education on new products. I could not comprehend how one person could talk about nothing but products 8 hours a day, 5 days a week! This subjective observation convinced me that staff development was not a viable career option.

Interestingly enough, the head nurse told there was a staff development position in critical care that she wanted me to consider. I was surprised to learn that the role encompassed more than just in-service education: I would be responsible for assessment, planning, conducting, and evaluating the critical care orientation program and other projects as assigned. I told her that I would give it some thought and get back to her.

After reviewing our conversation over the subsequent days, I decided that speaking to the director of staff development and the staff development educators might be insightful. The conversation with the educators was overwhelming. As a staff nurse, I had tunnel vision about what the educators did. I only saw the finished product, never realizing the hours it must have taken to research, plan, write, and so forth the educational offering. The educator made the presentation look so easy, which disguised the time, effort, and organizational skills that were required to present such a polished effort.

I met with the director for staff development to obtain her perspectives and expectations of the critical care educator. One of the high-priority needs for that service was to conduct a critical care orientation within 2 months. Two months did not seem like quite enough time to research and write the entire curriculum. The director eased my concern by saying that the curriculum used in the past would be suitable. The handouts, slides, overheads, equipment, and contact-hour applications were in place and available for use in this upcoming orientation. Ironically, I was offered and accepted a position I believed I would never want.

It took only a few weeks before I received my first educational challenge: the orientation curriculum that was in place was suddenly nowhere to be found! No matter where I looked, this infamous notebook was gone. There was no time to waste in searching further; a decision had to be made. My choices seemed to be the following: continue to mourn the loss of the notebook, resign and return to my staff position, or accept this as a challenge and move forward. I chose to accept the challenge and be ready by January 1, even though it was already November!

My previous experience teaching at a school of nursing and radiology prepared me to meet this challenge. I had been so fortunate to have faculty and directors who were willing to provide me with opportunities and experiences in education, even though I was a graduate of an associate degree program. It was those experiences that helped me complete this seemingly insurmountable task at 6 p.m. on Christmas Eve. It is a holiday I will never forget!

I have been privileged to practice in the specialty of staff development—critical care for over 10 years. Not a day, week, or month goes by without a new challenge emerging. It is that constant challenge that somehow keeps the educator going despite all odds. Resources diminish and roles may change, but the staff development educator continues to persevere and create strategies that educate staff to affect health care outcomes.

REFERENCES

Abruzzese, R. S. (1996). *Nursing staff development: Strategies for success.* St. Louis: Mosby.

Alspach, J. G. (1995). *The educational process in nursing staff development.* St. Louis: Mosby.

Alspach, J. G. (1996). *Designing competency assessment programs: A handbook for nursing and health-related programs.* Pensacola, FL: National Nursing Staff Development Organization.

American Academy of Nursing Writing Group of the 1996 Expert Panel on Women's Health. (1997). Women's health and women's health care: Recommendations of the 1996 AAN Expert Panel on Women's Health. *Nursing Outlook, 45*(1), 7–15.

American Nurses Credentialing Center (ANCC). *1996 certification catalog.* Washington DC: Author.

Aucoin, J. W. (1997). The comparison in participation in continuing nursing education between certified and non-certified staff development specialists. Unpublished doctoral dissertation, Louisiana State University.

Avillion, A. (1995). *Core curriculum for nursing staff development.* Pensacola, FL: National Nursing Staff Development Organization.

Belenky, M. F., Clinchy, B. M., Goldberger, N. R., & Tarule, J. M. (1986). *Women's ways of knowing: The development of self, voice, and mind.* New York: Basic Books.

Benner, P. (1984). *Novice to expert: Excellence and power in clinical nursing practice.* Menlo Park, CA: Addison-Wesley.

Benner, P., & Tanner, C. A. (1987). Clinical judgment: How expert nurses use intuition. *American Journal of Nursing, 87*, 23–31.

Benner, P., Tanner, C., & Chesla, C. (1992). From beginner to expert: Gaining a differentiated clinical world in critical care nursing. *Advances in Nursing Science, 14*(3), 13–28.

Bennett, N. L. (1990). Theories of adult development and continuing education. *Journal of Continuing Education in the Health Professions, 10*, 167–175.

Bille, D. A. (1982). *Nursing staff development: A systems approach.* Thorofare, NJ: Slack.

Carper, B. A. (1992). Fundamental patterns of knowing nursing. In Nicoll, L. H. (Ed.). *Perspectives on nursing theory*, pp. 216–224. Philadelphia: J. B. Lippincott.

Chinn, P. L., & Kramer, M. K. (1995). *Theory and nursing: A systematic approach*, 5th ed. St. Louis: Mosby.

Coye, D. (1976). *Guidelines for staff development.* Kansas City, MO: ANA.

Del Bueno, D. J. (1978). Competency-based education. *Nurse Educator*, May/June, 10–14.

Del Bueno, D.J., Weeks, L., & Brown-Stewart, P. (1987). Clinical assessment centers: An cost-effective alternative for competency development. *Nursing Economic$, 5*(1), 21–26.

Del Bueno, D. J. (1990a). Experience, education and nurses' ability to make clinical judgments. *Nursing and Health Care, 11*(6), 290–294.

Del Bueno, D. J. (1990b). Evaluation: Myths, mystiques and obsessions. *Journal of Nursing Administration, 20*(4), 208–211.

Del Bueno, D. J. (1993). Competence, criteria, and credentialing. *Journal of Nursing Administration, 23*(5), 7–8.

Del Bueno, D. J. (1995). Spotlight on ... Ready, willing, able? Staff competence in workplace redesign. *Journal of Nursing Administration, 25*(9), 14–16.

Dreyfus, H. X., & Dreyfus, S. X. (1986). *Mind over machine: Intuition in an era of artificial intelligence and the computer.* New York: Free Press.

Dubois, D. D. (1993). *Competency-based performance improvement: Strategy for organizational change.* Amherst, MA: HRD Press.

Glover, E. (1994). Education and the quality of banking. *Banking World, 12*(4), 22–24.

Jelinas, L. S., & Manthey, M. (1995). Improving patient outcomes through systems change. *Journal of Nursing Administration, 25*(5), 55–63.

Jeska, S. B., & Fischer, K. J. (1996). *Performance improvement in staff development: The next evolution.* Pensacola, FL: National Nursing Staff Development Organization.

Johnson, N. (1994). Education reforms and professional development of principals: Implications for universities. *Journal of Educational Administration, 32*(2), 5–20.

Kegan, R. (1994). *In over our heads: The mental demands of modern life.* Cambridge, MA: Harvard University Press.

Kelly, K. J. (1992). *Nursing staff development: Current competence, future focus.* Philadelphia: J. B. Lippincott.

Kelly, K. J. (1995). The nature of intuition among nursing staff development experts: A Heideggerian hermetical analysis. Doctoral dissertation, George Mason University, 1994. *Dissertation Abstracts International*, 55-11, B4786. (University Microfilms No. AAI95 10813).

Knowles, M. S. (1988). *The modern practice of adult education: From pedagogy to andragogy.* Englewood Cliffs, NJ: Cambridge Book Co.

Manecke, S. R., & Wild, J. (1994). Medical staff development plan a valuable resource. *Healthcare Financial Management, 48*(2), 66–67.

McLagan, P. (1989). Models for HRD practice. *Training and Development Journal, 43*(9), 49–59.

McLaughlin, F. E., Thomas, S. A., & Barter, M. (1995). Changes related to care delivery patterns. *Journal of Nursing Administration, 25*(5), 35–46.

McSweeney, J. C., Allen, J. D., & Mayo, K. (1997). Exploring the use of explanatory models in nursing research and practice. *Image: Journal of Nursing Scholarship, 29*(3), 243–248.

Meleis, A. I. (1997). *Theoretical nursing: Development and progress*, 3rd ed. Philadelphia: Lippincott-Raven.

National Nursing Staff Development Organization (NNSDO). (1994). *Getting started in nursing staff development.* Pensacola, FL: Author.

National Nursing Staff Development Organization (NNSDO). (1997). *Report of the task force on advanced practice in nursing continuing education and staff development.* Pensacola, FL: Author.

Nierenberg, A. (1996). Teaching managers to be trainers boosts morale and the bottom line. *Business Marketing, 81*(1), 20–22.

O'Connor, A. B. (1986). *Nursing staff development and continuing education.* Boston: Little, Brown.

Pfefferkorn, B. (1928). Improvement of the nurse in service: An historical review. *American Journal of Nursing, 28*(11), 700.

Portwood, D. (1993). Work-based learning has arrived. *Management Development Review, 6*(6), 36–38.

Schoenly, L. (1994). *Research priorities in nursing staff development: A Delphi Study.* Pensacola, FL: National Nursing Staff Development Organization.

Schultz, P. R., & Meleis, A. I. (1988). Nursing epistemology: Traditions, insights, questions. *Image: Journal of Nursing Scholarship, 20*(4), 217–221.

Simpson, M. (1990). Progression to peak performance model. In Kelly, K. J. (Ed.). *Nursing staff development: Current competence, future focus,* p. 23. Philadelphia: J. B. Lippincott.

Stream, P. A., & Herrin, R. M. (1990). *Characteristics of successful staff development specialists.* Personal communication.

Taylor, K., & Marrienau, C. (1995). Bridging practice and theory for women's adult development. *New Directions for Adult and Continuing Education, 65,* 5–11.

Tripp-Reimer, T., Woodworth, G., McCloskey, J. C., & Bulechek, G. (1996). The dimensional structure of nursing interventions. *Nursing Research, 45*(1), 10–16.

Tobin, H., Yoder-Wise, P., & Hull. P. (1979). *The process of nursing staff development: Components for change.* St. Louis: Mosby.

Wright, D. (1997). *The ultimate guide to competency assessment in health care.* Eau Claire, WI: Professional Education Systems.

4

Competence: The Outcome of Assessment and Development

KAREN J. KELLY-THOMAS

This chapter supports the premise that competence is the outcome of assessment and development. If clinical staff development specialists (SDSs) engage in systematic assessment of an array of clinical competencies using a variety of strategies that provide meaningful data about persons and groups, they can provide information about the capacity of the health care team and organization to provide quality patient care. Further, the assessment data generated can be used as part of an organized program to develop competent providers of health care services who are also capable of improving personal clinical performance and quality care.

The concept of competence will be discussed, along with perspectives and terms in common use in assessment and development activities. Several approaches to assess and develop competence are presented, and a few myths are debunked with reality checks.

The potential for continuous quality improvement is embedded in competence assessment and development activities; indeed, the entire clinical staff development (CSD) process is conducted against a backdrop of quality improvement.

COMPETENCE

Competence means many things to many people. The word has gained so much popularity in so many circles that its meaning must be clarified by anyone planning to profess it, measure it, assess it, or develop it. Therefore, definitions for several terms are offered to bring some consistency to the conversations that may start as a result of this text.

Some definitions are suggested in Table 4-1. SDSs should adopt a similar list acceptable to the administration, clinical managers, and clinicians in their organization.

What Competence Is

The word "competent," for the purposes of this text, is used merely as an adjective to describe the clinician who has demonstrated the ability to perform selected skills adequately. These skills were selected because they had been identified as important to the organization and the population of patients served.

Benner (1984) defined competent nurses as those in practice for more than 3 years or so who could perform a task with a desirable outcome in the context of the real world. The competent nurse, in Benner's lexicon, may progress to other levels of skill, such as proficient or expert, but may also remain at the competent level indefinitely.

TABLE 4-1	
SOME WORKING DEFINITIONS OF COMPETENCE	
Competence	A person's *capacity* to perform his or her job function
Competency	A person's *actual performance* in his or her specific job function or specified task
Competency or competence assessment	An appraisal that measures whether persons or groups have the knowledge and skills required to provide care; with the appraisal, focus is on making the technical, critical thinking, or interpersonal relationships visible or observable in some way—an organized staff development activity that systematically ascertains if the person or group has requisite knowledge and skills and can put them into action at the right time and place for the best reasons
Competencies	A new word developed through popular use; those identified skills considered necessary to perform a specific job or service
Standards	Authoritative statements, promulgated by the profession, by which the quality of practice, service, or education can be judged (ANA, 1994)

Del Bueno (1990) defined competence as the effective application of knowledge and skill in the work setting and identified the dimensions of competence as critical thinking skills, technical skills, and interpersonal skills applied in a given setting (see Fig. 6-1 in Chap. 6). The National Council of State Boards of Nursing (1996) defined competence as the application of knowledge and the interpersonal, decision-making, and psychomotor skills expected for the nurse's practice role, within the context of public health, welfare, and safety.

Organizations have sprung up as a result of the concern about competence. Most clinical specialty organizations and professional societies refer to competence in their charters or mission in some direct or indirect way. According to the National Organization for Competency Assurance (NOCA), it has been the leader in setting quality standards for credentialing organizations (NOCA, 1997a). NOCA's mission specifically promotes excellence in competency assurance for all occupations and professions. NOCA also develops standards and accredits the organizations that meet them. It lists more than 160 organizational members (NOCA, 1997b).

It seems that with all these organizations, groups, and people concerned about competence, there would be abundant evidence to support the belief that most health care providers are competent. There is. It is up to the SDS to reveal that competence and other findings through routine assessment and development activities.

Principles

Although the definitions in Table 4-1 have not been empirically tested in a randomized, controlled trial, they do offer a commonly held set of principles. These principles include competence as an outcome of:

- Learning
- Assessment
- Development
- Experience.

The outcome of competence can be achieved through any one of these four principles when the principles are applied in a systematic way. The principles may be evident alone as a single competency demonstrated by a person, the competence of a group or a person, or some other combination. For example, a learning activity that includes periodic feedback and final evaluation of skill acquisition is a combination assessment and development activity that may or may not be part of the person's or the group's previous experience. The SDS assesses, develops, and assesses learning again in a circular pattern and integrates the experience of the group to assess their readiness to learn and their motivation for learning. During a CPR class, for instance, recent cardiopulmonary arrest incidents may be discussed, further developing the skills of participants through their own experience and that of others.

The *outcome of learning as competence* is reflected in the data collected at the end of formal learning activities. Although some of these data may be suspect, aggregated scores of persons using valid and reliable measurement instruments form a piece of the fabric that makes up a competent person and a competent organization. Other data (*e.g.,* performance test results, direct observation using a data collection tool, or actual performance self-assessed using a tool or model answer) can also be used to help weave the cloth of competence of people, groups, and organizations.

The *outcome of assessment as competence* can be observed from the data collected during the activity and the subsequent judgment and analysis of those data. Any systematic assessment should be designed to collect data about the abilities of people, groups, and the entire organization. The systematic assessment is designed to produce data that is judged by the SDS and others to support or refute the claim of competence.

Data may be presented in the form of means, median, modes, yes/no percentages, averages of several variables, or higher-level statistical analysis, such as correlations or analysis of variance. The data may even be in the form of text, photos, or videos that can be analyzed using qualitative or interpretive methods. The important issue is the judgment of the person analyzing and reporting the findings. For example, an SDS or clinical manager may judge a set of high test scores assessing fire safety knowledge as adequate evidence that all staff can perform safety maneuvers in an emergency. In fact, the test scores illustrate only that the participants know what to do in the situation presented in the test; they do *not* prove that they can perform the skills, only that they know what to do and may be able to apply that knowledge in an actual emergency.

Although test items can be written in a sophisticated manner and can test critical thinking in presented situations, the test is only one part of assessing competence. The assessment activity provides data about the competence of the organization, group, and person related to the specific competency assessed. In other words, test scores do provide some evidence about the competence of the group and may predict its ability to perform. Data collected during assessment activities in laboratories or actual clinical situations also provide information about competence.

The *outcome of development as competence* is found in the data collected during the evaluation phase of the learning activity. Depending on the methods used by the CSD to evaluate a formal or informal learning activity, the level of staff confidence as well as the data analysis can add to the tapestry of competence. For example, say that a new technology will be introduced into the high-risk OB area that includes a change in the way a fetus is monitored. The developmental learning activity should be designed so that quantitative and qualitative data will be generated during the evaluation stage of the activity.

The *outcome of experience as competence* is found through the everyday stories of persons performing clinical patient care, including managers, SDSs, and clinicians. All have stories to tell that can inform others about their competence. How those stories are collected and analyzed determines how those data can be used to support or refute claims of competence in an organization or group. The SDS interested in using everyday experience as evidence of competence must still conduct that assessment activity in a systematic way. Display 4-1 gives a classic example of a data collection tool that can provide at least nominal (yes or no) data to support or refute one part of the person's or group's competence. The tool is derived from Del Bueno's performance-based development system (Del Bueno et al., 1987) and is modified for use by clinicians, managers, and SDSs.

What Competence Can Be

The problem with many clinical competence assessment and development programs is that they are set up only to meet regulatory body requirements, rather than considering the larger intent of the requirement. Quality care is the backdrop for these activities, and the competence assessment and development program should make significant contributions to the continuous improvement of quality in that organization. If it does not, then it is not a meaningful method for the organization, and patients do not benefit.

Long checklists in binders on shelves or files in drawers will not provide meaningful data for the organization to use to illustrate its commitment to quality care. A review of some of those lists, files, and other records demonstrating "compliance with mandatories" will show that many are merely "paper drills" because "so-and-so said we have to do it this way." Although a few regulations are very specific, most specify only that an organization must have a competence assessment and development system, leaving it up to the organization and its professionals to design, implement, monitor, evaluate, and improve such a system. When checklists in use are found to include procedures no longer performed (*e.g.*, application of Skultetis binders), this is evidence that the organization is not evaluating its system. This is where the SDS role comes into play to implement systematic improvement.

Competence assessment and development can take on many looks and designs. Dubois (1993) designed a competency-based performance improvement system and attempted to describe competency in its most generic form. Competency, he said, is any characteristic a person has and uses that leads to successful performance in a life role. He described approaches to develop a competence perspective, such as the modified task analysis approach, critical trait approach, and situational approach. His work emphasizes competency-based education and training processes and the measurement of the resulting competence. Dubois (1995) further developed this approach by introducing diagnostic checklists, planning and conducting data-collection activities, handling and analyzing data, and interpreting data for program implementation. Within the context of human resources development, he presented another approach to the development of a competency-based performance improvement system. What is relevant to the SDS in his work is the description of another approach that may work better in a given organization.

Staying licensed and meeting regulatory and accrediting body recommendations are

---

DISPLAY 4-1

Assessment Tool for Aggregating, Analyzing, and Reporting Data About Critical Thinking Skills

Competence Assessment Program
Skill: Critical Thinking
Unit:
Assessor:

During rounds, report, or other interactions with staff, create the following conversation and assess your staff's critical thinking skills.

Q1: What is this patient's priority health care problem or concern?
Q2: What nursing actions are you taking to manage the problem or reduce the risk?
Q3: Why (or what is your rationale)?

NAME	PT. ID	Q1	Q2	Q3	COMMENT

Summary/Judgment:

Action Plan:

Source: Author. Used with permission.

one way the organization demonstrates its commitment to the community. Serving the members of the community is the reason for being for every health care organization, whether it is a small rural community hospital or a large tertiary care complex on several campuses. A commitment to providing competent care providers is evident in established and systematic competence assessment and development programs.

PERSPECTIVES

A variety of motivators cause people, groups, and organizations to engage in competence assessment and development activities. Some of these activities are planned, organized endeavors designed to collect masses of data as efficiently as possible—hence, the growth of "skills fairs" to "check staff competence." Although skills fairs are efficient, they may not be as effective for long-term recall about selected topics. (Chapter 7 discusses mandatory education in more detail, and Chapter 11 discusses many design options available to the SDS.)

Motivators

Clinicians are motivated by many reasons and circumstances. Motivators to participate in activities designed to produce the outcome of competence are external or internal. External motivators include, "I was sent," "I don't know why I'm here," and "I'm here because I want to learn about my competence and improve it." The latter, which is music to the SDS's ears, can be brought about by continuous reinforcement by clinical managers and specialists; they can reiterate, frequently, that the purpose of clinical staff assessment and development activities is to produce data to support or refute the competence of the person and group and to improve that competence continuously for quality patient care.

Many clinicians are internally motivated to do the best job they can. Most professionals in health care fields entered the field because they had a strong desire to help people. Doing good work is motivated by this strong internal desire, and this internal motivation helps SDSs, too. SDSs and clinical managers who must provide participants with an incentive and compel them to assess and develop their competence are often frustrated by this need for external motivation. Although SDSs are often internally motivated, many learners need to be motivated externally.

Like people, groups and organizations may be internally motivated or externally motivated. Health care organizations with a commitment to quality, as evidenced by actions of the members of the organization, are internally motivated. In these organizations, there is a sense of purpose and focus on the patient that goes beyond the visions, missions, and goals set forth on the walls or in manuals. On the other hand, groups and organizations that are externally motivated often set up systems that meet requirements but do not necessarily improve care.

Agendas

Wright (1997) provided a practical and well-thought-through guide and listed five reasons why health care organizations initiate competence assessment activities. She says organizations may be:

1. Looking for ways to evaluate individual performance
2. Looking for ways to evaluate group performance
3. Meeting standards set by a regulatory agency
4. Addressing problematic issues within an organization
5. Enhancing or replacing performance appraisal (p. 2).

The National Council of State Board of Nursing (1997) adopted a landmark change for nursing regulation in August 1997 during its meeting in Chicago. The Delegate Assembly took a significant step forward in the advancement of nursing regulation and credentialing when it endorsed a mutual recognition model for nursing regulation. The effect of this endorsement on those states who consider accumulation of continuing education hours as a measure of competence will play out in interesting ways. The effect on health care system-based competence assessment and development systems may be momentous, too, depending on how the mandatory continuing education for relicensure rules are interpreted for the nurse who holds a license in one state and can practice in any state.

One reason often cited by SDSs for engaging in competence assessment and development activities is that they represent a true commitment to continuous improvement of care through improvement of the care providers. SDSs realize that all of these reasons serve as an agenda for designing a sound competence assessment and development system and use all agenda items to operationalize and improve their systems.

TERMS

As mentioned above, the terms "competence" and "competency" are problematic due to their popularity. To many contributors to this text and to the body of knowledge of CSD, "competency" is used most commonly to describe a person's actual performance of a skill in a particular situation. The situation may be in the real clinical setting with an observer assessing, or the competency can be self-reported by the person. The competency also may be measured in a classroom setting with a simulation set up to mimic the real world. A competency also can be measured in everyday clinical settings by peers, managers, and SDSs, depending on the system in place in the organization. Sophisticated SDSs recognize that competence assessment and development pervades most of the work performed by clinicians, managers, and specialists and is not something that has to be recreated in a bogus setting, such as a classroom, to take some measure of the particular competency.

"Competency-based education" is a term used to describe a philosophical approach to education. Outcomes, or what the learner can do as a result of learning, are more important than the path taken to get to competence. Emphasis is on the learning outcome rather than the process of teaching. The term emerged in the 1950s when teacher education was overhauled to emphasize student learning and application of that learning rather than how teachers should teach.

"Competency-based orientation" is a term that gained popularity in the 1970s in health care and challenged staff development specialists to reconsider the methods used to teach new employees. They noted the importance of competence as the outcome of teaching and learning and the need to use alternative strategies, including self-learning packages and modules, to provide information to new and continuing employees. Del Bueno (1993) underscored the importance of evaluating learning using a variety of strategies, some within the context of real-world patient care.

Competence, throughout this text, is meant to include the overall skillfulness and capacity of a person, group, or organization. The assessment of competencies, selected because they are important to the organization and the patients served, is the normal work of the organization, usually through SDSs, to accumulate various data sets that can serve as evidence that the clinicians are competent. The organization can show its overall competence through these assessment and development activities for all stakeholders, including patients, care providers, administrators, regulators, accreditors, and the community.

Competent is a word that describes clinicians, other employees, groups, or an entire organization as having demonstrated their critical thinking skills, technical skills, and interpersonal skills and having been deemed capable of demonstrating performance expectations. Evidence is available to support the application of this term to the person, group, or organization.

An outcome is the result of a staff development intervention. This "action" word is meant to illustrate that CSD is a dynamic and continuously developing field with many interventions available for assessing and developing the competence of clinicians. Chapter 8 provides additional information about this notion of competence as the outcome of a staff development intervention. SDSs who recognize this outcome and can demonstrate results and a track record will be successful in health care organizations today.

APPROACHES TO ASSESS COMPETENCE

As mentioned throughout this chapter and text, there are many approaches to assessing competence. In Chapter 5, Wolgin describes an approach grounded in quality management, performance evaluation, and development of competence within complex systems. In Chapter 6, Jeska describes a strategic thinking approach using organizational learning teams. In Chapter 7, Katz describes a competence assessment system that is built primarily on external organizational motivators such as regulatory bodies, while still integrating many of the hardy values of most established staff development programs. Other contributors also discuss staff development and its related competence assessment and development activities.

"Quality management" is another term that has lost its clarity through its popularity. The notion of quality and its management has taken on many forms in health care and other industries. Quality is viewed as a desirable state of an organization that is always seeking ways to improve its services, providers, and the processes used to provide those services. All efforts are devoted to helping the patient return to health. Health promotion, health maintenance, and health restoration are the primary goals, and quality management is the means to get to that state of health. Chapter 13 discusses quality management in CSD and how it fits into the larger picture.

Performance evaluation is another routine organizational activity in a health care facility that values quality as part of its mission. Data collected through assessment and development activities are used to build a case for (or against) individual or group competence. The formal activity in which the data are presented and analyzed is called performance evaluation. Improvement and continuous development activities are the ongoing items that feed data into a performance evaluation. The performance evaluation may be about a person, a group, a team, or the total organization. "Report cards" are a common approach to performance evaluation in health care today.

There is great disagreement about the role that competence assessment and development activities should play in performance evaluation. Most agree that data generated by the persons and groups engaged in competence assessment and development activities should be part of performance appraisal. The data contribute to the overall appraisal of performance, but they are never considered the full picture until they are put into context by the clinical manager, who measures individual or group performance against clinical outcomes.

Team development, along with its evaluation, is a new member of the competence assessment family. Competence assessment within the scope of overall performance of the team has been advocated (Human Technology, 1996). The model developed by this human resources group is in the form of a wheel, with commitment to a team approach as the central or core competency. Nine other competencies are clustered under three key areas:

- Team interpersonal skills
- Team management skills
- Team analytic skills.

Team competencies are defined and a survey is offered on disk for each team member to complete and pass to the next team member. After all team members have completed the survey, a report is generated by the team leader or administrator. This report is used as the basis for training and subsequent evaluation based on the initial competence assessment data. Is this competence assessment, performance evaluation, or staff development? Elements of all three are present. It simply serves as another tool for SDSs seeking to reveal and measure competence.

The term "staff development" is considered throughout this text to mean an organized program of systematic activities designed to assess and develop the competence of persons and groups for quality patient care within a defined organization. Data from many of the activities, which sample an array of competencies meaningful to the organization using a variety of strategies, are used to provide evidence about the overall capacity of the person or group within the health care facility to provide quality patient care.

Searches through the literature of education, business, law, and health care yield a great deal of information. The concept of staff development began to show up in the health care literature in the late 1920s (Pfefferkorn, 1928). The term "staff development" emerged in the health care and education literature in the early 1970s and as a subject heading in ERIC in 1980 and in Medline in 1991. Staff development became a subject heading in CINAHL in 1983. Competence as a value, concept, principle, theory, and area of inquiry has quite a different history, but competence and staff development have traveled within the same spheres for decades, continuously spinning around each other. Other concepts often linked with CSD are learning activities, learning laboratories, and data generation methods. "How-to's" for CSD abound in the literature today, often with different underlying thoughts and theories than those discussed here. This phenomenon may be frustrating to the novice SDS but serves as evidence of CSD's dynamic nature.

DEVELOPING COMPETENCE

Established CSD programs have certain traditions. Some are probably rituals or "sacred cows" that ought to be evaluated under the light of competence. Orientation, in-service education, and continuing education continues to be the model used by some (ANA, 1994). Today, however, programs must show patients that their care providers are competent, and this evidence is generated by persons and groups engaged in competence assessment and development programs.

CSD programs are a symbol of a competent health care organization. Care providers should know what their customers, actual and potential, expect from them; this is no easy feat today, given the myriad of managed care plans. The confusion and complexity in health care about who expects what of whom will not be solved. Indeed, it may continue to serve as the greatest challenge for SDSs. SDSs can address this by returning to the core values of the health care organization and ringing the quality care bell loudly or softly, depending on the situation.

The field of CSD, the organized program or set of activities designed to assess and develop the competence of clinicians, will also continue to develop; if it doesn't, it is not alive and changing with evolving health care systems. New and fresh approaches to assessing and developing competence should be pursued. Attempts to clarify and test models, methods, systems, and strategies are a welcome component of the field and serve as evidence of its liveliness.

CSD processes are the strategies and methods that make up an alive program. Much activity can be observed in organizations with vigorous staff development programs. Work teams always include or are led by a SDS. SDSs lead or are included in organization-wide project teams assigned tasks to improve quality. Clinical ladders or clinical career development programs include industrious and productive clinicians readily recognized as participants in this staff development activity. SDSs form formal or informal groups and work teams to get the jobs done that flow toward the common goal of quality care for patients.

OUTCOME EVALUATION

If competence is the outcome of clinical assessment and development, then evaluation of that outcome deserves attention. Chapter 8 addresses outcome measurement and how to appraise and report it, but some information is provided here to show the connections between these ideas.

A Few Gurus

In the public sector, particularly the Agency for Health Care Policy and Research, new names and ideas are emerging in the field of outcome evaluation. The Center for Outcomes and Effectiveness Research was formed specifically to address this issue in health care. Through patient outcomes review teams and evidence-based practice centers, the agency hopes to demonstrate methods, approaches, and outcomes that can be replicated in other settings and used to established evidence-based guidelines for health care. This old idea is receiving fresh thinking.

Rossi and Freeman, who are evaluation research investigators, addressed outcome research in their classic text about evaluation (1993). They wrote that outcome research (using the term "impact assessment") is directed at establishing whether or not an intervention is producing its intended effects, within an estimated certainty. The basic aim of impact assessment is to produce the estimated "net effect" of an intervention—that is, an estimate from which the effects of other processes have been removed. This approach requires well-articulated objectives.

Berk and Rossi (1990) described outcomes in the context of social programs. They proposed that policy-makers and other interested parties (stakeholders) and the environment ("policy space") were part of common-sense program evaluation. They also acknowledged the existence of evaluation research and other empirical generalizations from social sciences. They wrote that successful evaluation attains practical perfection when it provides the best information possible on the key policy questions within the given set of real-world constraints. They also suggested strategies to pose evaluation questions and select empirical techniques and offered chronological perspectives in designing evaluations for new and ongoing programs, with questions at each suggested stage.

Garbin (1991) provides a slightly dated but still relevant conference report in which the theoretical and societal background of the assessment and evaluation movement was discussed in relation to outcomes in higher education. Approaches and future directions were suggested. Novella Keith (1991), in the keynote address on which this conference report was based, proposed dual concepts of assessment as measurement and assessment as conversation. Keith also proposed, through metaphor, that to link assessment and improvement, assessments must:

1. Answer questions people care about.
2. Be owned by the faculty (managers, educators, other stakeholders).

3. Be specifically linked to the curriculum and the classroom (performance expectations).
4. Be a means to an end and not an end in itself.
5. Involve collaboration.
6. Occur in a context that facilitates change: the culture of an institution or department, its values, and its system of rewards.

Mohr (1992) used the term "impact evaluation" and defined it as determining the extent to which one set of directed human activities (X = programs, classes, skill assessments) affects the state of some objects or phenomena (Y = change in skills, behaviors, knowledge, attitudes, or any one of many possible outcomes) and, at least sometimes, determining why the effects were as large or small as they were. Further, he wrote that all program theories can be reduced to mean that the program's activities will have certain specified results in terms of Y. Testing this theory is what impact (or outcome) evaluation is all about: what matters is only that someone is interested in the truth or falsity of the theory that X results in Y and is willing to devote some resources to it. Mohr proposed an evaluation framework:

1. The program theory has component elements; impact analysis consists largely of making observations about these elements and relating them to one another. The primary elements are the problem, the activities, the outcome of interest (sometimes called an objective), and the subobjectives.
2. There must be some means of determining if the theory is correct (also called a design, as most of Mohr's book deals with advantages and disadvantages of impact analysis designs).
3. There must be some way of quantifying the program's effectiveness.

Mohr makes a strong case for using statistical approaches in designing impact evaluations and recognizes the complexity of program activities' effect on objectives and subobjectives. He acknowledged the crux of impact analysis as a comparison of what did happen after implementing the program with what would have happened had the program not been implemented. He called this term the "counterfactual" and suggested some rather complicated approaches toward determining outcomes as ratios. He also suggested the scope of an integrated evaluation task:

1. Comprehensiveness in the presentation of outcomes
2. Correct choice of the outcomes to be submitted to actual research
3. Quality of selection and execution of research designs
4. Formative evaluations, in most cases.

Mohr did not emphasize the politics, diplomacy, and policy-making aspects of program evaluation. Puetz did this in her *Evaluation in Nursing Staff Development* (1985), as did Berk and Rossi (1990), Rossi and Freeman (1993), and Kirkpatrick (1959). Kirkpatrick's classic proposal, based on the meta-analysis of training evaluation methods, is still in common use and is applied in other chapters of this text. In the 1950s, Kirkpatrick found that training outcome methods fell into one of four levels:

- Level 1. Reaction: how well participants like training, or their reaction to the learning activity.
- Level 2. Learning: an objective determination to measure if learning has taken place. Kirkpatrick suggested pretests and posttests and the use of control groups when possible to measure classroom (or time-limited learning activity) performance changes.

- Level 3. Behavior: measurements of whether behavioral changes have taken place on the job as a result of training. This has also been called the transfer of learning. Kirkpatrick suggested using a systematic approach completed by the participant, peers, subordinates, and superiors. Posttraining appraisals are made at least 3 months after training.
- Level 4. Results: examples are reduction of costs, reduction of turnover or absenteeism, reduction of grievances, increase in quality or quantity of production, or improved morale as leading to stated results (observable business results). This was described as the most difficult level, and few models exist. A technical difficulty is the separation of variables.

Kirkpatrick's work has generated a whole new dialogue about outcome evaluation, and today some refer to outcome evaluation as "level 4" evaluation. Shelton and Alliger (1993) wrote an article entitled, "Who's afraid of level 4 evaluation?" They suggested that the lack of level 4 evaluations was due to data collection and interpretation difficulties, which are time-consuming and expensive. They suggested routine collection of data that can be used for results evaluation, such as number of hours worked, units produced, or defects, and then obtaining, organizing, and analyzing already existing data. They proposed a list of questions that can serve as a guideline to help plan evaluation:

1. Should I conduct a level 4 evaluation?
2. Is a level 4 study feasible in relation to business measures (or the variable or outcome of interest), time, extraneous factors, and costs?
3. Which design should I use?
4. What will the training cost?
5. How do I analyze the data?
6. How do I report the results?

McIntosh et al. (1993) presented a proposal of some merit for the SDS. They tied management training values to training and development by aligning training and education's performance with business-unit operations, ensuring that the products and services of education added value, and gauged education's effectiveness through measured results. They recognized three stakeholders: consumers, sponsors, and clients.

Hamilton (1993) differentiated between evaluation research and research methods. "Evaluation provides an overview; research is a biopsy" is a philosophy that has some application to CSD. Evaluation refers to routine assessment of the worth of programs; evaluative research implies the use of scientific research methods and techniques for performing an evaluation. Hamilton identified four models: goal- or objective-based, systems evaluation, responsive evaluation, and goal-free evaluation. She suggested that outcome and impact analyses are evaluation strategies that focus on whether a program is effective; she also called these analyses "summative evaluations."

Evaluation is sometimes seen as threatening to the people involved in the program. Hamilton refers to "fourth-generation evaluation" as qualitative methods used in responsive evaluation that seek the questions and methods that emerge during program evaluation. Others have called this approach naturalistic or perhaps hermeneutical.

Del Bueno in 1993 wrote an article entitled, "Outcome evaluation: Frustration or fertile field?" According to her, competence and positive health status are outcome measures, the former leading to the latter. She discussed what can be evaluated and the frustrations of outcome evaluations. She advocated having a high tolerance for ambiguity and the messiness of outcome evaluation. She suggested that "control within context" and fuzzy answers to right questions rather than precise answers to wrong questions are attributes of sound outcome evaluation. She reaffirmed this approach to evaluation as an open and intellectually stimulating field (and a possible way to stay young!).

Jones (1993) provided an excellent review article of approaches commonly used in health care for outcome measures. The novice SDS will find this a good article for collaborating with managers on "training values."

A recent review of the health care literature from 1990 to 1996 about outcomes in staff development found that the terms were used at least 68 times. In journals as diverse as *Health Manpower Management*, *Medical Group Management*, *Health Systems Strategy Report*, *Health Care Finance Review*, *Health Library Review*, and *Brain Injury*, the terms "outcome" and "staff development" were linked. This is today's reality as well as an omen for the future.

Orest (1995) presented an interesting study about clinicians' perception of self-assessment in clinical practice. Using in-depth interviews with four practicing physical therapists, three themes emerged: self-assessment of competence, patient outcomes, and professional development. Clinical outcomes linked with competence and staff development are here to stay.

The savvy SDS will learn and develop skills in outcome measurement. Display 4-2 lists a series of statements that SDSs can use to evaluate their organization's competence assessment system. All "yes" answers must be qualified and "no" answers improved. Chapter 8 provides specific measurement and appraisal strategies for outcome measurement.

Ⓓ ISPLAY 4-2

Self-Assessment Questions for Competence Assessment System Evaluation

Competence Assessment System Evaluation©

   I. New employee competence assessment is completed during the initial orientation process.
  II. Employee orientation is based on assessed competencies and the knowledge and skills required to deliver patient care services.
 III. New employee competence assessment is completed at the conclusion of the (total) orientation process.
  IV. Clinical staff participate in ongoing educational activities to acquire new competencies that support patient care delivery. These activities are minimally based on QI findings, new technology, therapeutic or pharmacologic interventions, and learning needs of nursing staff.
   V. Mangement or leadership staff participate in competence assessment activities (*i.e.*, clinical knowledge, skills, technology).
  VI. Management or leadership staff participate in ongoing educational activities to acquire new competencies for patient care management (*i.e.*, management development).
 VII. The performance evaluation system addresses staff competence.
VIII. When competency deficiencies are noted, a plan for correction is initiated and implemented.
  IX. Reassessment of competence occurs as necessary.
   X. Summaries of competence assessment findings are available by individual, by patient care unit, and by department.
  XI. Plans for competence maintenance and improvement are documented.
 XII. An annual report is submitted to the governing body.
XIII. Policies and procedures exist to define the process of competence assessment.

Karen J. Kelly-Thomas, © 1994.

A Practical Exercise

The following exercise can be used to evaluate the outcomes of a clinical competence assessment system.

A series of statements is given, and questions follow each statement. Not all the answers may be readily available, and some questions may have to be asked in the organization for the first time. These questions provide a practical and time-tested way to assist the SDS with system evaluation.

1. A competence assessment system is a management tool that measures and monitors an array of competencies using a variety of strategies to collect data that are meaningful to the organization for the purpose of continuous improvement and quality patient care outcomes.
   a. Does this match your understanding of a competence assessment system?
   b. Is it like the one on your unit, department, or division?
2. The world of clinical practice is made up of traditions, theories, knowledge, beliefs, tasks, reflections, relationships, and more, and the whole world of patient care is more than the sum of its parts. We have a rich heritage of descriptions of our health care universe. Every organization with groups of clinicians has added to this heritage and developed a nursing culture specific to the organization. This legacy is often found in "artifacts" such as policy and procedure manuals, standards of practice, performance standards, job descriptions, skills lists, and others. These documents also describe the expected competencies of the persons they refer to.
   a. In your organization, what documents are available to describe expected competencies?
   b. Do your documents reflect your expectations regarding competence for the people providing care on your unit, department, or division?
3. These artifacts describe the world of clinical practice. A competence assessment system attempts to make visible those areas of expertise that are meaningful to the organization and the patients served. It is not necessary (or possible) to measure the entire universe of clinical practice; it is more important to support a sampling of meaningful clinical care activities to measure competence.
   a. Given your patient population, what competencies are important to you as a clinician, manager, or specialist concerned about quality care? Why?
   b. What competencies are measured in your division or unit? Why are they meaningful to you? Should you be measuring something else?
   c. Are there some expected competencies across units that you can collaborate with others about, assess together, and learn more about through the experience?
4. A competence assessment system includes a plan to collect data at various points. There is no set answer as to how often or how many; you set that out as part of your plan. As a clinician, manager, or specialist concerned about patient care quality, you are responsible for assessing the competence of care providers in a systematic way. You can deputize others to assist you with some of this task, but the responsibility for the quality of care remains with you, as does the judgment about the competence of your care providers. As you are developing your competence assessment plan, consider your environment and typical workloads and assignments. Also consider that some relevant data may already be available to you from other departments, such as CSD, medical education,

human resources, or others. In addition, consider what you are *not* going to do to balance your workload to include competence assessment activities.

    a. What are some logical and sensible data collection points on your unit, department, or division?

    b. Whom will you deputize to help you develop the competence assessment system?

5. There are many and varied strategies used to collect data: credential appraisal, experience evaluations, self-assessments, skills lists, written tests, performance tests, performance evaluations, certifications, and others. All are useful and all can be improved. For example, a skills list of more than several criteria becomes meaningless, more so if it measures performance in a simulation rather than the actual situation. A classic example is the expert venipuncturist who can't start an IV on a rubber arm. The more situated the assessment, the better the data, and the better judgment you will be able to make.

    Besides these measures, there is another competence assessment approach that you may want to try. It has been called "assessment as conversation," in contrast to "assessment as measurement." This approach advocates an ongoing dialogue with care providers and can include the following three questions about critical thinking advanced by Del Bueno (1993): What is your patient's priority health care problem or risk now? What nursing actions will you take to reduce the risk and manage the problem, in priority order? What is your rationale?

    To use this approach as part of your system and show evidence that you are using it, you can use a data collection tool such as that shown in Display 4-1. It is important to include your overall judgment of your findings.

    a. What variety of strategies are you using to collect worthwhile data about the competence of your staff?

    b. What strategies are you using to assess critical thinking competence?

6. Your data collection tools should be set up to help you analyze the data and make a judgment about the overall competence of your clinical staff. Grids are the most common and sensible approach. Confidentiality of data is a consideration as you present your findings to others. To compare your findings to expected outcomes, consider central limit theorem and other analysis strategies. Reconsider the mean (or average) as the standard of quality; this does not mean you should not move the mean forward or advance the standard. Remember, the purpose of your competence assessment system is to collect meaningful data as measures for quality patient outcomes. Incompetence is not rampant! This is how we engage in data-driven continuous improvements for quality patient care outcomes.

    a. What do your data collection tools look like now? Do they help you make a judgment about the overall competence of your staff?

    b. What improvements will you make to help you with this work?

7. Now that you have had the opportunity to evaluate your competence assessment system, you have the elements, knowledge and ideas for improvements. Consider the next few months and the next 3 years, and draft your plan. Your final plan should not be more than one side of one piece of paper! Implementing and then evaluating your plan is where you will spend your time.

    a. What is your plan for the next 3 years regarding the continued development of competence assessment activities in your assigned area of responsibility?

    b. What will you have accomplished by December 31 of this year, next year, and the next?

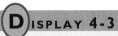

ISPLAY 4-3

Self-Assessment Exercise for Measuring Clinical Staff Development Outcomes

Outcomes and Measurements
Self-assessment exercise

1. Name at least three staff development outcomes you can already observe.
2. Describe a measurement method for one.
3. Delineate the issues surrounding the data collection process.
4. Refine the data collection process.
5. Develop a scheme or tool (use back of page to sketch).
6. Make a plan—list steps to implement outcome measurement.
7. Write down what you will do tomorrow with this project.

Source: Author. Used with permission.

This self-assessment approach toward evaluation is a time-honored one and illustrates an individual SDS's commitment to a quality system. The self-assessment questions can also be used by a group or team interested in or charged with evaluating an entire system or parts of it at various levels.

Display 4-3 gives another series of self-assessment questions that may be useful to SDSs, managers, and others concerned with quality care of patients in various health care settings. The focus of this exercise is on outcomes.

MYTHS AND REALITIES

Despite efforts to reach a common understanding of what competence is and why and how it is meaningful to quality patient care, there will continue to be different approaches. What is important is the quality improvement programs and processes of the organization, often led by SDSs, in which questions are asked and answered that will represent the specific organization's belief and value of competence among its care providers and how the organization goes about assessing that outcome. Many myths are and will continue to be propagated by various people who understand competence and its assessment from diverse perspectives. Many of these people are in search of (or believe they have found) the one best or right way to assess and develop competent health care providers. The reality of competence and its assessment and development is that it can be measured and improved for the pure purpose and desire of continuously improve the care we provide.

SUMMARY

This chapter has addressed the concept of competence: what it is, and what it can be. Some definitions have been proposed to help novice SDSs apply these concepts to their individual settings. Various perspectives and terms were considered. Approaches to assessing and developing competence were discussed and put in context with the remainder of this text. SDSs will want to consider these ideas and proposals while assessing and evaluating their organization's programs.

Bringing the Outcome of Competence to Life

FREDDICA L. BRUBAKER

During my 20 years in the nursing profession in Washington, DC, New York, and Miami, I have worked in emergency departments, a surgical intensive care unit, and staff development. I have witnessed numerous instances of poor communication and lack of trust between nurses in emergency departments and critical care units due to misperceptions of each other's workloads. Because of this, I was skeptical when I was asked to help develop a single course that would include the competency assessment requirements for the emergency department and critical care nurses at our hospital. Even though these nurses have similar job responsibilities and levels of expertise, I had never experienced or developed a cohesive joint program. We were hopeful that this course would encourage communication and trust between the two units.

The Joint Commission on Accreditation of Healthcare Organizations (JCAHO) was scheduled to visit our hospital in the fall of 1995. JCAHO requires several different competencies for critical care and emergency department nurses. With this in mind, we developed a 1-day course—offered 12 different times that fall—in which we attempted to instruct more than 100 nurses as a single group. We felt, however, that at times it still would be necessary to divide these nurses into two groups because the critical care nurses already had completed some of the competencies.

Because all nurses are faced with the challenge of caring for dying patients and helping their families cope, we scheduled a morning lecture for all nurses on death and dying. JCAHO requires hospitals to cover this topic in its educational programs for all nurses. Then we decided to send the critical care and emergency department nurses to separate sessions. The latter attended lectures on fire and safety, central line management, and Accu-Chek blood glucose monitoring. The former, meanwhile, attended sessions on mechanical ventilation and rehabilitation in critical care.

In the afternoon, we brought all the nurses together and divided them into small, mixed groups. All nurses were required to rotate through ACLS mock code blue, external pacemaker, and pulse oximetry stations. Critical care nurses—from the ICU, CCU, and intermediate care unit—were sent to an internal pacemaker station while the emergency department nurses rotated through a pediatric mock code station. By the end of the afternoon, each group had rotated through three competency stations.

The nurses from the emergency department, ICU, and CCU were required to pass a written exam that included questions on defibrillation, thrombolytic therapy, and interpretation of 14 EKG rhythm strips. We administered a separate exam to the intermediate care unit nurses that excluded questions on thrombolytic therapy because these nurses are not responsible for administering thrombolytic drugs. Naturally, the two exams had to be scored separately.

By offering separate sessions, it was our hope that the majority of these nurses would complete their required competencies before the JCAHO visit. We achieved that objective. However, when the course was later evaluated by myself; Maria Dawson, our hospital's emergency department clinical specialist; and Vickie Sears, our critical care clinical educator, who coordinated the program, we recognized that the sessions had sometimes been confusing and cumbersome to some nurses as well as faculty. This was due to several factors.

For example, study books had been offered to all nurses a month before the start of the course. We had instructed each of the nurses to review this information and come to class prepared to demonstrate their competencies. However, it quickly became obvious that many nurses had not reviewed the information. Some nurses told us they didn't know the books were available. This lack of preparation by nurses changed the instructors' focus at the competency stations: instead of simply testing competencies, instructors found themselves teaching them.

The rotation assignments through the competency stations were confusing because the stations had to be dispersed throughout the hospital due to space limitations. Some nurses reported to the wrong stations and later told us their rotation assignments had not been made clear to them. Furthermore, due to limited faculty and equipment, some nurses had to wait up to 30 minutes for their turn at the mock code blue competency station. In the end, the course required nine faculty members for the lectures and competency stations and proved to be very resource-intensive.

Despite these problems, the course was rated highly on the participants' written "reactionnaires." But the coordinators, including myself, decided that some major restructuring was needed. In January 1996 we went back to the drawing board, planning a revised critical care competency assessment course in which all emergency department and critical care nurses would go through the entire course together.

In this revised course, we focus only on the competencies required for both groups of nurses. Competencies required only for emergency department or critical care nurses will now be taught by the clinical educators for these units. The new course also will be offered to nurses in our telemetry and post-anesthesia care units, whose JCAHO requirements are similar to those of the emergency department and critical care nurses.

As before, the 1-day course will be offered 12 times in the fall. The morning session will focus on fire and safety as well as bioethics and organ and tissue donation—all JCAHO-required subjects. In the afternoon—unlike in the first course—all nurses will take the same written exam. Then the entire class will demonstrate their competence at an ACLS mock code blue station, where instructors will use standardized checklists and scenarios. Unlike in the first course, no instruction will be offered at the competency station, thereby reducing the waiting time. If participants do not successfully complete the station, they will be required to retest within 2 weeks. As before, we will distribute study books, but this time we will require nurses to initial their receipt of the books.

Unlike the original course, classes will be scheduled in only two areas of the hospital (as opposed to four). For the new course, we also will stress to the nurses that this is a competency—not education—class, so teaching should not be necessary.

We are confident this course will be more effective. In the end, my fear that there would be friction between the emergency department and critical care nurses was unfounded. In early 1996, after the original course had been completed, nurses from these two groups began planning a holiday party for December—together, I am pleased to add.

REFERENCES

American Nurses Association. (1994). *Standards for professional development: Continuing education and staff development.* Washington DC: Author.

Benner, P. (1984). *From novice to expert: Excellence and power in clinical nursing practice.* Menlo Park, CA: Addison-Wesley.

Berk, R. A., & Rossi, P. H. (1990). *Thinking about program evaluation.* Thousand Oaks, CA: Sage.

Del Bueno, D. J., Weeks, L., & Brown-Stewart, P. (1987). Clinical assessment centers: A cost-effective alternative for competency development. *Nursing Economic$, 5*(1), 21–26.

Del Bueno, D. J. (1990). Experience, education and nurses' ability to make clinical judgments. *Nursing & Health Care, 11*(6), 290–294.

Del Bueno, D. J. (1993). Outcome evaluation: Frustration or fertile field? *Journal of Nursing Administration, 23*(7/8), 12–19.

Dubois, D. D. (1993). *Competency-based performance improvement: Strategy for organizational change.* Amherst, MA: HRD Press.

Dubois, D. D. (1995). *Competency-based performance improvement: Organizational assessment package* (administrator's handbook). Amherst, MA: HRD Press.

Garbin, M. (1991). *Assessing educational outcomes.* New York: NLN Press.

Hamilton, G. A. (1993). An overview of evaluation research methods with implications for nursing staff development. *Journal of Nursing Staff Development, 9,* 148–153.

Human Technology, Inc. (1996). *Performance skills teams: Competency assessment training program.* Amherst, MA: HRD Press.

Jones, K. R. (1993). Outcomes analysis: Methods and issues. *Nursing Economics, 11*(3), 145–152.

Keith, N. Assessing educational goals: The national movement to outcomes education. In Garbin, M. (1991). *Assessing educational outcomes.* New York: NLN Press.

Kirkpatrick, D. L. (1959). Techniques for evaluating training programs. *Journal of the ASTD, 3,4.*

McIntosh, S. S., Page, S., & Hall, K. B. (1993). Adding value through training. *Training and Development Journal, 48*(7), 39–44.

Mohr, L. B. (1992). *Impact analysis for program evaluation.* Thousand Oaks, CA: Sage.

National Council of State Boards of Nursing. (1996). *Definition of competence and standards for competence.* Chicago: Author.

National Council of State Boards of Nursing. (1997). Boards of nursing adopt revolutionary change for nursing regulation. *Issues, 18*(3), 1, 3.

National Organization for Competency Assurance. (1997a). *NOCA Home Page.* Retrieved November 7, 1997, from the World Wide Web: http://www.noca.org.

National Organization for Competency Assurance. (1997b). *NOCA Organizational Members.* Retrieved November 7, 1997, from the World Wide Web: http://www.noca.org/omembers.htm.

Orest, M. R. (1995). Clinicians' perception of self-assessment in clinical practice. *Physical Therapy, 75*(9), 824–829.

Pfefferkorn, B. (1928). Improvement of the nurse in service: An historical review. *American Journal of Nursing, 28,* 700.

Puetz, B. E. (1985). *Evaluation in nursing staff development.* Rockville, MD: Aspen Publications.

Rossi, P. H., & Freeman, H. E. (1993). *Evaluation: A systematic approach*, 3rd ed. Thousand Oaks, CA: Sage.

Shelton, S., & Alliger, G. (1993). Who's afraid of level 4 evaluation? *Training and Development Journal, 47*(6), 43–46.

Wright, D. (1997). *The ultimate guide to competency assessment in health care.* Eau Claire, WI: Professional Education Systems.

5

Competence Assessment Systems and Measurement Strategies

FRANCIE WOLGIN

Since 1994, evidence of competence has been a requirement for accreditation by the Joint Commission on Accreditation of Healthcare Organizations (JCAHO). Competency is seen as actual performance in real situations. It describes how well health care workers integrate their knowledge, attitudes, behaviors, and skills in delivering care according to expectations. In the 1996 *Comprehensive Accreditation Manual for Hospitals*, competence is described as capacity equal to requirement, referring to the person's capacity to perform his or her job duties. JCAHO Standard HR.3 states, "Leaders ensure that the competence of staff members is assessed, maintained, demonstrated, and improved continually." McCrone (1995) described competence as knowledge, skills, and judgment and their application. The application is considered the crucial component: it is immaterial if health care workers have all the knowledge and skills and judgment in the world if they cannot apply them effectively in the actual practice setting.

CONCEPTS

Competence Assessment as a Quality Management Tool

Quality management systems can be set up in health care organizations to resemble quality control systems in industry. The desired outcome of a quality management system is measurement of the quality of the organization's product. In health care the desired product is quality patient care provided by caring and competent personnel. To support this objective, a competency assessment system can serve as a useful quality management tool. The system should be based on techniques and strategies familiar to and understood within the organization but still grounded by objective methods or a scientific process.

Variety of Strategies

There are various ways to assess competency. Competency measurement is a complex task that should not rely on only one approach. Each hospital or other agency must decide how to structure its assessment, evaluation, and appraisal process in building a competence assessment process. There are two requirements:

- The hospital must use a combination of ongoing competence assessment and educational activities to maintain staff competence.
- An objective, measurable system must be used periodically to evaluate job performance, current competencies, and skills.

In other words, health care organizations must have in place written job descriptions for each job category, a competence assessment and development system, and performance evaluation processes (JCAHO, 1996, p. 389).

Performance is something a person or organization does (processes, procedures) or achieves (outcomes). For purposes of this discussion, the term "performance" is used to represent overall competence. Performance can be quantified to produce neutral numbers to which qualitative meaning is attached. The performance data are evaluated to determine if they represent predeterminant levels of quality. Accurate, complete, and relevant performance data can provide managers and users of organizational services with objective evidence on which quality judgments can be made.

Array of Competency Statements

A variety of innovative approaches can be used to demonstrate an objective competence assessment or performance evaluation system. JCAHO surveyors seek supporting data demonstrating that the needs of the patient population served have been assessed and an adequate number of qualified persons are recommended by the staffing plan. Supporting evidence can be found in departmental budget documentation, staffing plans, minutes of governing body or board meetings, or medical executive committee meeting minutes. It is important that these two factors—assessment of the patient population served and the number of recommended qualified persons—are reflected in the development, implementation, and assessment of specific activities. For example, a geriatric unit is staffed by persons qualified to assess and treat older adults. Each staff member would have documentation of unit competencies to care for older adults.

JCAHO Standard HR.3.1 states, "The hospital encourages and supports self-development and learning for all staff." This standard recognizes that job performance is the result of both individual competence and the work environment created by leadership. Regular communication and feedback between leaders and staff provide a continuous loop between the identified needs, the plans developed in a coaching session, and the evaluation of the process outcomes. Examples of evidence for performance of HR.3.1 are:

- Staff interviews
- Senior and department leadership interviews
- Performance evaluations or competency assessment process
- Contracts
- Employee personnel files and job descriptions
- Hospital or department policies and procedures
- Staffing plans
- In-service, staff development, and continuing education records
- Orientation curriculum
- Meeting minutes and written reports
- Employee handbook or human resources brochures
- Description of licensure, certification, privileges, and activities for verifying credentials.

Data Collection

Data collection is the gathering of information on which a discussion or inference can be based; examples are documentation in a patient's medical record, an employee's permanent record or file, or unit quality indicators. Once the data are collected, they can be analyzed and displayed in a format from which valid conclusions and decisions can be made.

Meaningful to the Organization

Competency models can provide the basis for implementing performance improvement strategies. Anderson and McCafferty (1996) wrote:

> Although for many organizations getting through the JCAHO accreditation process is challenging enough, we only achieve maximum benefit when we exploit the power of competencies to help our organization achieve its strategic goals. (p. 3)

While working to integrate competencies into the performance improvement process, staff development specialists should remember that competencies must be meaningful to both the staff and administration if they are to achieve any performance improvement goals. They can be tied to the organization's business strategies and initiatives and to patients' needs.

Improve Care Outcomes

There are a variety of ways in which acquiring competencies or targeting persons to acquire a skill set or competency can lead to improved patient satisfaction and a reduction in complications or adverse events. One example is a low-volume, high-risk procedure such as chemotherapy administration. In a large medical center, usually it is not cost-effective to educate and validate 2,000 nurses to administer many chemotherapy drugs. On the units where patients infrequently receive treatment, a core group can be taught to perform the procedure and administer IV chemotherapy medications to children or adults. On the oncology units, it would be reasonable for the entire nursing staff to have this skill set, because they would easily be able to maintain their competence. Table 5-1 is a validation tool for administration of intravenous push chemotherapy via peripheral IV. Targeted education results in better-prepared nurses who can provide expert care to patients and serve as resource persons to their colleagues; it also reduces adverse reactions and medication administration errors. All these goals serve to improve care outcomes.

Another example is training staff members who work with patients at high risk for injuring themselves and others with violent behaviors. Staff members in psychiatry, emergency services, and security are taught physical crisis management skills and techniques. When implemented in one setting (Wolgin, 1990), there was a 65% reduction in the number of injuries to staff and a 92.7% reduction in calls to security. The use of seclusion or restraints to manage patients fell from 57.8% to 23.6%, and this improvement was maintained over the 3-year follow-up period.

DESIGN

There are four basic elements of a competency system (Fig. 5-1):

1. Pre-employment qualifications and assessments
2. Orientation assessments
3. Targeted interval assessments and annual performance appraisals
4. Response to appraisals.

Pre-Employment Qualifications and Assessments

The employing agency must review each applicant's education, training, appropriate licensure, and previous experience. This holds true for all employees, from environmental service workers through to the CEO. Assessment of competence begins with evaluating

TABLE 5-1

COMPETENCY VALIDATION: ADMINISTRATION OF INTRAVENOUS PUSH CHEMOTHERAPY VIA PERIPHERAL IV

Name: _____   Date: _____

Preceptor: _____   Drug: _____

Completed chemotherapy administration course: _____ Post test score: _____
Completed module(s): Adult _____   Pediatric _____

Before Administration	Yes	No
1. Verifies MD order for IVP chemotherapy		
2. States antidote, if applicable, for chemotherapy. If drug is not a vesicant, states difference between administering vesicant and nonvesicant drug		
3. Assures availability of antidote, if applicable		
Setup for Administration	**YES**	**NO**
1. Obtains IVP medication(s) and verifies drug(s), dosage(s), and applicable lab results on MD order form with another RN		
2. Gathers equipment		
3. Washes hands		
4. Correctly identifies patient		
5. Identifies self and procedure to patient		
6. Prepares all equipment before venipuncture		
Administration of Chemotherapy	**YES**	**NO**
1. Applies tourniquet properly		
2. Selects site for venipuncture with regard to patient preference, previous venipunctures, history of mastectomy/lymphadenopathy (when applicable)		
3. Cleanses area according to policy without subsequent contamination		
4. Successfully performs venipuncture using butterfly		
5. Backflushes butterfly tubing with blood, connects to primary IV line, removes tourniquet, and sets IV rate		
6. Dons protective gown and prepares needed equipment (gloves, blue pad, alcohol wipes, 2 × 2s)		
7. Verifies IV placement (site condition, positive blood return)		
8. Cleanses side port of IV line with alcohol and protects with 2 × 2 gauze pad		
9. Injects syringe into side port of IV line		

(continued)

TABLE 5-1 (Continued)

COMPETENCY VALIDATION: ADMINISTRATION OF INTRAVENOUS PUSH CHEMOTHERAPY VIA PERIPHERAL IV

Administration of Chemotherapy	YES	NO
10. Pushes 1 ml vesicant drug and observes for signs/symptoms of extravasation		
11. Completes IV push, verifying IV placement after every 2 ml of drug		
12. Pulls syringe out, protecting with a 2 × 2 gauze pad to avoid splatter of drug		
13. Disposes of chemo equipment properly		
14. Discontinues IV line/maintains with ordered IV solution (when ordered after IVP medication has sufficiently flushed through); documents in patient record		

Source: St. Joseph Mercy Health System, Ann Arbor, MI. Used with permission.

each applicant's qualifications and ability to perform the job. The degree of pre-employment screening often influences the "match" between the employee and the organization. If the person hired demonstrates the qualifications and technical skills desired and has interpersonal skills, personality, ethics, and values that are compatible with those of the organization, the match is a good one.

It is routine to find requirements that direct caregivers be able to lift 50 pounds and be able to bend, stoop, and stand for long periods of time. For a person not involved in direct patient care, however, reasonable accommodations would be required if the person could not meet these job expectations due to a disability.

LICENSURE

A license provides evidence that a person has command of a given profession's relevant body of knowledge and has met standardized entry requirements. The staff development specialist must verify that the applicant's license is current and valid in the given state (or, if applicable, any other states) to ensure there are no problems or restrictions of the license.

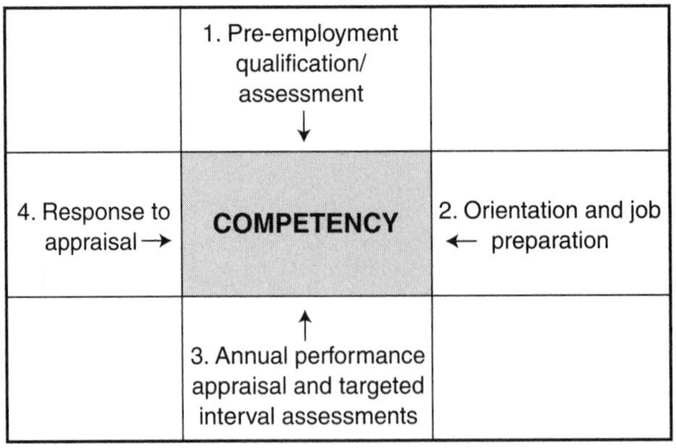

	1. Pre-employment qualification/ assessment ↓	
4. Response to appraisal →	**COMPETENCY**	2. Orientation and job ← preparation
	↑ 3. Annual performance appraisal and targeted interval assessments	

FIGURE 5-1. Four elements of a competency system.

Even after gaining licensure, however, practitioners continue to develop their expertise and gain new knowledge. Given the explosion of technology and new information, the skills and competencies actually needed in practice may bear only a faint resemblance to those a practitioner has at the beginning of his or her career.

States generally do not impose specific requirements on licensed professionals to demonstrate their continuing competence to practice or achieve license renewals. In 1996, about half of the states required attendance at continuing education courses or contact hours to maintain licensure. There is minimal review of whether the courses chosen are related to the person's specific practice needs or if the person could apply the information in appropriate practice situations. Attending continuing education programs is no guarantee of competence. Gross (1994) concluded that there was little evidence of any relation between participation in continuing education programs and job performance or clinical outcomes.

EDUCATION

Evidence of graduation or completion of courses or programs must be confirmed, particularly if this is a requirement for the position. Telling the applicant that it is the organization's policy to call and confirm graduate degrees may reduce the number of inconsistent findings or avoid later dismissals. Many employers require a copy of the diploma or other evidence of required education or certification before extending a job offer.

CERTIFICATION

Certification is the process in which a nongovernmental agency grants recognition to persons who meet certain predetermined criteria or standards for their practice specialty. There has been some confusion within nursing resulting from the casual use of the term "certification," particularly in terms of verification of particular skills. Certification is a relatively new phenomenon, so it is easy to understand how this developed. However, staff development specialists must be aware of the correct use of the term and must be able to explain the concept.

The Committee for the Study of Credentialing in Nursing (1979) views certification as a process signifying "competence for entry into specialized professional practice based on the acquisition of additional knowledge" (p. 678). Initial licensure, in contrast, addresses competence for the general practice of nursing.

Credentialing is a mechanism of providing accreditation, certification, and licensure (O'Connor et al., 1979). Webster's Dictionary (1983) defines a credential as a letter or certificate given to a person to show that one has the right to a certain position or authority.

Certification in nursing began in 1946, when the American Association of Nurse Anesthetists (AANA) established certification as the entry criterion to practice nurse anesthesia. The American College of Nurse Midwives followed suit in 1971. In 1974, the ANA began to offer certification programs. Many nursing specialty groups and associations also began to offer certification. Currently cards or evidence of certification are awarded by certifying bodies such as the American Nurses Credentialing Center, the National Certification Corporation, and others. By December 1995, the American Nurses Credentialing Center had listed over 113,000 nurses certified in 25 speciality areas.

When hiring, the staff development specialist should ask to see this card or should have applicants include a copy of the card with their application. Some positions require current ACLS, CPR, basic trauma life support, pediatric advanced life support, or other training; verification can be handled the same way.

There is a need for research on certification. To date, there are no studies showing that certification is correlated with improved practice. Del Bueno (1990) raised the concern that certification does not ensure competence. Therefore, many facilities have developed their own methods when asked to provide evidence of staff competency. The need to provide this documentation has led institutions to develop programs and skill checks to validate numerous competencies or "certifications" recognized only within that facility. This is confusing and can be misleading to both nurses and persons outside the facility.

EXPERIENCE

Transferring similar skills from one position to another, or acquiring new skills, is possible with staff development support. Agencies may use different job titles for a similar position. When there are major differences between the person's former job and the one he or she is applying for, it may be helpful to obtain a job description outlining the areas of responsibility or duties performed in the previous job.

QUALIFICATIONS

Qualifications are the traits, knowledge, skills, licenses, degrees, experiences, or character-istics deemed necessary for a certain role. JCAHO HR Standard 2 states that each employee and contracted staff member must show:

- Verification of any education or training required by law, regulation, or organization or facility policy
- Evidence of current licensure, registration, or certification, as appropriate to the position
- Knowledge and experience for assigned job duties.

Orientation and Job Preparation

All new employees must undergo a thorough orientation to their job responsibilities specific to the organization. Orientation to a new facility, or to a different position in the same facility, is the time when the new associate is introduced to the work environment, the culture of the organization, the job benefits, the expectations and responsibilities of the position, general work rules, and policies and procedures. Most employers have a probationary period during which the employee and employer can evaluate if there is a mutually rewarding match. During this time, necessary job-related and interpersonal skills are demonstrated and competencies are validated or verified. In a successful orientation process, skills are modeled in a precepted experience.

When designing new orientation programs or reviewing current ones, the specialist should consider including the following:

- Provide each employee with a copy of his or her job description.
- Review age-specific considerations for all populations the employee will be expected to care for or interact with on a regular basis.
- Review departmental and organizational policies and procedures.
- Provide education about information management for everyone who makes decisions or generates, collects, or analyzes data and information. Computer and software application skills can be taught if applicable.
- Review the performance improvement process.
- Review JCAHO mandatory education requirements of life safety, back safety, infection control, and so forth.

The formal education presented in classrooms varies among institutions. In addition to the core information included in a comprehensive orientation, opportunities to assess skills and performance expectations in the classroom portion of orientation are scheduled. There is also the opportunity to test appropriate cognitive knowledge or acquisition of necessary skills in a simulation, followed by validation in the clinical setting. For example, an experienced nurse might attend a percutaneous inserted central line insertion class and then be scheduled for the skill validation by a preceptor. The nurse would then perform three insertions in the practice or clinical setting.

During orientation, clinical skills are assessed by the preceptor, educator, or manager. Through the actual performance of the skills in the practice setting, competence can be assessed. The specific expectations to be achieved are included on a checklist, or a more elaborate competency-based orientation process can be used.

TIME LINES

Time lines are established to provide consistent expectations for the completion of a training program or orientation. Display 5-1 shows a critical path for orientation used in one facility. The path also has been incorporated into prehire assessment activities.

A clear statement about when the organization expects the employee to complete the orientation also must be made—for example, "All clinical and support staff are expected to complete the defined orientation process in 3 months." Clinical staff development specialists (SDSs) monitor this aspect of orientation along with managers.

Many organizations expect that after 4 to 6 weeks, an experienced nurse will be able to meet job expectations. For new graduates, this time line may extend to 12 weeks in noncritical care areas and 6 months in critical care units. Whatever time line is established, it must be known and deemed reasonable by everyone involved in the process.

Some persons may require an extension of the preset time lines. In these cases, clear, specific expectations and time lines are set with the person, and the consequences of not meeting the expectations are made clear. Organizational policies related to coaching, counseling, and disciplinary actions may also be used.

After the new employee has completed orientation and demonstrated expected minimum competencies to practice in the clinical area, appropriate documentation is placed in his or her file. Plans are made with the employee to complete any additional skill acquisition required of the role; frequently, needed experiences are not available during the initial orientation. The manager and employee meet to set goals for the coming 6 months or 1 year. An educator or preceptor may be involved if such expertise or schedule coordination is needed. Although a person can remain competent to perform all job duties over time, it is uncommon in most health care institutions today.

TRANSFEREES

When an employee is transferred to a new unit or work setting, the transfer should be documented and an evaluation conducted for the employee at that time. Alternatively, a summary can be written, shared with the employee, signed, and forwarded to both the new manager and the employee's permanent file. A transfer to a new or similar position should be treated like a new hire. Orientation to the new area or assessment of additional competencies should occur at the time of transfer. A written orientation plan should be shared with the employee. It may be unnecessary for the transferred employee to attend organization-wide orientation if he or she has already participated in these programs, depending on the length of his or her service. A preceptor or other person determines the employee's learning needs; once the plan has been implemented and evaluated, the employee's newly required competencies are documented, and successful completion of the orientation is placed in his or her file.

PROMOTIONS

Historically in health care, persons have been promoted to management positions because they were expert clinicians. However, the skills that contributed to their expertise were not necessarily those needed in the new role. In recent years, increased attention has been focused on providing needs assessments, orientation, and skill development for those

(*text continues on page 102*)

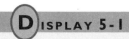

Critical Path for Orientation for Medicine/Surgery Divisions

CRITICAL PATH FOR ORIENTATION
PHASE I
PROJECTED COMPLETION - ON OR BEFORE ORIENTATION DAY # _____

OBJECTIVE: Become familiar with the environment, unit resources, and expectations.

PATIENT ASSIGNMENT SUGGESTION: Bowel Resection, Lap, Chole, or 23 hour (less complex patients) (need med x)

INSTRUCTIONS: This Phase is "Complete" when orientee practices "COMPETENTLY" - able to state theory, performs independently, acknowledges limitations, but may need to increase speed = #3.

When this Phase is complete, move orientee to Phase II.

Interpersonal • communication • motivation • accountability • attitude • cooperation	_____ Introduction to interdisciplinary team members (Case managers, Physician Assistants, Clinical Nurse Specialist, Nutritionist, Social Worker, Enterostomal Therapist, Wound Care Specialist, Pastoral Care, PCA I, PCA II, PCT, LPN, Clerk, RN, Pharmacy resource, Physical Therapy, Nurse Clinician)
Critical Thinking • assessment skills • documentation skills • organization • prioritization • decision making	_____ Observe general report and assignment _____ Listen to individual report with your RN "Buddy" _____ Observe RN "Buddy" interaction with peers, MDs, etc. _____ Observe RN "Buddy" fill in the charting forms _____ Differentiate roles and responsibilities of the team members

Technical
• skill performance
• speed in performing skills and procedures
	_____ Look at the patient room layout (CODE 33 button, equipment on wall, mouth to mask, fire blanket, equipment in drawers).
	_____ Identify paperwork (nursing flow sheet, MAR, Adult Functional Assessment, Anesthesia Patient Questionnairre, Risk for Falls).
	_____ "Buddy" with Desk Clerk/E.C. - describe/demonstrate use of the following:
	  • pneumatic tube system
	  • dry erase board (surgeries, admissions, on-call, clerk communication board)
	  • patient stamper machine
	  • nurse call system
	  • telephone capabilities (hold, transferring, park, conference call)
	  • location of incident report, medication error forms, conscious sedation forms
	  • role of clerk with admit, transfer and discharge of patient
	  • process with patient death (include location of death packet)
	  • patient referrals
	  • log book
	  • communication admit clipboard
	  • ANSOS staffing sheet
	  • patient arm band and how to make one
	  • PCIS "Downtime Box"
	  • role of the Unit Coordinator and how to contact
	  • visiting hours and rules
	  • family waiting room
	  • McAuley Inn (location, rates, etc)
	  • location of physician "on call" list
	  • use of patient charge stickers
	_____ Locate lab resource book
	_____ Look through a patient chart to observe its' organization
	_____ Do "Unit Scavenger Hunt" (attached)
	_____ Schedule and Request book (includes staff phone numbers)

DISPLAY 5-1 (Continued)

Critical Path for RN Orientation
Critical Care Phases I–V

PHASE 1 - Become familiar with the environment, unit resources, and expectations	PHASE II - Develop a beginning competency with basic assessment skills, usage of "common" equipment, documentation and less complex patient populations	PHASE III - Develop expertise with more acutely ill patients and with more technical equipment, in collaboration with the interdisciplinary team	PHASE IV - Demonstrate expertise with the hemodynamically and/or physiologically unstable acutely ill patients and with more technical equipment in collaboration with the interdisciplinary team	PHASE V - Demonstrate ability to assume role of coordinator for assigned patient's care, integrating interpersonal, critical thinking, and refined technical skills
Shows a beginning awareness of unit and divisional resources (paper and people)	Demonstrates awareness of unit routines and expectations	Demonstrates awareness of unit routines and expectations	Demonstrates compliance with unit routines and expectations	Demonstrates compliance with unit routines and expectations
Developing familiarity with the environment	Follows policies, procedures, basic safety and infection control principles	Follows policies, procedures, basic safety and infection control principles	Follows policies, procedures, basic safety and infection control principles	Follows policies, procedures, basic safety and infection control principles
	Administers meds safely using the 5 Rs	Administers meds safely using the 5 Rs	Integrates care of the patient with administration of meds appropriately	Integrates care of the patient with administration of meds appropriately
Developing familiarity with work flow process (reports, etc.)	Skill in performing basic head-to-toe assessment	Developing skill in performing advanced head-to-toe assessment; begins to identify real/potential indicators of patient instability and discusses appropriate interventions	Demonstrates skill in performing advanced head-to-toe assessment; identifies real/potential indicators of patient instability and responds appropriately	Integrates findings from complete patient assessment (e.g., hemodynamic, lab, x-ray findings); responds to situations utilizing appropriate clinical judgment and decision-making skills
Becoming familiar with paperwork/ documentation system	Beginning familiarity with documentation	Demonstrates familiarity with documentation	Exhibits an understanding of critical pathways	Demonstrates skill and comfort with nursing process and documentation
	Considers cultural diversity, maturation level, and developmental age when providing care	Considers cultural diversity, maturation level, and developmental age when providing care	Considers cultural diversity, maturation level, and developmental age when providing care	Considers cultural diversity, maturation level, and developmental age when providing care

(continued)

DISPLAY 5-1 (Continued)

	Acknowledges self-limitations/ growth needs	Acknowledges self-limitations/ growth needs	Acknowledges self-limitations/ growth needs	Acknowledges self-limitations/ growth needs
Becoming familiar with unit and patient room layout (supplies, etc.)	Able to set up, use, and trouble-shoot basic equipment	Demonstrates competency in using basic equipment	Demonstrates a beginning ability to set up, use, and trouble-shoot technical equipment	Demonstrates competency in using technical equipment
	Uses method of organization	Uses/refines method of organization	Demonstrates a beginning ability to prioritize and reprioritize; exhibits efficient organization skills	Demonstrates ability to prioritize and reprioritize as needed, while maintaining organization skills

Source: St. Joseph Mercy Health System, Ann Arbor, MI. Used with permission.

promoted to new roles. In situations like this one, it benefits both the employee and the manager to:

- Assess areas for growth and development
- Identify a preceptor or resource person during the transition
- Clearly define role expectations
- Share the evaluation process that will be used.

CONCLUDING THE ORIENTATION PROCESS

Once an employee completes orientation and has acquired and demonstrated desired competencies, there should be a meeting to conclude this process. At this time the manager, SDS, or preceptor solicits feedback from the employee as to what worked and what could be improved in the process. If there are further developmental needs, a plan can be agreed to in writing, along with expected dates for completion. The process for any planned interval assessments can be reviewed, as well as the overall performance system. Goals can be established to be met and evaluated at the employee's next evaluation or annual review.

Targeted Interval Assessments and Annual Performance Appraisals

The third element of a competency system includes targeted interval assessments and annual performance appraisals. These evaluations include:

- Assessment of competence in job-related knowledge and skills
- Management skills (for those who supervise or manage others)
- Safe use of appropriate job-related equipment
- Compliance with annual reviews of lifesaving techniques and other mandatory education requirements (CPR, Clinical Laboratory Improvement Act, infection control, Occupational Safety and Health Administration, and others designated by the organization).

Patient care staff must demonstrate competence in obtaining, understanding, and interpreting patient information regarding human growth and development. Treatment needs appropriate to the ages of the populations served, as well as professional performance, judgment, and clinical and technical skills.

SKILLS

The three types of skills vital to competency assessment are technical skills, clinical judgment, and interpersonal skills (Del Bueno et al., 1987).

Technical skills are those pertaining to an art, science, handicraft, or profession, or tasks performed manually by clinicians. Technical skills include maintenance of equipment and usually require some psychomotor or manual activity to operate. Table 5-2 lists common skills assessed during orientation. Skills requiring manual dexterity make up the

---

TABLE 5-2

COMPETENCY VALIDATION CARD FOR RNs

Completed Competency Validations

Name/Title: _____ , RN

❑ Medication Administration—Adult
❑ Medication Administration—Peds
❑ IV Fluid Administration—Adult
❑ IV Fluid Administration—Peds
❑ IV Starts—Adult
❑ IV Starts—Peds
❑ Blood Draw—Adult
❑ Blood Draw—Peds
❑ Chemotherapy—Adult
❑ Chemotherapy—Peds
❑ Blood Administration
❑ PCA
❑ Infusion Control Device
❑ Syringe Pump
❑ IVAD
❑ Blood Glucose Monitoring

External Pacemaker ❑
Basic Dysrhythmias Test ❑
D/C Central Line ❑
D/C Arterial Line ❑
Withdraw Blood—Arterial Line ❑
Arterial Puncture ❑
Defibrillation ❑
Epidural Analgesia ❑
Cardiac Output Determinations ❑
PA Catheter Insertion ❑
PA Pressures ❑
PA Catheter Withdraw for Position ❑
Pericardial Aspiration ❑
Umbilical Line ❑
Surgical Debridement ❑

Completed Competency Validations

Name/Title: _____ , LPN

❑ Medication Administration—Adult
❑ Medication Administration—Peds
❑ IV Fluid Administration—Adult
❑ IV Fluid Administration—Peds
❑ IV Starts—Adult
❑ IV Starts—Peds
❑ Blood Draw—Adult
❑ Blood Draw—Peds
❑ Chemotherapy—Adult
❑ Chemotherapy—Peds
❑ Blood Administration
❑ IV Push Administration
❑ PCA

Infusion Control Device ❑
Syringe Pump ❑
Bedside Glucose Monitoring ❑
Basic Dysrhythmias Test ❑
Central Line Management ❑
Right Atrial Catheters ❑
IVAD's ❑
Withdraw Blood—Arterial Line ❑
D/C Arterial Line ❑
Arterial Puncture ❑
Peritoneal Dialysis ❑

Source: Shulby, G. A. (1993).

majority of any skill checklist or CBO system, but these skills are only one component of clinical competence.

Clinical judgment is a complex skill involving several cognitive phases and integrative processes. Del Bueno (1990) argued that the ability to think critically and make appropriate clinical judgments is the most important dimension of nurses' work. It is through the use of clinical judgment that nurses make decisions and master the complex process of integrating simultaneous cues, forming hypotheses, and generating options. Other clinicians use similar decision-making processes. Video simulations and case scenarios are helpful teaching tools, but actual clinical experience over a period of time (about 8 months to 1 year) appears to be the foundation needed for new graduate nurses to achieve acceptable levels of clinical judgment. In general, additional clinical experience leads to improved clinical judgment in most clinicians over time.

Interpersonal skills are the actions and words used when interacting with other persons. For example, courtesy, caring, and compassion, and behaviors showing these, are required of competent clinicians. Good interpersonal skills enable people to work together in a productive and satisfying manner, and good working relationships and communication among the nursing staff and physicians lead to improved patient outcomes.

CONTEXT

Many variables influence learning, and it is important to take into consideration the basic principles of adult learning when putting programs into place. It is critical for both the patients' well-being and outcome and the organization's potential liability that staff can process information, make the right decisions, and implement and evaluate the necessary steps or the plan of care.

When a new skill needs to be learned or practiced, it is helpful to allow the learner to become familiar with the equipment, practice the procedure, develop the technical skills, and process the skill in a predictable environment like that of a simulation or learning laboratory. The goal is to help the learner gain familiarity with the equipment or technique in a controlled setting. Once specific criteria are met—for example, three successful IV insertions or starts on an IV practice arm or willing clinician—the learner may be deemed ready to advance to performing the skill on patients in the more complex and challenging clinical setting.

The next phase of acquiring the skill is to observe a preceptor or skilled clinician perform the skill on patients, where difficulties are more likely to be encountered. Once a "comfort level" is achieved, the learner can perform the procedure a specific number of times under the supervision of the preceptor or an expert clinician. As appropriate, follow-up can be arranged.

SAMPLING

Sampling of skills is usually done to determine safety rather than to generate new knowledge. The sample size and method used depend on the item or skill to be sampled or the times something such as a procedure occurs in actual practice or in the natural setting. Sampling can be used to look at any given procedure or aspect of care to assess if expected outcomes are evident. A preset percentage of charts, procedures, or persons are evaluated, in theory representing the whole.

To assess a person's ability to perform a new skill—say, IV insertion—a random sample of charts could be pulled or a random group of his or her patients examined. A review of patients whose IVs infiltrated or needed to be restarted, or cases where there were other complications, would be a more focused way to identify problems and take appropriate steps when indicated.

DATA ASSESSMENT FOR ANNUAL APPRAISALS

When evaluating personnel, it is best to use a sampling of work performance over time. For example, patient care records can be prospectively or concurrently reviewed on a consistent basis by the manager. In this way, a trend becomes apparent.

Nurses involved in clinical ladder programs are often asked to supply a list of five or 10 patients for whom they have provided care. A committee of peers reviews these charts to determine if established criteria were met or if there is documentation to support desired interventions. The various work samples may be summarized at regular intervals (annually or twice yearly) to represent performance competence in selected areas.

Individual data can be obtained from self-assessments or from the data from other assessment activities. For example, nurse practitioners or nurse midwives can be evaluated using standards of their professional societies and associations. The information obtained through self-reports, chart review, or other means can be used to develop a performance development or enhancement plan.

Group data reflect the combined efforts of a team, unit, department, division, or institution, aggregated in some way that provides information for clinical managers and others about the quality of the group's practice. Examples include patient satisfaction data, medication error rates, and documentation of trends and patterns related to staff competency. The data can be compiled at the unit level, summarized at the department or division level, and finally merged into a report reflecting the entire organization. At the aggregate level, patterns and trends can be identified. Two useful purposes of this data are to identify staff learning needs for planning ongoing education and development programs and to keep the governing body informed about staff competence and the education provided to enhance staff performance.

For a manager's evaluation, data used could include percentages of employees compliant with their annual competencies and evaluations completed. A vice president of patient care services could be evaluated on meeting budget targets for the total number of cost centers within his or her control.

Several peers could evaluate a given person; the data then serve as peer review group data. Reviewing group data is useful to identify trends or learning needs for designing and planning continuing education offerings or other staff development learning activities.

Response to Appraisals

The fourth element of a competency system, response to appraisals, includes feedback from the person evaluated as well as the manager's subsequent coaching and counseling.

Conducting an annual appraisal does not in itself ensure overall competence. What is most significant is identifying the conclusions reached or the action steps that resulted from the discussion with the clinician or staff member. Consistent with the concept of continuous quality improvement, the appraisal should emphasize assessing and improving the employee's ability to develop knowledge, technical skills, and interpersonal skills and to function in an ever-changing, complex environment.

Employees are expected to be accountable for identifying their own developmental needs. Programs to provide the necessary education or training to perform specific job duties are made available to employees who identify them. Organizations are accountable to provide patients and the public who use their services with competent employees. The ongoing assessment process increases the likelihood that competency needs will be identified, improvement plans implemented, and outcomes of planned activities documented.

DATA

Data are the facts on which a discussion or inference is based. Examples include documentation in the patient's medical record, quality indicators, and compliance with competency validation. Data-based performance measurement can change the way groups deal with issues and problems. Having complete, accurate data can lead to insights and answers not usually obtained with more subjective approaches. For example, physician specialty groups may uncover a difference in patient outcomes between two or more speciality groups when comparing patient outcomes. While analyzing the data, they may discover that patient outcomes are influenced more by individual practitioner competence, severity of illness, or the quality of support or management services provided by the organization (JCAHO, 1993).

Reports

Reports are formulated for various audiences, including:

1. Organizational boards expect to receive reports on a quarterly or more frequent basis. These reports allow this oversight body to monitor trends or identify issues that need their attention or require intervention.
2. Regulations stemming from the Clinical Laboratory Improvement Act of 1988 ensure standardization of the testing and monitoring of laboratory equipment, as well as the competency of the persons who perform tests. Data supporting competence assessment and development of persons and groups is routinely organized into these reports.
3. State health departments require evidence of compliance with standards and regulations for specific specialties or practice areas, such as mother-baby, psychiatric, or rehabilitation units. Their purpose is to ensure consistent levels of quality care rendered within the state.
4. The Occupational Safety and Health Act has established guidelines and regulations to ensure a safe environment for patients and employees. Specific training is required for all employees to familiarize them with these requirements; there should be an annual review of defined content.

A variety of reports may be compiled using various assessment data to demonstrate progress toward or compliance with regulations, requirements, budget targets, and other purposes:

1. Safety education is required to reinforce employees' ability to manage a fire, to use oxygen and other potentially dangerous substances (*e.g.*, cleaning agents or chemicals) safely, and to use electrical equipment appropriately. Safety reports addressing accidents, needle sticks, and crimes committed on the premises are generated quarterly and summarized annually to spot trends, measure compliance with regulations, and alert administrators or board members to the need for corrective action or potential areas of liability. SDSs may contribute data to these reports or be responsible for organizing and coordinating the reporting mechanism and generated data. Table 5-3 is an example of a quarterly or annual safety report.
2. Quality assessment reports are generated quarterly and summarized to demonstrate trends in established monitors at the targeted unit, division, or organization levels. The goal is to identify ways to improve both processes and patient care outcomes.

3. Infection control reports are generated to review infection rates, the incidence of specific organisms or hospital-acquired infections, the appropriate use of antibiotics, sterilization effectiveness, and other factors specific to the organization. Through the use of standard or universal precautions, staff, patients, and the community are better protected from possible infections.
4. Medical privileging reports demonstrate physicians' compliance with organizational requirements. Physicians are expected to undergo the same scrutiny as all other employees. Mandatory education requirements apply to them, as well as a peer review process through which they are awarded practice and admitting privileges.

In 1987 the National Practitioner Data Bank was established to collect malpractice judgments and settlements as well as disciplinary actions taken by state licensing boards and hospitals. The data bank has made it easier to identify high-risk practitioners. Physicians' credentials, references, and practice record are reviewed by the organizational committee initially and usually about every 2 years. The review is done to ensure the competence of medical practitioners and also provides an opportunity to examine the organization's potential or real liability issues.

Most of the reports related to staff competency and regulatory compliance, safety, and infection control are prepared on a quarterly basis and presented to appropriate committees, the executive team, and the board at their meetings. Should action be necessary, a plan is developed, approved, implemented, and monitored to achieve expected levels of compliance.

Usually in response to some untoward event, it is sometimes necessary to monitor a given situation. An example is two or more critical incidents or unexpected patient deaths resulting from perceived faulty equipment. It may be difficult to pinpoint the cause quickly. Generally, the monitoring plan includes closer observation of other patients using the same equipment, competence assessment of staff using the equipment, and reviews of the safety records for the equipment more frequently than quarterly.

Meeting Many Needs

In the ever-changing health care environment, there is seemingly no end to the demands on the system to provide reports, surveys, and comprehensive data ensuring competence of staff and quality of care provided. There is little likelihood that there will be any reduction in these expectations.

Quality monitors can be used to demonstrate improvement and to serve as benchmarks for selected information for payors. Care must be consistent and available in today's increasingly high-tech and complex environment. In more mature managed care markets, reimbursement rates will be fixed and competition for contracts will focus on quality. An organization can establish a quality indicator to measure and track the competence of personnel. Each department will need to report its quarterly compliance rates and develop corrective plans when indicated.

Societal expectations have come to play a significant role in health care. As patient satisfaction and response to discharge planning and patient education are studied and compared, there is increased sensitivity to the role of the health care provider as a service provider. Ethical issues and expectations that advance directives be reviewed and honored within the organization are necessitating more individualized care.

Legal considerations are involved in compliance in many areas, including the fire code, nondiscrimination practices in hiring, documentation of review of advance directives,

(text continues on page 110)

TABLE 5-3

QUARTERLY OR ANNUAL SAFETY REPORT

St. Joseph Mercy Health System
Safety Mandatory Education/Competency Summary

Department: _____ Service/Area: _____ Quarter: _____

Person Completing Report: _____ Phone: _____ 199 ____

INSTRUCTIONS

1. Please include number of associates completing the education as well as total number of associates.
2. All associates are to be considered except those on LOA.
3. If participation is below 95%, please indicate rationale and action plan on reverse side.
4. Submit quarterly report to the Safety Office.
5. Include total number staff completing education and % completion in your QI Report.

Department/ Service Area	# Completing		%	# Completing		%	# Completing		%	# Completing		%
	Total #		Completion	Total #		Completion	Total #		Completion	Total #		Completion
Infection Control												
Emergency Procedures and Codes												
Electrical Safety												

Fire Safety							
Right-to-Know/ Hazardous Materials							
Back Care							
Patient Confidentiality: How Do You Plead?							
Safe Medical Devices Act							
Workplace Violence							
Totals							

Source: St. Joseph Mercy Health System. Used with permission.

organ donation regulations, patients' rights to confidentiality, and reporting employee substance abuse to some state boards. Helping employees learn the information they need to know to avoid legal problems is essential.

The marketing department may compare its benchmark data with those of other organizations in the country, region, or targeted service area to determine if there are new market opportunities or areas for improvement. Adding a new service area or product line usually requires teaching personnel additional skills and competencies. Assessment data generated through routine CSD activities or other data collection strategies may also be useful when marketing a new service.

Certification data may be used to position an organization as competent because a certain percentage of its clinical staff are certified by their respective professional group. Certification in a given area of speciality can serve as a method to demonstrate knowledge acquisition, professional commitment, or professional growth. Some clinical ladder programs suggest certification as one means of meeting certain program requirements. Others view it as an optional way to demonstrate proficiency or to meet a requirement or qualification for a given step on the ladder.

Staff members may identify professional or learning goals beyond those needed in their job; these are reflected in their personal goals. Examples might be a scheduling coordinator who is taking courses toward an MBA, or a staff nurse enrolled in a nurse practitioner program. Both these examples demonstrate the person's commitment to learning new skills or information that enhances his or her ability to contribute. These data also may be useful to the organization attempting to take a position about the educational levels of staff.

QUANTITATIVE AND QUALITATIVE MEASUREMENTS

Whether conducting formal research, planning a quality monitor, assessing employee competence, or collecting information for a report, it is helpful to determine in advance the purpose, method, perspective, and intended use of the generated information. In addition, the investigator's skills and other factors should be considered. Rather than classifying a design as strictly qualitative or quantitative, it is more useful to view these terms only as approaches to the process. The qualitative paradigm is descriptive, subjective, and naturalistic in approach; in contrast, the quantitative approach seeks facts or causes in a controlled and more objective way.

Quantitative Measurements

Quantitative measurements involve data that can be counted, such as the number of yes or no answers, rankings on scales, test scores, or ratios of one variable to an established standard (*e.g.*, temperature or heart rate).

TEST SCORES

Test scores serve as a quantitative means of measuring knowledge, using an examination or a series of questions to ascertain a person's ability to identify correct responses. Examples are a standardized medication test, a keyboarding or typing test, basic arrhythmia recognition, and knowledge needed for selected procedures such as chemotherapy administration. Testing can be used to assess a large number of staff members in a short period of time and allows the cognitive level of knowledge to be assessed. Other tests commonly constructed by SDSs are those to measure a nurse's ability to calculate medication doses or a clerical staff member's ability to define medical terms. Chapter 11 discusses test construction in more detail.

CENTRAL LIMIT THEOREM

A useful approach to determine the sample size needed to assess practice patterns or competency can be supported by the central limit theorem. This theorem states if we draw samples of equal size from a nonnormal distribution, the distribution of the means of these samples will still be normal as long as the samples are large enough. The more the subjects in a population resemble each other, the smaller the sample size needs to be to find reliable information. Norman and Streiner (1994) wrote that when populations closely resemble each other, 10 or 20 could be a large enough number. A sample size of 30 can work in many circumstances. When assessing organization or division compliance with documentation standards, a random sample of 30 charts would reveal areas of strength or opportunities for improvement. For an individual practitioner's chart review, a sample size of two to five similar cases may be large enough to validate documentation patterns.

PERFORMANCE LISTS

Performance lists, another quantitative tool, focus on validation of skills or observed demonstration of important functions or processes. A sample external defibrillation performance checklist is shown in Table 5-4. The nurse is "checked off" by an SDS or preceptor as the procedure is being performed.

COMPETENCY-BASED ORIENTATION

In the past 10 years, many SDSs have developed CBO programs, particularly for use in documenting new employees' ability to perform required tasks. CBO includes the skills, knowledge, and behaviors necessary for minimal safe levels of independent practice in a clinical area. This is accomplished within a particular time or orientation period. The new employee is "checked off" or evaluated on his or her ability to perform the tasks required by agency policy, procedure, or standards. A sample CBO assessment tool can be found in Table 5-5.

The purposes of CBO are to:

- Delineate the skills, knowledge, and behaviors expected in the new position
- Provide a means of tracking the skills acquired and demonstrated during orientation
- Provide some flexibility in designing individual orientation plans, while aligning the plan with the needs of the organization or the learner
- Serve as an orientation checklist.

CHART AUDITS

Chart audits can be used to demonstrate compliance with requirements, regulations, and policies and to help determine areas for improvement. Audits can be done on an individual, unit, division, or organization-wide basis. Chart audits can provide:

- A review process for clinicians in career ladder programs
- A way to establish the practice patterns of clinicians
- Evidence for patient discharge teaching, planning, or the use of restraints.

(*text continues on page 114*)

TABLE 5-4

EXTERNAL DEFIBRILLATION PERFORMANCE CHECKLIST

Lake Hospital System
Nursing Service
Competency Skill Sheet

EXTERNAL DEFIBRILLATION

Operator: _____   Date Completed: _____

SS#: _____

Competency statement: Registered nurses practicing in the critical care areas will demonstrate appropriate steps and safety in defibrillation techniques.

Performance Criteria	Met	Not Met	Comments
1. Recognizes Vfib/VTach on monitor.			
2. Assesses patient for LOC, presence of pulse.			
3. Calls for help and ER cart.			
4. Turns defibrillator ON.			
5. Identifies appropriate joules for defibrillation.			
6. Turns selector switch to defib and check synchronizer switch off.			
7. Applies defib patches to appropriate location on chest.			
8. Selects joules on monitor and charges.			
9. Applies paddles over the defib pads.			
10. Verifies presence of Vfib/VTach on monitor.			
11. Calls "All clear."			
12. Discharges paddles depressing both buttons simultaneously.			
13. Checks patient for return of pulse, identify cardiac rhythm.			

Verified by: _____

Source: Lake Hospital System. Used with permission.

TABLE 5-5

CBO ASSESSMENT OF LEARNER OUTCOMES

Expected Performance	Learner Outcome Assessment	Self Assessment	Practiced/ Reviewed	Demonstrates Competency Date/ Preceptor
Maintains IV in central lines	Administers medications through line Changes dressing Flushes line Changes cap			
Maintains IV therapy: IVADs, Portacath, Infusaport	Initiates infusion Administers medications through line Flushes Withdraws blood Accesses Removes needle			
Maintains IV therapy: right atrial catheter, Hickman, Broviac	Administers medications through line Changes dressing Flushes Changes cap Withdraws blood			
Performs venous access for IV start	Successfully passes IV course test Starts and secures IV			
Collects blood specimens—venous access	Successfully completes blood specimen collection module/skill validation Withdraws blood from patient Monitors patient after blood withdrawal			

FOLLOW-UP

The application of new knowledge is reinforced when there is follow-up, particularly when the clinical setting provides challenging opportunities for application different from those encountered in the classroom setting.

Qualitative Measurements

Qualitative research refers to the inductive, holistic, subjective, and process-oriented research methods used to observe, document, describe, understand, analyze, and interpret or develop a theory pertaining to a phenomenon, group, or setting. The goal of qualitative research is to understand a phenomenon or develop theory by exploring a topic of interest or a neglected or little-understood phenomenon. Qualitative research plays an important role in knowledge development by producing theory that guides a discipline. Because the theory is inductively derived, it is quite likely to be accurate or right (Morse & Field, 1995). In nursing, for example, a qualitative theory may provide insights that can be used to revise clinical practice. Qualitative findings may also provide rich descriptions that enable clinicians to understand a clinical reality or an otherwise incomprehensible situation or behavior.

Qualitative research is data-driven and as such provides data-based theory that should be valid and able to withstand external challenge, even more so than quantitative theory developed from incomplete data sets or the status quo. Qualitative data, rather than numbers, are words on paper, audiotape, or videotape. In clinical practice, qualitative "conversations" prove an ideal way to assess an employee's grasp of situations encountered in daily practice.

SELF-REPORTS

Self-reports are individual assessments of personal knowledge, skill, or ability. These can serve as efficient ways to focus education and training efforts on the areas identified for improvement, but some researchers have found inconsistencies between self-reports and actual practice skills. Cruden (1991) tried to determine why nurses would appraise their resuscitation skills unrealistically; the results suggested that unrealistic self-appraisal arose from poor or infrequent resuscitation training. Cruden noted in a study of nurses participating in CPR training that self-reports were hampered by their inability to assess their own skills or performance. The nurses' attempts to identify with roles they perceive they should fulfill, as well as their past performance in cardiac arrest situations, influenced their perceptions. Cruden concluded that current resuscitation training is inadequate, inappropriate, and inconsistent with the needs of practicing nurses.

SDSs are faced with the challenge of developing methods to focus needed education and create an environment where it is safe for clinicians to identify their own development needs. If there are negative consequences for those who report that their skills are lacking, few will participate in self-reports.

EXEMPLARS

An exemplar is a clinical experience that conveys more than one intent or outcome and can be easily translated to other clinical situations with different objective characteristics. Benner (1984) wrote that a paradigm case can serve as a clinical exemplar. Kuhn (1970) used the word "exemplar" for scientific experiments that guided subsequent scientific works. Benner argued that the term conveys an active stance in clinical situations. Exemplars can be used in a situation-based interpretive approach to assessing competence by identifying and describing the knowledge embedded in clinical practice, that hybrid of theory and experience (Benner, p. 40). She wrote that in the context of the whole, we can begin to base nursing theory and nursing research on a well-charted background of clinical knowledge (p. 41). Exemplars are particularly useful to assess clinical judgment and critical thinking skills.

WAYS OF KNOWING

Brockopp and Hastings-Tolsma (1995) defined ways of knowing as the variety of modes available to find new knowledge. There are a variety of ways to gain new knowledge (Kaplan, 1964), including intuition, problem solving, practical experience, and scientific inquiry.

Del Bueno et al.'s (1987) proposal of competence is example of how competence exists in the real world. The three overlapping circles categorize competence as technical skills, critical thinking skills, and interpersonal skills. All three types of skills are required to provide clinical care in most situations.

INTEGRATING PARTS

A competence assessment system is not complete unless the four components described earlier are integrated. Component integration is done by evaluating and continuously improving the system.

When evaluating the competence assessment system, it is important to look objectively at what is required for the system to be used. Questions to ask are:

- If this competency assessment system were not in place, is this the way it would be set up?
- Is there an easier way to accomplish the same goal?
- Are other colleagues doing something else that requires less work and still accomplishes the desired outcome?
- Is the system providing the data needed by various stakeholders?

Health care providers face the challenge of continuously improving the delivery system and the health services provided. Quality is a perception made by patients, providers, purchasers or third-party payors, and other interested persons. Perceptions of quality result from a variety of inputs, from the perceived compassion of a physician or caregiver to hard performance data comparing patient outcomes and costs across the system over time. Competence assessment systems are always grounded in continuous quality improvement.

Many synergistic effects can be realized by SDSs who develop sound competence assessment systems. Persons, groups, or organizations can join forces to achieve mutual goals. Group synergistic effects can lead to competence assessment or development of skills beyond what each person alone may envision or implement.

WHERE TO BEGIN

The first step is to identify time-intensive functions, programs, or processes important to the organization. Examples commonly implemented are training in IV chemotherapy administration, percutaneous central line insertion, training and competency validation for advanced-level patient care technicians, ACLS, and BTLS. Novice SDSs are encouraged to try the examples given in this text.

Building coalitions to accomplish common goals is an efficient approach to CSD. One example of coalition building is the establishment of regional training for basic and advanced arrhythmia recognition and interpretation. By establishing standards and eliciting cooperation from several organizations, consistent expectations and regional models of competence assessment can be realized. The cost of offering the training programs is shared by those who use the program.

Generally, collaborative programs are a "win-win" situation for all involved. Often, large organizations must provide the training programs because of their high volume of

---

DISPLAY 5-2

Age-Specific Competency Tool

Confidential

AGE-SPECIFIC CRITERIA-BASED PERFORMANCE APPRAISAL (FOR PATIENT CARE STAFF ONLY)

The associate has been ***observed demonstrating*** the knowledge and skills necessary to provide care appropriate to the age of the patients served in his/her assigned service area. The skills and knowledge needed to provide such care may be gained through education, training, or experience. Supporting documentation is retained in department files for at least 3 years. *NA* means that the associate does not perform this competency as a part of his/her job.

	Demonstrates at least the minimum knowledge skills and abilities for the following patient groups: Indicate date observed in "Met," "Not Met" columns.											
	Neonatal *Birth–6 mos*			*Pediatrics & Adolescence* *6 mos–17 years*			*Adult* *18–64 years*			*Geriatric* *65+ years*		
Competency	*Met*	*Not Met*	*NA*	*Met*	*Not Met*	*NA*	*Met*	*Not Met*	*NA*	*Met*	*Not Met*	*NA*
1a. Patient Care: Collect data utilizing age appropriate technique, tool or equipment.												
1b. Patient Care: Interprets data and modifies care appropriate to age of the patient.												
2. Communication: Uses communication techniques appropriate for the age of the patient.												

A *Not met* response above must be reflected in the associate's overall performance rating and must be established as a development goal for improvement through additional training or education.

Observer signature: _____ Date signed: _____

Source: St. Joseph Mercy Health System, Ann Arbor, MI. Used with permission.

learners. Smaller facilities can have their employees participate in a more efficient and effective experience than they might be able to provide themselves, with reduced costs and fewer staff resources needed to assess or develop the skill.

Another example of coalition building is formation of a group from two facilities to achieve consensus about how to document demonstration of compliance with age-specific competency. The goal of each facility is to develop a simple tool to document age-specific competency for all levels of direct caregivers. Each facility wants to avoid the time-consuming process of developing different mechanisms. Consensus on the goal, process, and desired outcomes allow the work to proceed, with a tool jointly developed to achieve the overall purpose of documentation of competency. Display 5-2 is a sample of one health care system's coalition for assessing age-specific competency.

SUMMARY
● ●

This chapter presented competence assessment system concepts. Four integrated elements of a sound system were suggested: pre-employment qualifications and assessment, orientation and job preparation, targeted interval assessments and performance appraisals, and response to appraisal. Methods were discussed by which SDSs can use the data generated through competence assessment activities to meet their specific needs. Quantitative and qualitative measures and methods were compared. Suggestions for building coalitions were offered to help the SDS evaluate and improve competence assessment systems.

Real-Life Steps Toward a Competency Assessment System
MITZI T. GREY

In a small community hospital of 110 beds, I am an overwhelmed, unappreciated educator reviewing the JCAHO human resources standards because the joint commission is coming to survey the hospital in 8 months. I feel frustrated as I focus on the competence assessment standards. Each department in the hospital is doing something different or nothing at all to validate the competence of its staff. We have to go to three different files to get all the information—the personnel file, the education file, and the departmental file. No one seems to have a sense of the big picture for a competence assessment system. Our process is fragmented, disorganized, and cumbersome.

I have been asked to lead a process improvement team to address these issues. We will need to identify the process to be improved and what we hope to accomplish, organize a team of stakeholders, clarify our current process, measure variation in the process, and then develop and implement strategies to improve our process.

Several department managers are invited to attend our first meeting and are asked to bring examples of how their department validates and documents competence assessment of staff. Our first task is to identify what we hope to accomplish, our expected outcome. After discussion, we agree that our goal is to improve our competence assessment system for validating initial and ongoing competency. Our goal is to develop a consistent hospital-wide approach to competence assessment that is accessible and organized. We also want all department managers to be knowledgeable about the system and able to implement it at their departmental level.

At our second meeting, the team members have brought information from their departments and are waiting to share.

Fred (all names have been changed), the dietary manager, isn't sure why he has been included in this meeting; his position is that "this whole competence assessment thing" is the educator's or the personnel manager's problem, not his. He has brought a sample performance evaluation and one quality control checklist for cleaning the hood above the stove.

Mr. Davis, the personnel manager, is a highly dedicated and meticulous man with a mission: to organize, guard, and defend the hospital personnel records. He takes his job very seriously. I had asked him to bring personnel files for us to review during the meeting, and he has reluctantly brought one file. He is patiently waiting to caution us about maintaining the confidentiality of personnel records.

Anxious to share her wisdom is Ms. Primm, the laboratory manager. Sitting open before her is a 3″ binder with initial and ongoing proficiency testing and education records for each of her staff members. She has been managing quality control and competence validation in her lab for years and is eager to tell us the "right way" to develop a competence assessment system for the rest of the hospital.

Karen, the pharmacist, nervous and frequently checking her watch, has brought several file folders that contain evidence of licensure verification and a pharmacy orientation checklist for each pharmacist and technician.

The nurse administrator, Sally, has brought cookies to share and is smiling broadly at the team members while wondering how exactly to facilitate this team process. She has brought with her a policy on licensure verification, competence assessment worksheets for each job category in nursing, and a list of annual competencies that are validated in nursing such as defibrillation, CPR, and blood glucose monitoring.

I have brought a notebook full of resources and samples that I have compiled over time. I have also provided each team member with a copy of the JCAHO's human resources and leadership standards and the competency assessment review form found in the JCAHO "Guidelines for Survey" manual. We had all brought pieces of a competence assessment system, but none of us had a complete package.

We share our examples and develop two flowcharts: one for assessing initial competency and one for validating ongoing competence (Figure 5-2). We plan the next agenda and future steps. We need to plan for measuring the process. I suggest that the department managers

conduct an audit of their staff's personnel records using the JCAHO's competency assessment review form. The personnel manager agrees to this if the department managers complete the audit in the personnel department and do not remove any records from the department. We agree to look at all the quality indicators we are currently measuring to see if any related to staff competency. We are sure that we will find several areas for improvement after completing these measurements.

I conclude the meeting by sharing some strategies that we might implement to improve our process of competency assessment in the future:

- Develop a standard competency assessment worksheet format
- Reorganize personnel files into sections such as licensure verification, initial hire and orientation documents, competency validation, education records, performance evaluations, and correspondence
- Develop a process for department managers to identify relevant competencies to be validated each year, including high-risk, low-volume, and problem-prone procedures; new equipment or processes; mandatory in-services; and age-specific competence
- Redesign hospital orientation and mandatory in-services to make them competency-based rather than just a set of lectures.

Looking around the table, I realize that many of the faces are blank or overwhelmed. I assure them that we are at the beginning of a journey to recognize what we already have in place and identify what we need to improve for our competency assessment system. I thank them for coming, and we evaluate the meeting. The participants express what they feel went well and what we need to improve about the meeting or team process.

After the meeting, Sally and I review the meeting and recognize that some of the team members know what to do, but others are going to need some guidance to do their homework. We agree to talk to each team member before the next meeting.

This brief story is a common occurrence in health care organizations today, and staff development specialists can learn much from our experiences.

Initial Competency Flowchart

Ongoing Competency Flowchart

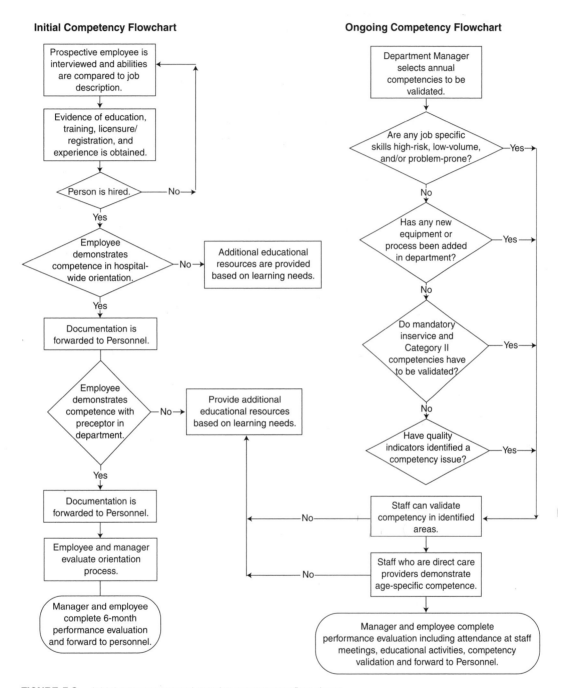

FIGURE 5-2. Initial competency and ongoing competency flow charts.

REFERENCES

Anderson, R., & McCafferty, J. R. (1996). Competencies: A tool for continuous learning and change. *Aspen's Advisor for Nurse Executives, 11*(9), 1, 3–6.

Benner, P. (1984). *From novice to expert*. Menlo Park, CA: Addison-Wesley.

Brockopp, D.Y., & Hastings-Tolsma, M. T. (1995). *Fundamentals of nursing research*. Boston: Jones & Bartlett.

Committee for the Study of Credentialing in Nursing. (1979). Credentialing in nursing: A new approach. *American Journal of Nursing, 79*(4), 674–693.

Cruden, E. J. (1991). An investigation into why nurses inappropriately describe their own cardiopulmonary resuscitation skills. *American Journal of Nursing, 16*(5), 597–605.

Del Bueno, D. J., Weeks, L., & Brown-Stewart, P. (1987). Clinical assessment centers: An cost-effective alternative for competency development. *Nursing Economics, 5*(1), 21–26.

Del Bueno, D. J. (1990). Experience, education, and nurses' ability to make clinical judgments. *Nursing & Health Care, 11*(6), 290–294.

Finocchio, L. J., Dower, C. M., McMahon, T., Gragnola, C. M., & the Taskforce on Health Care Workforce Regulation. (1995). *Reforming health care workforce regulation: Policy considerations for the 21st century*. San Francisco: Pew Health Professions Commission.

Gross, S. J. (1994). *Of foxes and hen houses: Licensing and the health professions*. Westport, CT: Quorum Books.

Joint Commission on Accreditation of Healthcare Organizations. (1993). *The measurement mandate*. Oakbrook Terrace, IL: Author.

Joint Commission on Accreditation of Healthcare Organizations. (1996). *Comprehensive accreditation manual for hospitals*. Oakbrook Terrace, IL: Author.

Kaplan, A. (1964). *The conduct of inquiry*. New York: Thomas Y. Crowell.

Kuhn, T. S. (1970). *The structure of scientific revolutions*. Chicago: University of Chicago Press.

McCrone, E. (1995). Focusing on competence. Presentation at Council on Licensure, Enforcement, and Regulation 15th annual meeting, San Antonio, TX, September 6–9, 1995.

Morse, J. M., & Field, P. (1995). *Qualitative research methods for health professionals*. London: Chapman & Hall.

Norman, G., & Streiner, D. (1994). *Biostatistics: The bare essentials*. St. Louis: Mosby.

O'Connor, K. F., Soukup, M., Brown, S,. & Burnes, B. (1979). Certification within specialities. *Oncology Nursing Forum, 6*(4), 28–31.

Shulby, G. A. (1993). Getting started: Communicating float staff competency validation. *Journal of Nursing Staff Development, 9*(5), 246–247.

Webster's new 20th-century dictionary of the English language (unabridged). (1983). McKechnie, J. (Ed.). Springfield, MA: Merriam-Webster, Inc.

Wolgin, F. (1990). Focus on outcome: Perspectives on research. *Journal of Nursing Staff Development, 6*(3), 151–152.

BIBLIOGRAPHY

Alspach, G. (1996). *Designing competency assessment programs: A handbook for nursing and health-related professionals*. Pensacola, FL: National Nursing Staff Development Organization.

Joint Commission on Accreditation of Healthcare Organizations. (1995). Staff competency is the foundation of excellent care. *Joint Commission Perspectives*, May/June.

Leininger, M. (1985). *Qualitative research methods in nursing*. Orlando: Grune & Stratton.

6

Competence Assessment Models and Methods

SUSAN B. JESKA

The design of a rational model for competence assessment (CA) requires a very deliberate and thoughtful process. Like any other major organizational change initiative, strong leadership and passionate championship are needed to sustain the long and sometimes arduous process that begins with model design. Most organizations want to jump-start this work and move right to implementation. However, time and again, evidence suggests that without the critical thinking and commitment that occurs during model design, efforts fail due to the lack of core tenets and philosophical underpinnings.

When faced with the challenge of a major change initiative such as establishing a CA model, many look to help from the outside. This may come in the form of consultation, conference attendance, or a review of the available literature and reference books. Any of these approaches may be helpful to the beginning work with model design, but none of these strategies in isolation is sufficient. For instance, attending a conference to learn more about CA models and methods may give the participant an overview of approaches used in the field. During the conference, a participant is likely to be exposed to a variety of preferred approaches. But for someone at the beginning stages of competence model design, this information may seem overwhelming. Similarly, a review of the literature could prove unwieldy, given the thousands of citations on CA, many of which date back as far as the early 1960s (Pollock, 1981; Scott, 1982).

These kinds of experiences are likely to cause disappointment and frustration to those with limited exposure to CA models. This often leads to desperate calls for outside consultation. And although a consultant may prove to be worthwhile in advancing organizational thinking, he or she is likely to offer a packaged approach or preferred model. These packaged products typically undervalue the critical elements of model design and thereby place an emphasis on the use of specific tools and techniques. We have only to look to the field of quality management to learn why this does not work. No packaged program will meet the exact needs of an organization.

The key "to successful use of competencies is building a model with characteristics that best fit the organization's strategies, business objectives and culture" (American Compensation Association, 1996, p. 19). Therefore, the best models for CA are developed from within. They are created by organizational leaders and change agents to reflect the fundamental thinking regarding staff development and organizational performance. They are based on a clear purpose and intended results. They often take a year or more to develop and implement (American Compensation Association, 1996).

Organizations that appear to have the most successful models move from very deliberate reflection and planning to implementation. These models have a logical flow from conceptual design to operational details. The following process steps are suggested to ensure a similar movement.

PHASE I: DESIGNING THE MODEL

First, the model infrastructure must be created and several key decisions must be made, including:

- Who will have overall accountability for the CA model and process
- The working definition of competence
- The domains of practice to be measured by the CA model
- The operating philosophy to be used.

These decisions lead to the fundamental thinking and belief system that permeate the model and drive all other decisions. These critical first steps are often overlooked by those charged with establishing a CA model.

Identifying Accountability

Overall accountability for the CA model and methods must be given to a person who can champion an organizational change initiative, has credibility throughout the organization, and is perceived to be able to influence a strategic human resource effort. This person must be able to influence the chief executive and senior leadership staff to the merits of CA and work with them to set the tone for the organization. He or she must be able to work with service area directors and managers to promote understanding and support of CA and to enlist their participation in the identification of relevant competencies.

The person assigned accountability for CA should, in turn, be able to identify a group who can spearhead and oversee the organization's model. Group members should be selected based on their willingness to lead organizational change, ability to look beyond traditional departmental and discipline boundaries, and ability to demonstrate commitment to the development of a competence model and process that will meet the intended results. Once identified, this group should be ready to accept the appropriate authority and responsibility consistent with leading an organizational change initiative.

Understanding the Purpose

The group's first and most important step is to gain an understanding of why CA is needed—in other words, to answer the question, "What is CA really intended to accomplish?" The group must understand its purpose to be able to spearhead the change. If the group is not clear as to what it is trying to achieve and why, it will probably not get there. Both the "why" and the "what" of CA must clearly be understood from the beginning.

In essence, CA is a tool to drive organizational performance. At its best, it is the foundation from which all other human resource functions flow. CA is the framework that defines:

- What employees must demonstrate when hired
- What employees must demonstrate to remain employed
- What new performance is expected based on strategic directions of the organization
- How work settings are staffed and work assignments managed
- What developmental offerings are provided
- How employees are supported in their career planning
- How performance is measured
- How employees are rewarded and recognized.

At its best, CA is directly tied to the organization's mission, vision, values, and strategies and is a dynamic process that changes along with any organizational change.

When it isn't working so well, CA is the process of sending staff through skills laboratories and testing stations to measure rote memorization and technical skills that have been evident in practice for years. At its worst, it measures the status quo and costs the organization hundreds of thousands of dollars annually to create checklists and skills stations that bring no return on investment.

The purpose of CA is to prepare people for the future. It advances the human resource potential and is essential for organizational survival.

Defining Competence

Once the purpose and intent of CA are understood, the next step is to determine a working definition of competence. This helps to clarify what is to be accomplished.

The literature is replete with definitions of competence (Jeska et al., 1995). In general, these references describe competence as the composite of knowledge, skills, and abilities needed to perform in a role. As such, there is an assumption that competence is the interplay of interpersonal and technical skills with critical thinking—in other words, it is the integration of cognitive, affective, and psychomotor domains of practice.

Some organizations have selected Benner's (1982) definition of competence for their models: "the ability to perform the task with desirable outcomes under the varied circumstances of the real world" (p. 304). Others prefer the definition by Del Bueno et al. (1990): "the effective application of knowledge and skills in the work setting" (p. 135). Under either definition, competence is not simply the ability to do well on a cognitive test or to perform well in a structured environment such as a skills laboratory; rather, it is the ability to integrate knowledge, skills, and abilities into actual practice.

With the operating definition of competence in place, the oversight group may find it helpful to clarify some of the terminology likely to be used during the CA process. Without this clarity, employees may be confused by inconsistent language and mixed messages. In general, proponents of CA use the following terms and general understandings in their models:

COMPETENCY A broad statement describing an aspect of practice that must be developed and demonstrated

COMPETENCE The achievement and integration of many competencies into practice; the overall ability to perform

COMPETENT An adjective used to describe a person who has met all identified role-related competencies.

A competency statement measures just one dimension of a person's overall ability to perform; thus, for any given role, there are many competencies that must be achieved and demonstrated. Some competencies identify and measure a person's ability to relate to patients and colleagues, others test specific technical skills, and still others assess the ability to use critical thinking. When a person has demonstrated the ability to meet all the identified role-related competencies, he or she is deemed competent to perform in that role.

Many organizations further define competencies into various types. Depending on organizational preference, it is possible to find any of the following (or other) terms used in practice: core competencies, critical competencies, universal competencies, initial competencies, ongoing competencies, developmental competencies, and threshold competencies. There is no commonly agreed on practice.

To illustrate why an organization might choose to delineate competencies into various types, the University of Minnesota Hospital and Clinic (UMHC) model can be used as an example. UMHC uses the terms "core competencies" and "critical competencies."

Core competencies measure a person's ability to perform the core functions of the role. For instance, the core competencies of a nurse measure the ability to do patient teaching, discharge and transition planning, and care delivery skills, among others. In contrast, the core competencies of a clinical nurse specialist address advanced practice knowledge and skill, research use, and ability to promote staff development. A manager's core competencies reflect the fiscal, operations, and people management responsibilities inherent in a management role.

Critical competencies are those that change over time, reflecting the dynamic nature of the health care environment. Each year, critical competencies are identified based on changes in care and practice, findings from quality improvement, and organizational issues and directions. Critical competencies are considered essential in maintaining a viable and responsive organization within a changing work environment. The following hypothetical example is given to highlight why UMHC believes critical competencies are important:

> Tom, a 45-year-old manager of a clinical laboratory, has been employed in the same organization since he began his career 23 years ago. He has followed his desired career path and worked his way to a management position after several clinical practice roles. Tom has always been known for his ability to solve problems and improve systems for efficiency. For this, he has received very positive performance reviews and acknowledgments from the laboratory administrator.
>
> One year ago, the hospital's CEO identified the need for major change. Significant budget reductions and re-engineering efforts were deemed critical for the hospital to survive the emerging managed care environment. The CEO asked all managers to work across traditional departmental and discipline boundaries to cut costs and improve service. He developed as a critical competency for all the managers "Establishes and builds bridges across departments and work settings to achieve new organizational goals."
>
> Most of the managers rallied to the cause and began to develop cross-functional work teams focused on addressing issues, creating new approaches to practice, and reducing operating expenses. However, none of this behavior was evident in Tom. He seemed to understand the expectation but was not initiating any activities in support of this expectation. Tom's boss, the laboratory administrator, noted that Tom was still able to meet the core competencies of his management role but was not demonstrating this critical competency.
>
> The administrator sat down with Tom to discuss his performance and his obvious inability to achieve this critical competency. During the conversation, Tom acknowledged his lack of attention to it. He shared his fear of working with groups outside the laboratory because of his obvious lack of experience beyond his own department. Tom was concerned that he would have no credibility with other groups and was worried that his skills and abilities were not transferable.
>
> The administrator discussed Tom's concerns with him and reinforced the need for him to demonstrate an ability to work beyond his departmental boundaries. He and Tom developed an action plan to create developmental opportunities and build Tom's confidence.
>
> Today, Tom is an active, contributing member of various organizational initiatives. He has demonstrated his ability to maintain core competencies for the manager role and at the same time has developed and demonstrated the new critical competencies for his position. Tom and others have seen the merit of identifying and measuring new role-related critical competencies each year.

UMHC has further delineated critical competencies as universal competencies, area-specific competencies, and role-specific critical competencies. Universal competencies apply to everyone in the organization, regardless of position. These typically address broad-based needs and directions. They may address stress and change management during times of major organizational change, or they might focus on customer service if patient satisfaction surveys show less-than-desirable results. In contrast, area-specific competencies apply only to staff members in a particular department or work area, role-specific competencies only to staff within a specific role.

This delineation of critical competencies can be very effective because it recognizes that data from a variety of sources are used to determine the need for organizational attention and change. It is possible, for example, that quality monitoring may lead to the identification of a problem with clinical outcomes within one patient population that is not evident in another. By identifying a critical competency to address this deficiency, improvements may be made in the appropriate arena. Similarly, if data regarding employee injuries show escalated rates within one employee group and not another, a role-related critical competency on specific personal safety measures is warranted for the affected group only.

Other organizations have chosen models based on developmental competencies and threshold competencies. Threshold competencies come with the person and are demonstrated at the time of hire or during orientation. In contrast, developmental competencies must be developed and demonstrated after hire.

Determining Domains of Practice

Another important decision to be made in model design is determining the domains of practice. Domains are the dimensions of performance deemed essential for the role. Historically, only one domain of practice was emphasized: psychomotor skills. An undue amount of attention was placed on this aspect of practice, as evidenced by the voluminous skills checklists and procedures that emphasized the technical dimension of performance. More recently, however, there has been a growing recognition that psychomotor skills are not enough; equally important are the affective and cognitive domains of practice, which recognize interpersonal skills and critical thinking. A brief look at a few practitioners helps to point out the importance of all three of these domains.

Sally, a 30-year-old nurse, has worked in orthopedic surgery for 7 years. The surgeons are very appreciative when she is working because no one else in the operative area is as technically adept. She is proficient with all the equipment and instruments, anticipates the surgeons' preferences and needs, and can stay focused on the case at hand. However, the other nurses and technicians view Sally differently. They note her inability to work with them as a team on operational issues within perioperative services. They feel resentful because the surgeons praise Sally for her technical skills but see no evidence of her commitment to other team members or an improved work environment.

Lizzy, a young, outgoing, friendly nurse, has worked in pediatrics for just 1 year. She is known for her ability to develop rapport with children and their parents quickly; consequently, she signs up to be primary nurse for several patients at the same time. Lizzy's colleagues have noted that her technical skills are satisfactory and her interpersonal skills are certainly unquestionable, but they have become concerned regarding her ability to set priorities and use sound judgment in emergent situations. On several occasions, Lizzy has not followed through on her accountabilities as a primary nurse.

Ahmad, who came to the hospital 5 years ago from another country, works as a respiratory therapist in a medical/surgical area. Ahmad has very strong technical skills and his colleagues are impressed by his ability to respond to acute situations and anticipate patient needs. However, he has difficulty communicating with others. He is shy and self-conscious about his imperfect English and consequently does not participate in staff meetings, group projects, or other team activities. A few patients have complained about his limited communication. He arrives on time for work and promptly leaves when the work is done.

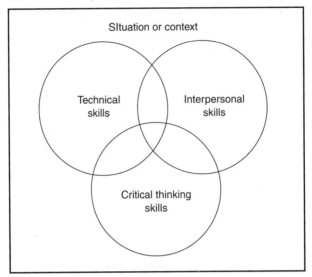

FIGURE 6-1. Dimensions of competent performance. Reprinted with permission of Janetti Publications, Inc., publisher, *Nursing Economic$,* Volume 5, Number 1 (January/February, 1987), p. 23.

These examples show that competence in any one domain of practice does not guarantee competence in the other domains. A weakness in any one domain may have profound implications. The person with questionable technical skills quickly loses the confidence of patients, families, and colleagues. The person with weak interpersonal skills has difficulty establishing relationships and working on teams. The person with limited critical thinking ability typically has difficulty setting priorities and responding in acute situations and often makes inappropriate assumptions.

Therefore, the most comprehensive assessment of competence is one based on the confluence of psychomotor, affective, and cognitive dimensions of practice. This integration is best captured by the familiar diagram in Figure 6-1 (Del Bueno et al., 1987).

Developing an Operating Philosophy

A final element in model design is developing an operating philosophy. Typically, organizations do not bother to discuss or develop a philosophy about CA. Although some organizations may have gotten along fine without one, many have found the absence of a philosophical approach to be a problem. Philosophy statements are generally used to describe and define an operating belief system. Without attention to philosophy, entire models may be developed that fail to meet the defined goals.

A philosophy statement for CA need not be elaborate, but it must be clear and to the point. For instance, UMHC's philosophy statement regarding CA succinctly defines its operating beliefs and assumptions. This operating philosophy for CA was not difficult to produce; it naturally flowed from the organization's overall philosophy regarding staff development. Documents illustrating this belief system can be found in Appendix B.

For this organization, the philosophy statement helped to guide discussions during the difficult stage of competence model development. For example, when it was time to create forms to record the assessment of staff competence, it was important to develop a tool that would reflect the operating belief regarding shared accountabilities for the achievement and documentation of competence. Similarly, because this organization held a firm belief that their model should be dynamic, the process established for the annual identification of competencies reflected the results of quality monitoring, changes in work environment, and new strategic directions.

Developing Operating Guidelines

Once the fundamental decisions regarding accountability, definition of competence, domains of practice, and philosophy have been made, the next order of business is to determine the operating guidelines. These guidelines might include such things as overall directions regarding how the CA process will be handled for new employees in contrast to current staff, how CA will relate to systems for performance management, and how competencies should be developed and assessed from an organizational, work setting, and role-specific perspective.

At this point in the process, it is common for the oversight group to face questions for which, in essence, they have no answers and which stimulate more questions and further deliberation. They might be asked, "If my staff are required to have a license, certification, or registration to work here, can't I assume they are competent?" This question and others like it often lead to a lengthy discussion about what licensure, certification, or registration implies. The group will need to grapple with what credentials mean in relation to core competence or continued competence in a role. More often than not, the group will determine that these credentials provide supporting evidence of some aspects of core competence but are insufficient evidence of continued role-specific competence. However, it would depend on what competencies have been identified and how the organization has chosen to articulate competence.

Definitely at this stage of model development, there will be many more questions raised than answers provided. Instead of causing major frustration, however, the oversight group should consider this a healthy and natural by-product of an evolutionary process and organizational change initiative.

Creating the Template for Competency Identification

The final steps of model design are determining how competency statements will be written and how competencies will be assessed in practice.

A review of the literature shows that competency statements may be organized within a variety of frameworks (Gurvis & Grey, 1995). Depending on organizational preference, competencies can be written to reflect novice-to-expert practice (McGregor, 1990), nursing practice standards, nursing diagnoses, medical diagnoses, or any other preferred approach (Display 6-1). The organizing framework provides a backdrop for decision making regarding how competency statements will eventually be written.

Proponents of CA models generally recommend using a very simple structure of five to 12 statements to describe the core competencies for any given role. They recommend that these statements be written broadly to define aspects of performance associated with success in the role. More specifically, Alspach (1984) recommended that competency statements should have five essential characteristics; they should:

- Describe a general category of behavior
- Be focused on the learner
- Be behavioral and measurable
- Be free from performance conditions
- Be validated by experts.

DISPLAY 6-1

Types of Competency Statements

Medical diagnoses	Provides nursing care for patients with adult respiratory distress syndrome
Nursing diagnoses	Provides nursing care for patients with altered mental status
Nursing practice standards	Implements nursing practice standards for patients undergoing cardiac catheterization
Nursing process	Obtains clinical data that accurately reflect patient status
Phases of the health continuum	Provides nursing care for patients from labor through the postnatal phase
Therapies	Manages and organizes care for patients receiving hemodialysis

From McGregor, R. J. (1990). Advancing staff nurse competencies: From novice to expert. *Journal of Nursing Staff Development, 6*(6), 287–290.

Alspach recommended that competency statements integrate all the domains of performance and not distinguish between cognitive, affective, and psychomotor competencies. She provided examples of possible competency statements for critical care nurses, as shown in Display 6-2.

In a nutshell, competency statements are best when they reflect broad and measurable aspects of practice and when they are clear and understandable to the persons demonstrating and validating the competencies. To achieve this clarity, Alspach and others have advocated the identification of critical behaviors or criteria sets for each competency statement.

Critical behaviors, simply put, are what must be done to validate the competency. With a new employee, the critical behaviors may be more focused on process and psycho-

---

DISPLAY 6-2

Examples of Competency Statements

1. Provides all appropriate components of nursing care for patients with actual or potential neurological dysfunction.
2. Documents physiological and psychosocial assessment data that reflect pertinent trends in the patient's condition.
3. Provides safe nursing care for patients recovering from general anesthesia.
4. Meets all written and behavioral performance criteria for certification in basic cardiac life support.
5. Communicates assessment data to appropriate members of the health care team as the patient's situation warrants.
6. Provides all essential components of nursing care for patients with documented or suspected acute myocardial infarction.
7. Meets nursing practice standards that are related to care of the patient who requires hemodynamic monitoring.
8. Sets appropriate priorities among elements in work assignment.

From Alspach, J. G. (1984). Designing a competency-based orientation for critical care nurses. *Heart & Lung, 13*(6), 658.

DISPLAY 6-3

Sample Criteria for the Competency "Provides All Essential Aspects of Nursing Care for a Patient Undergoing Elective Cardioversion"

1. Describes the general rationale for cardioversion (cognitive).
2. Identifies the clinical indications for elective cardioversion for assigned patient (cognitive).
3. Assembles all necessary equipment in preparation for the cardioversion procedure (cognitive and psychomotor).
4. Prepares all medications for use during the cardioversion procedure (cognitive and psychomotor).
5. Verifies that the defibrillator is synchronizing appropriately (cognitive and psychomotor).
6. Prepares the patient/family for the cardioversion procedure (cognitive, affective, and psychomotor).
7. Adheres to all electrical safety precautions throughout the cardioversion procedure (cognitive, affective, and psychomotor).
8. Assists the physician with electrocardiographic waveform interpretation during the cardioversion procedure (cognitive and psychomotor).
9. Supports the patient throughout the cardioversion procedure (cognitive, affective, and psychomotor).
10. Documents all pertinent aspects of the cardioversion procedure (cognitive, affective, and psychomotor).

From Alspach, J. G. (1984). Designing a competency-based orientation for critical care nurses. *Heart & Lung*, *13*(6), 659.

motor skills. With other employees, critical behaviors are likely to emphasize the integration of all domains of practice. The example in Display 6-3 demonstrates how a set of critical behaviors is used to clarify the competency "Provides all essential aspects of nursing care for a patient undergoing elective cardioversion." This delineation of critical behaviors is particularly helpful for staff who may be new to caring for a patient undergoing a specific procedure. Display 6-4, taken from a model for medical/surgical nursing competencies, shows how competency statements and the critical behaviors may be written based on specific patient populations served.

DISPLAY 6-4

Competency: Provides Safe and Skilled Care to the Patient With an Acute Spinal Cord Injury Based on Presenting Nursing Diagnoses

Assesses, monitors, and intervenes in all aspects of respiratory care
Provides for a safe environment
Monitors and implements appropriate interventions to enhance mobility and prevent complications
Monitors skin integrity to prevent breakdown
Monitors and intervenes to promote evacuation of the bladder and prevent complications
Monitors and intervenes to promote evacuation of the bowels and prevent complications
Promotes the patient's feeling of self-worth
Teaches the patient and family procedures and techniques to care for the patient at home

From Buszta, *et al.* (1993).

A common misconception about the identification of competencies and their related critical behaviors is that they should reflect all aspects of performance and job expectations. This is clearly not the case: competencies should address only the critical aspects of a role deemed essential for success. These should be captured within the five to 12 core competency statements.

Creating the Template for Competence Assessment

The final step in model design is to determine how competencies will be assessed in practice. Each competency should have its own method of validation. Depending on the organizational model, any given competency may be assessed and validated using a number of different means. Models that encourage many different methods of verification recognize individual differences in learning styles, demonstration preferences, and experience bases from which to demonstrate competence. A role-related critical competency for a nurse, for instance, might be demonstrated and verified through the use of clinical exemplars on one unit, peer review on another unit, and case study on a third. Methods of verification should directly correlate with the competencies to be measured and the perceived performance level of the staff. The purpose of CA is developmental; therefore, methods of assessment should gradually increase in sophistication each year.

PHASE II: IDENTIFYING COMPETENCIES AND DETERMINING ASSESSMENT METHODS

The second phase of creating a CA model is to begin identifying competencies and assessment methods. This occurs in three steps:

1. Determining relevant core competencies
2. If appropriate to the organizational model, determining critical competencies
3. Establishing verification or assessment methods.

Determining Core Competencies

Various methods are available to identify competencies. In nursing, a typical process used to identify competencies is a consensus-based approach of expert practitioners. The assumption behind this method for identifying competencies is that expert practitioners have the best understanding of how practice should occur. As Alspach (1984) noted:

> Individuals who are already considered competent in . . . role and setting represent a logical source of information to identify the most salient competencies. Such a . . . panel of experts can systematically analyze the major components of their daily role. (pp. 657–658)

This approach generally involves a focus group process where expert practitioners are asked to respond to events and reflect on their practice. Out of this discussion, themes are identified and clustered to produce a potential listing of core competencies and critical behaviors. The list is validated and further refined through subsequent discussions. This process can be effective but lengthy, because it can take 2 or more months to complete. Another commonly used approach is the direct observation of staff by peers, supervisors, or job analysis experts.

Some organizations do not rely on either of these approaches and instead look to existing job postings, job descriptions, or performance standards to help identify competencies. These documents generally include behavioral statements related to the core functions of a job and, as such, provide a beginning foundation for thinking about core competence. In addition to these types of internal documents, professional standards or other practice guidelines may be available for some roles.

A recent research study conducted on CA models found that the most common techniques used to collect information and identify competencies are focus groups, critical incident or behavioral interviews, surveys, and other types of interviews (American Compensation Association, 1996). The study showed that the most common sources for competency identification are senior management, high performers, and functional experts. This study of health care, business, and industry practices found that most organizations identify competencies that address performance behaviors (93%) and personal attributes (83%). Competencies that reflect knowledge (61%) and technical skill (55%) are not identified as often.

It is often helpful to have some basic guidelines when identifying competencies. The following suggestions are offered to help with the process (Parry, 1996):

- Focus on generic competencies applicable across settings. Core competencies for persons in the same role typically do not change because of work settings.
- Avoid the obvious. If a role requires a license to practice, some competencies do not need to be listed; they may be taken for granted.
- Make sure each competency is observable and measurable.
- Illustrate the desired behavior with examples.
- Use familiar and simple language to ensure understanding.
- Keep the core competency list short. If the list is long, it probably includes specific skills instead of generic competencies.
- Keep competencies mutually exclusive.
- Focus on future needs whenever possible.
- Work backwards from the desired results to the desired behavior to competencies.
- Adapt the competency list to levels of performance (such as novice-to-expert) if desired.
- Avoid including personality traits.
- Group competencies into like clusters whenever possible.

As previously noted, it is very important to know how competence has been defined and what organizing framework is to be used before competency identification actually begins. Once this is determined, the steps to competency identification need not be difficult. For instance, when identifying competencies for a clinical manager role, the following might be the first steps:

1. Clarify the role. Is there a brief description or job summary that broadly defines the role? If so, it might read something like this:
   This advanced practice role is responsible for establishing an environment of collaborative, integrated care delivery for a clinical program or several patient populations. The person in this role uses advanced knowledge, skills, and abilities to direct the patient care operations. This leadership role includes responsibility for establishing a vision, creating a climate for collaborative care delivery, establishing meaningful communication systems, and ensuring the competence and development of staff, effective stewardship of limited resources, and continuous quality improvement efforts.

2. Determine if there are professional practice standards, job descriptions, or other documents available. If so, they are likely to provide guidance regarding possible competency statements. For instance, if the clinical manager role has been defined as a traditional management role, there will probably be a need for

competencies that address personnel management, financial management, and operations management. If it has been defined as a leadership role, specific leadership competencies should be identified.

3. Consider who might be identified as an expert clinical manager. Gather the experts together to reflect on their performance. Use a focus group approach to identify themes and patterns in responses. This information can then be used to generate a list of possible competencies. For example, out of this process five clusters of competencies might be generated: role model, vision and communication, environment and climate, stewardship of resources, and continuous improvement and evaluation. These competencies can then be validated, further refined, and eventually made clear with the addition of critical behaviors. The end product might be a list of five to 12 core competencies and their respective critical behaviors (Display 6-5).

As the identification of role-related competencies in health care evolves, there will probably be more sharing of information across organizations. The literature since 1993

DISPLAY 6-5

Sample Core Competencies

Cluster	Competencies
I. Role Model	• Supports the mission, goals, and objectives of the department and hospital, and through own behavior leads and motivates others to do so also. • Sets example for personal and professional development. • Demonstrates leadership competencies.
II. Vision/Communication	• Establishes shared vision. • Creates meaning through communication. • Maintains constancy of purpose toward vision.
III. Environment/Climate	• Establishes environment for collaborative care delivery. • Creates culture of shared values. • Establishes environment that promotes individual growth, and job satisfaction, and nurtures professional practice.
IV. Stewardship of Resources	• Develops and directs the patient care unit budget. • Establishes systems and processes to support unit operations and ensure care delivery goals. • Serves the public and community through effective stewardship of limited resources.
V. Continuous Quality Improvement/Evaluation	• Evaluates and communicates patient care delivery, systems, processes, and outcomes. • Integrates continuous quality improvement efforts. • Acts as change agent.

begins to show evidence of this trend. For instance, a 1993 article by Farrell and Robbins described the new leadership competencies needed for physicians. In 1994, after an extensive study of nurse leaders, information regarding core competencies for nurse executives was published (Jeska, 1994). This work highlighted the executive's need to establish vision, create meaning for others, build trust, and demonstrate integrity, among other things. Subsequent study of nurse executive practice in managed care environments (Jeska, 1996) has led to additional competencies deemed essential for nurse executives practicing in these complex environments.

Determining Critical Competencies

If an organization has chosen a model that includes critical competencies, the next step of the process is to identify them. Critical competencies are generally identified on an annual basis and are used to respond to quality management findings, changes in care and practice, and organizational directions. They reflect the contextual aspects of practice, which change over time even when core competencies do not.

With the advent of managed care, it is not uncommon for critical competencies to address heightened expectations for clinical outcomes and fiscal responsiveness. For instance, a critical competency and related behavior for a manager within a managed care environment might read, "Involves staff and stakeholders in ongoing work analysis using benchmarking studies to determine service improvement, clinical outcomes, and cost reduction opportunities." A critical competency for a social worker in the same environment might read, "Facilitates discharge planning to support patient movement across the continuum of care in accordance with the identified clinical pathways."

Some organizational leaders may believe they are exempt from critical competencies, but this is clearly not the case: these must be identified for all roles. Today's leaders must also grow and develop to respond to new expectations and the ever-changing world of health care. In an organization plagued by old practice patterns and operating methods, a critical competency for organizational leaders might be developed that reads, "Leads system or process design or redesign using continuous quality improvement tools and techniques." In another organization where layoffs have occurred and employees' fear and anxiety have escalated, a critical competency addressing the leader's role in managing stress and dealing with "survivor syndrome" would be appropriate.

All in all, the best competencies are those that parallel the organization's strategic directions and are developed and critiqued by top performers within their respective roles and disciplines. So although a nurse may be able to suggest specific critical competencies for a pharmacist, these suggestions should not be used in isolation; rather, they should be integrated into other source information and data. The core and critical competencies for pharmacy should be developed by expert pharmacists with the guidance of others to ensure a fit with the philosophy and direction of the organization's CA model.

Determining Methods of Assessment

Once competencies are identified, decisions can then be made regarding appropriate methods of assessment. Each competency should have its own method of assessment because it measures only one aspect of performance.

The optimal measure of a competency occurs during job performance (Alspach, 1984, citing Ebel, 1981), so the best models are those that measure competencies in the real world. Unfortunately, however, this is not the usual practice. The vast majority of CA processes in health care occur outside of the practice setting because they are easier to organize and control. The desired outcome is usually sacrificed in the process.

Common assessment approaches are described in Chapters 2 and 10. The ultimate decision of which processes to use should rest with the practice setting, based on the competency to be measured.

It is always important to ask, "What do we really want to measure?" For some competencies, the intent is to measure discrete psychomotor skills and sequential process steps. In this case, direct observation is best, and it may occur in a skills laboratory or in the practice setting. Most organizations lean toward observation in a skills laboratory because it is relatively easy to control this setting and process. On the other hand, it can be argued this type of observation is insufficient because it merely measures a person's ability to demonstrate a technical competency in a controlled environment. The importance of direct observation in actual practice situations cannot be stressed enough. Clinical nurse specialists and other expert practitioners can be invaluable in the direct observation of skills as they occur at the bedside.

Indirect observation may also be used. This technique may be employed by managers, charge nurses, and others through patient rounds (Castleforte & Dunlap, 1995) and medical record reviews. With indirect observation, there is generally no witness of the specific process skills involved; however, there is a presumption that the process skills are correctly followed when the desired outcome is achieved. Clinical rounds can measure competencies as well as improve the standard of care and practice in the practice setting.

To assess specific critical thinking dimensions, verification methods should capture the ability to set priorities, make sound judgments, integrate and analyze data from a variety of sources, and ask critical questions to test and validate assumptions (Display 6-6). This assessment can also be done using a variety of methods. A cognitive test, although common, is less than effective: the ability to perform well on a test does not necessarily correlate with application of knowledge and critical thinking in practice. Instead, case studies or other methods that ask employees to respond to likely scenarios are better at measuring the capacity to respond to actual events.

Some organizations value an assessment center, defined by Del Bueno et al. (1987) as "a comprehensive standardized process by which multiple sampling techniques are used to determine a person's actual or potential ability to perform skills and activities vital to success on the job" (p. 21). Assessment centers are often used with new managers. For instance, to test a new manager's critical thinking skills, he or she may be asked to respond to an "in basket" containing several memos and documents (Crow & Ezell, 1996). The manager triages the information and identifies how he or she would respond. This process measures the ability to triage work and set appropriate priorities. Assessment centers can be very effective, but like all other simulation exercises they occur away from actual practice and merely measure the ability to perform in controlled situations. There is no guarantee that competence in a simulated environment translates to competence in actual practice.

Obviously, interpersonal competencies address a person's ability to relate to others. In general, interpersonal competencies are intended to measure the ability to empathize and to demonstrate effective communication, willingness to work as a team member, and commitment to others. Interpersonal competency assessment is best done from the perspective of others. It may come from indirect feedback gathered by a manager for performance appraisal purposes, or more appropriately through the use of a peer review process. A peer review tool, when properly structured, can be a very effective way to provide evidence of a person's ability to meet the identified competency.

Another means to assess interpersonal competency may come in the form of a customer survey. A customer survey structured to provide feedback about employees may provide ample evidence for meeting an identified competency. In a customer survey, it is not uncommon to ask patients to identify staff members they believe have specifically helped

DISPLAY 6-6

Critical Thinking Dimensions

Clinical Decision Making
- Ability to identify a priority risk to a patient's health.
- Ability to describe nursing interventions to correct or minimize identified risks.
- Ability to identify nursing interventions that may prevent potential risks.
- Ability to defend decisions using scientific knowledge principles or proven practice.
- Ability to make decisions related to urgent risks within a predetermined time limit.

Priority Setting/Revising
- Ability to differentiate the priority of both independent and dependent nursing activities required by a specific patient.
- Ability to determine the relative priority of specific uncontrolled events that occur in clinical units.
- Ability to describe or demonstrate interventions that will correct or minimize harm from specific uncontrolled events.

Problem Solving/Troubleshooting
- Ability to identify malfunction problems of specific invasive monitoring devices.
- Ability to describe/demonstrate nursing actions to be taken in response to malfunction problems.
- Ability to determine variables causing specific interpersonal problems and subsequent outcomes.

Care Planning
- Ability to develop or revise a nursing care plan for a specific patient based on a primary and secondary data base.
- Ability to develop a discharge plan to manage actual and potential health risks for a specific patient.

From Del Bueno, D., Weeks, L., & Brown-Stewart, P. (1987). Clinical assessment centers. *Nursing Economic$*, *5*(1), 24. With permission of Janetti Publications, Inc.

them during their hospitalization. A review of this information may be rich with examples of staff empathy and concern and information regarding the overall ability of staff to assist patients and families through their health care experience. This may be used to deem an employee or a group of employees competent in specific interpersonal competencies.

Although the above information may provide guidance for assessing specific competencies, it assumes that any given competency discretely measures technical skills, interpersonal skills, or critical thinking skills. However, as noted previously, it is the integration of all three that is important. Therefore, measurement approaches that assess this integration are far more effective than those that do not.

Consider this situation. Most organizations assess the competence of clinical practitioners regarding CPR. They focus on the technical skills of resuscitation and deem staff competent to perform this skill with an effective return demonstration. However, this approach merely measures the ability to do process steps of resuscitation. It does not measure the critical thinking ability that precedes an event, nor the analysis and processing that follow an arrest. It certainly does not demonstrate the elements of teamwork and interpersonal skills that are essential during a critical situation. A far more effective means to assess staff competence is to observe practice, debrief after the event, and analyze the effectiveness of the team. This approach provides a wealth of information regarding technical, interpersonal, and critical thinking skills of physicians, nurses, and cardiopulmonary staff. It measures what happened in actual practice, something that can never be simulated in its entirety in a skills laboratory. It measures something dramatically different than what happens when staff are asked to demonstrate the technical process steps of resuscitation: it measures the ability to make decisions based on the presenting information of the patient and it shows how staff work effectively as a team members during critical events.

PHASE III: ASSESSING COMPETENCE IN PRACTICE

A common error in competence models is to assume that competencies can be assessed in predetermined time slots, such as defined calendar months of the year. This assumes that CA can mirror the process of annual retraining. Although this may appear to be a logical way to organize a mammoth effort, it does little to meet the real intent of CA. After all, CA at its best is a developmental process. At its worst, it is a process of herding staff through predetermined skills stations. If all the steps in phases one and two have been carefully and deliberately followed, the actual assessment of competence becomes an ongoing process within practice settings.

In the beginning, the assessment of competencies will probably require assistance from members of the oversight group or other expert staff. Area managers generally struggle with the concept, wanting to hurry the process "so we can just get back to running the unit." However, after reminding them of the purpose and intended results of CA, they can become very active proponents. Managers first need to see the relevance to practice and tangible signs of its ability to advance performance. After that, they willingly offer suggestions regarding new competencies and how performance can be improved to match the strategic directions.

During this implementation phase, the work of the oversight group changes from model designers to champions for change. Group members are likely to be called on to consult in areas that are having problems and to help some understand the intent and purpose of CA—in other words, why the model was designed the way it was. Many questions will arise from staff. Some may say, "After all these years, why do I have to suddenly prove I'm competent? Just look at my performance appraisal. This is just one more thing to take me away from my patients. I can't get everything done as it is!" The oversight group must play a critical role in ensuring a common understanding and shared meaning about CA. Group members must be champions of and teachers about the concept and process to ensure ultimate success.

Finally, when the fundamental learning has occurred and there is evidence of CA at work in practice settings, the oversight group has an opportunity to reflect on the model design and can construct a description of the current operating practice. This is necessary so that the Joint Commission on Accreditation of Healthcare Organizations (JCAHO) and other accrediting bodies can measure the organization's ability to perform according to standards and internal expectations for CA. It is customary to use policies and procedures to describe the approach. However, a few organizations have seen the merit of using a narrative to describe their model. Narratives tend to be more descriptive and conducive to defining the operating philosophy and critical elements of competence model design. Either method is acceptable to the JCAHO. What is most important is that it describe the organization's model for CA so that it can be understood and evaluated for effectiveness. An example of a descriptive narrative, released with permission of the UMHC, is provided as Appendix B.

PHASE IV: INTEGRATING COMPETENCIES INTO PRACTICE

By now it should be obvious that effective integration of competencies into the practice environment is an evolutionary process. It is full of bumps and bruises along the way, but these are the natural by-products of any organizational change initiative. The absence of these growing pains may be the first symptom of a weak model and questionable process. But as experience is gained, evidence suddenly appears that justifies all the effort and begins to stimulate the excitement that comes with positive change.

A few brief success stories follow. They are not given in complete detail, but they demonstrate the potential of a well-conceived model and process. These stories have come from anecdotal comments of managers across a variety of practice settings.

1. The leadership staff of a patient care unit identified that nursing documentation in the medical record was substandard. A review of several records showed that the "story" of the patient was not consistently being told. The records were complete regarding documentation of physical care and nursing interventions, but many lacked evidence of discharge planning and patient teaching. In discussion with the primary nurses, it was learned they had followed through on their defined accountabilities but were inconsistent in reflecting this in the chart. A competency regarding documentation was generated, and staff were required to submit written evidence to the nurse manager and clinical nurse specialist to meet this competency. If the documentation was substandard, as identified by the practice guidelines, it was returned. Until sufficient evidence was presented on a consistent basis, staff were not deemed competent in this aspect of practice. Within 6 months, a marked improvement in documentation was evident through unit-based quality monitoring.

2. Aggregate results from patient satisfaction surveys showed that pain management was rated by patients as less than desirable. A critical competency was developed for nursing staff on all practice settings that read, "Demonstrates effective pain management and comfort interventions in daily practice." Many different learning opportunities were offered to improve nurses' knowledge and skill regarding pain management, and each practice setting was then asked to develop the appropriate tools to measure staff competence based on the patient population it served. A medical/surgical oncology unit chose a case study approach using actual unit-based scenarios. Nurses were asked to review the cases and to respond how they would manage each patient's pain. At the conclusion of the process, the nurse manager commented, "I used to think competency assessment was just more paperwork, but not anymore. It was obvious by the documentation staff submitted that they really didn't know effective pain management! We were able to put a developmental plan in place to increase staff knowledge and skill in this area. We raised the overall competence of staff in pain management, and patient satisfaction data improved."

3. In a pediatric area, an increasing number of patients were being seen with latex allergies. Staff identified their lack of knowledge in this area and agreed that a competency was needed to help improve practice. One staff member volunteered to create a learning module, which she dubbed "Latex Learning Lore." It was such an effective educational approach that staff quickly learned how to handle patients with latex allergies and could subsequently demonstrate the relevant competency in their practice. The learning tool has since been made available to other areas of the hospital. This high-risk safety issue is being appropriately

managed with the integration of education, CA, and quality monitoring through the nursing practice committee.

4. It was customary for laboratory staff of a large hospital to have their competence reviewed by means of the quality improvement collection processes they had established in the past. But for 1996, they decided they would use a different approach. They began using a peer review process and found themselves unprepared for the surprising results. Staff were more open and honest than they had ever been and provided effective feedback regarding each other's competence. This process created secondary benefits: staff learned what their barriers to effective work and job satisfaction were and how their work could be enhanced to create a more effective work environment, and they identified specific process improvements in work flow. Staff considered peer review to be an excellent idea that should be continued as part of their CA process.

5. An organization with several labor unions noted increased concern on the part of labor leaders when a CA process was initiated. Noting this discontent, the woman assigned accountability for the organizational CA process began meeting with the union leaders. She knew that the key to gaining their commitment was to hear their concerns and try to develop a mutually agreeable approach to the matter. During one discussion, it became apparent that an issue identified by one labor unit regarding CA was not the same as that identified by two other labor units, and a fourth labor unit had no concerns at all. As she listened to the comments, she noted several misperceptions about the CA model. There was also a primary concern regarding the use of peer review as a method to verify competence; labor leaders considered this to violate existing contracts regarding supervisors' responsibility to review performance. The woman assigned accountability for CA used this as an opportunity to increase their knowledge regarding the purpose and intent of CA and to address their primary concerns. By the end of a few meetings, she was able to advance their understanding and support of the concept. They worked together to develop an action plan and agreed that the unionized staff were not yet ready to use peer review as an assessment method; other approaches were selected to verify staff competence.

6. A state department of health received a complaint regarding the care delivered to a male patient admitted on a psychiatry unit. Immediately thereafter, the Health Facilities Complaint Office conducted an unannounced survey that included review of the patient's medical record, the patient care unit operations, personnel files of all involved staff, and the quality management program reports. Fortunately, no evidence was found to substantiate the claim, but during the survey process the reviewers commented that the personnel records were quite current and that the unit-specific critical competencies identified to ensure quality care were excellent.

7. The leadership staff of a large critical care area found it increasingly difficult to keep up with performance appraisals, CA, and annual retraining expectations for its 100-plus employees. After considering many approaches, a pilot program was initiated. Staff were divided into two groups (fall and spring) and assigned a day to try to capture all the above expectations. On the identified day, staff were to bring evidence that supported their achievement of competencies for the year, as well as feedback to be shared during a peer review process. The day was organized so that staff would be able to pass through various skills stations and learning modules to meet their annual retraining requirements, meet one-on-one with their manager to review evidence of their competency achievement and performance appraisal, and meet in small groups for peer review. The pilot project was such an overwhelming success that staff did not want to leave. They

had been allowed to dress in their street clothes and really appreciated spending the day in a relaxed but rewarding process of interfacing with their manager and colleagues. Staff who had not been part of the pilot process heard such wonderful comments that they asked to speed up the time line so they could benefit as well!

PHASE V: EVALUATING AND IMPROVING COMPETENCE ASSESSMENT

The last phase of CA is evaluation. As with other steps, it is a critical but often overlooked step. Most people just assume that the only work to be done is to record compliance data for JCAHO purposes and to report this information to the governing board, but this is clearly not true. As with other major initiatives, the CA process and model must be reviewed on an ongoing basis to determine its effectiveness and any opportunities for improvement.

An annual evaluation of the CA model and process is recommended to identify—simply speaking—what works, what doesn't, why it doesn't, and how it can be improved. This evaluation may take a very formal approach through survey methodology and interviews or a less formal approach, such as asking for subjective data and feedback from key people and groups. In any case, four evaluation steps are recommended.

First, quantitative data must be gathered and analyzed. The JCAHO expects that an annual report will be given to the governing body (JCAHO, 1996). At a minimum, this report should reflect the number of staff employed, the number of staff whose competence was assessed, and of those the percentage of staff deemed competent to perform in their roles. It is helpful if the report also includes any findings from the analysis of data, any reference to benchmarking data if available, and any plans to improve the overall competence of staff. An executive summary or brief narrative can help the governing board understand the purpose and desired outcomes of CA. This summary might highlight the intent of CA, any unusual findings in the data, how the overall staff competence rate compares with that of other organizations, how competencies were identified for the past year, any improvements in the CA model planned for the coming year, and what competencies have been identified for the next year and why.

Second, a qualitative approach should be used to gather subjective data regarding how well the current CA process worked for persons and groups, and any suggestions for improvement. This need not be extravagant. A broad organizational perspective can easily be determined with a short interview of department managers or delegates. Three simple questions can provide a wealth of information: "What worked about this year's CA process? What got in the way? What competencies should be advanced for next year?"

Third, a more focused review of how the CA model really worked in practice should be considered. A "biopsy" can be done by randomly selecting employees from various work settings, reviewing the documentation regarding their competency achievement, and asking the employee to describe how the specific competencies were established and measured in the work setting and what his or her feelings were regarding the process. It is usually an enlightening process! It is not uncommon to hear staff say, "I couldn't believe I had to prove my competence after all these years" or "I'm so happy we're moving away from an emphasis on technical skills. That never made a good nurse." These qualitative data can prove invaluable in validating efforts or identifying opportunities for further learning and development.

Finally, after the above steps have been taken, the fundamental beliefs and operating assumptions of the competence model should be reviewed for any needed changes. This is a good job for the oversight group because it is not uncommon to identify a need to

(text continues on page 142)

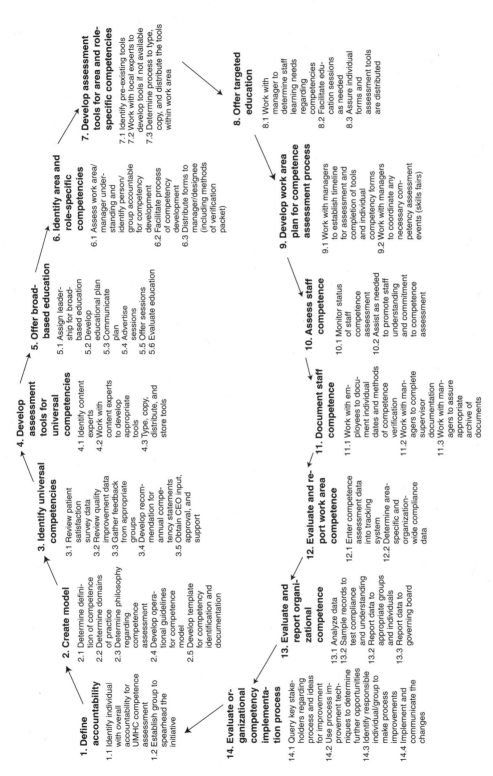

1. Define accountability

1.1 Identify individual with overall accountability for UMHC competence assessment

1.2 Establish group to spearhead the initiative

2. Create model

2.1 Determine definition of competence

2.2 Determine domains of practice

2.3 Determine philosophy regarding competence assessment

2.4 Develop operational guidelines for competence model

2.5 Develop template for competency identification and documentation

3. Identify universal competencies

3.1 Review patient satisfaction survey data

3.2 Review quality improvement data

3.3 Gather feedback from appropriate groups

3.4 Develop recommendation for annual competency statements

3.5 Obtain CEO input, approval, and support

4. Develop assessment tools for universal competencies

4.1 Identify content experts

4.2 Work with content experts to develop appropriate tools

4.3 Type, copy, distribute, and store tools

5. Offer broad-based education

5.1 Assign leadership for broad-based education

5.2 Develop educational plan

5.3 Communicate plan

5.4 Advertise sessions

5.5 Offer sessions

5.6 Evaluate education

6. Identify area and role-specific competencies

6.1 Assess work area/manager understanding and identify person/group accountable for competency development

6.2 Facilitate process of competency development

6.3 Distribute forms to manager/designee (including methods of verification packet)

7. Develop assessment tools for area and role-specific competencies

7.1 Identify pre-existing tools

7.2 Work with local experts to develop tools if not available

7.3 Determine process to type, copy, and distribute the tools within work area

8. Offer targeted education

8.1 Work with manager to determine staff learning needs regarding competencies

8.2 Facilitate education sessions as needed

8.3 Assure individual forms and assessment tools are distributed

9. Develop work area plan for competency assessment process

9.1 Work with managers to establish timeline for assessment and completion of tools and individual competency forms

9.2 Work with managers to coordinate any necessary competency assessment events (skills fairs)

10. Assess staff competence

10.1 Monitor status of staff competence assessment

10.2 Assist as needed to promote staff understanding and commitment to competence assessment

11. Document staff competence

11.1 Work with employees to document individual dates and methods of competence verification

11.2 Work with managers to complete supervisor documentation

11.3 Work with managers to assure appropriate archive of documents

12. Evaluate and report work area competence

12.1 Enter competence assessment data into tracking system

12.2 Determine area-specific and organization-wide compliance data

13. Evaluate and report organizational competence

13.1 Analyze data

13.2 Sample records to test compliance and understanding

13.3 Report data to appropriate groups and individuals

13.3 Report data to governing board

14. Evaluate organizational competency implementation process

14.1 Query key stakeholders regarding process and ideas for improvement

14.2 Use process improvement techniques to determine further opportunities for improvement

14.3 Identify responsible individual/group to make process improvements

14.4 Implement and communicate the changes

FIGURE 6-2. UMHC organizational learning team competency assessment planning process 1995–96.
© 1996. Reprinted with permission. University of Minnesota Hospital & Clinic.

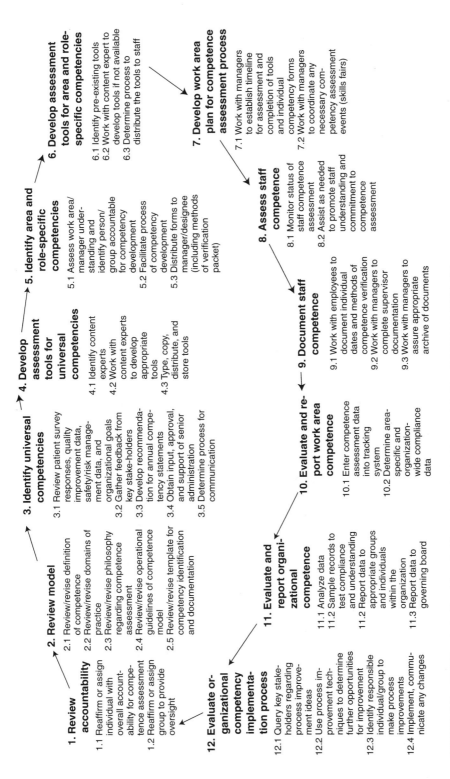

1. **Review accountability**
   1.1 Reaffirm or assign individual with overall accountability for competence assessment
   1.2 Reaffirm or assign group to provide oversight

2. **Review model**
   2.1 Review/revise definition of competence
   2.2 Review/revise domains of practice
   2.3 Review/revise philosophy regarding competence assessment
   2.4 Review/revise operational guidelines of competence model
   2.5 Review/revise template for competency identification and documentation

3. **Identify universal competencies**
   3.1 Review patient survey responses, quality improvement data, safety/risk management data, and organizational goals
   3.2 Gather feedback from key stake-holders
   3.3 Develop recommendation for annual competency statements
   3.4 Obtain input, approval, and support of senior administration
   3.5 Determine process for communication

4. **Develop assessment tools for universal competencies**
   4.1 Identify content experts
   4.2 Work with content experts to develop appropriate tools
   4.3 Type, copy, distribute, and store tools

5. **Identify area and role-specific competencies**
   5.1 Assess work area/manager understanding and identify person/group accountable for competency development
   5.2 Facilitate process of competency development
   5.3 Distribute forms to manager/designee (including methods of verification packet)

6. **Develop assessment tools for area and role-specific competencies**
   6.1 Identify pre-existing tools
   6.2 Work with content expert to develop tools if not available
   6.3 Determine process to distribute the tools to staff

7. **Develop work area plan for competence assessment process**
   7.1 Work with managers to establish timeline for assessment and completion of tools and individual competency forms
   7.2 Work with managers to coordinate any necessary competency assessment events (skills fairs)

8. **Assess staff competence**
   8.1 Monitor status of staff competence assessment
   8.2 Assist as needed to promote staff understanding and commitment to competence assessment

9. **Document staff competence**
   9.1 Work with employees to document individual dates and methods of competence verification
   9.2 Work with managers to complete supervisor documentation
   9.3 Work with managers to assure appropriate archive of documents

10. **Evaluate and report work area competence**
    10.1 Enter competence assessment data into tracking system
    10.2 Determine area-specific and organization-wide compliance data

11. **Evaluate and report organizational competence**
    11.1 Analyze data
    11.2 Sample records to test compliance and understanding
    11.2 Report data to appropriate groups and individuals within the organization
    11.3 Report data to governing board

12. **Evaluate organizational competency implementation process**
    12.1 Query key stakeholders regarding process improvement ideas
    12.2 Use process improvement techniques to determine further opportunities for improvement
    12.3 Identify responsible individual/group to make process improvements
    12.4 Implement, communicate any changes

FIGURE 6-3. UMHC organizational learning team competency assessment planning process 1996–97.
© 1996. Reprinted with permission. University of Minnesota Hospital & Clinic.

modify the philosophy or add operational guidelines. At this point, it is always helpful to ask a pointed question regarding why the organization is bothering with CA: "Does the CA model actually improve practice, and how do you know?" or, more specifically, "What difference is being made because of CA?" If the answers to these questions are limited, major improvements are likely to be needed in the model design and process. If the answers are more significant, the organization is well on its way to a model for staff and organizational development within a dynamic health care environment. In this case, only minor process improvements may be warranted.

During an evaluation process such as that identified above, the UMHC decided to capture the process steps associated with the design and delivery of their CA system. The CA group members chose a top-down flow chart to record the major process steps and activities associated with their model so that they could better look at opportunities for improvement (Fig. 6-2). By so doing, they determined the process steps that could be improved and also discovered the magnitude of what they were trying to accomplish. It was rewarding to look back and see all that had been put in place.

After discussion, the oversight group at UMHC quickly identified opportunities for process improvement for the next year. They began this work and modified their process flow chart accordingly (Fig. 6-3). They learned that their work would never end; there would always be room for improvement.

SUMMARY

From the information presented in this chapter, it should be apparent that creating a model for CA is no small task. When done correctly, it is comparable to any major organizational change initiative. As such, it requires very deliberate and thoughtful processing, design, and implementation and continuous evaluation and modification to ensure that the intended results are consistently achieved.

Across the country, organizations in and out of health care have begun to use competency-based approaches to improve employee and organizational performance. Although it is premature to tell just how effective competency models really are, the overall reaction to the effectiveness of competencies is "largely positive" (American Compensation Association, 1996, p. 8).

For those at the beginning stages of CA planning, it may be helpful to know that there are many lessons that have been learned by others. A review of these lessons (American Compensation Association, 1996) may provide the necessary insight to keep the vision of CA clear and reachable:

- Get senior management support to ensure the high-level buy-in that is critical to CA success.
- Take a systematic approach that includes careful planning and focuses on making a strategic connection between competencies and business objectives.
- Conduct more training to ensure a broad understanding of CA for both managers and employees.
- Improve communication about the identified competencies, why they are being implemented, and what must be done to succeed within the competence model.
- Establish clearer definitions so that employees see the link between competencies and their individual performance.
- Obtain employee buy-in by using as broad a participation in the design process as possible.

When all is said and done, CA should be the tool that drives staff and organizational performance. How close are you coming?

Competence Assessment and Development at Work in the Army

GRAHAM G. WILSON

Before moving to the United States, I was in the British Army. As training officer for a battalion (1,000 personnel), I was tasked to lead a 3-week intensive First-Aid Instructor's Course. This course would provide a nationally recognized civilian qualification (St. John's Ambulance—similar to the American Red Cross).

As a proponent of competency-based (mastery) learning, I was determined to see all 35 students successfully complete the course. Also, I wanted the training activities to expose the potential instructors to competency-based training. I defined competence assessment and development as organized learning over a specific period of time to improve performance.

My first task was to identify essential student prerequisites, and I broke these down into three areas:

1. What the students need on the job
2. What I will give them in the training program
3. What they must bring with them.

As the course content had already been established by the St. John's Ambulance and the Army Medical Services, my next task was to establish the course prerequisites for all students. These included:

- Senior Non-Commissioned Officer (SNCO) status
- completion of the Presentation Skills Course (3 weeks)
- completion of the Basic and Intermediate First Aid Courses (3 weeks each).

Next, because the terminal objectives had been set for me by the standards of the St. John's Ambulance, I had to design and try out performance and written tests and lesson plans.

I believe that assessment plays a crucial role in the competency-based approach to training. Four of the most important uses of competence assessment tests include:

1. diagnosing entry-level competencies
2. providing immediate feedback to students

3. assessing students' mastery of each task
4. evaluating the effectiveness of training materials.

After I had designed the assessment tests and put the learning packages together, the course could commence. The students—who were all straight-A students—were introduced immediately to mastery learning and were stunned to hear that neither traditional teaching methods nor traditional grades would be used. The only grades would be Pass or Fail, although I hoped there would be no failures. Requiring each student to demonstrate mastery of each task before moving on to the next task is perhaps the single most significant difference between competency-based training and the more traditional approach to training. This method also increases the students' chance of success.

As each student progressed at varying speeds, the three instructors who were providing the training with me experienced increased stress. No longer were they allowed to simply lecture and leave the learning up to the student. Now they were also responsible for ensuring the success of each student; they had to become actively involved with each student.

After a few days, the students divided themselves into self-directed study teams, with the more able students assisting those who were having difficulty. After an initial degree of resistance, the students began to see the value of mastery learning, and soon the lights in the study rooms were burning late into the night.

The course continued and the students progressed, at different paces, to mastery level. However, in order to satisfy the Medical Services criteria, final written and skill tests were administered, and—yes—everyone passed.

Initially the students' reaction to the training was skeptical, because they were accustomed to the traditional structured training methods of the military. It took course participants some time to realize that a norm-referenced approach is inappropriate in competency-based training. Norm-referenced reporting does not really reflect whether or not each individual student is competent in a task at some predetermined minimum level of competence.

Most learners found themselves working much harder than they anticipated (the instructors did too). Because I employed the students as coaches and aides to each other, the experience was richer for all involved. The course reinforced my belief in competency-based learning. Incidentally, I became a convert when, as an instructor at a tank-gunnery school, the pass rate on the "Enemy Tank Recognition Test" was 85%. My Commanding Officer asked me if I would like to be sitting in one of the 15% of tanks mis-recognized. As you may imagine, the pass level elevated quickly to 100%.

I believe strongly that if the prerequisites are appropriate, given enough time (within reason) and enough training, all students will achieve mastery learning. However, as a reality, I acknowledge that often this is quite impractical—but there is always hope...

REFERENCES

Alspach, J. G. (1984). Designing a competency-based orientation for critical care nurses. *Heart & Lung, 13*(6), 655–662.

American Compensation Association. (1996). *Raising the bar: Using competencies to enhance employee performance*. Scottsdale, AZ: Author.

Benner, P. (1982). Issues in competency-based testing. *Nursing Outlook, 30*(5), 303–309.

Buszta, C., Steward, P., & Chapin, J. (1993). Developing core competencies for medical/surgical nursing. *Journal of Nursing Staff Development, 9*(5), 236–239.

Castleforte, M. R., & Dunlap, M. (1995). Clinical rounds: A measure of competence. *Journal of Nursing Staff Development, 11*(6), 321–322.

Crow, C. S., & Ezell, H. F. (1996). Developing management skills: An experiential exercise. *Journal of Nursing Staff Development, 12*(3), 155–158.

Del Bueno, D. J. (1990). Evaluation: Myths, mystiques, and obsessions. *Journal of Nursing Administration, 20*(11), 4–7.

Del Bueno, D., Weeks, L., & Brown-Stewart, P. (1987). Clinical assessment centers: A cost-effective alternative for competency development. *Nursing Economic$, 5*(1), 21–26.

Ebel, R. L. (1981). Issues in testing for competency. *Measurement Education, 12*(2).

Edwards, M. R., & Ewen, A. J. (1996). 360° feedback: The powerful new model for employee assessment and performance improvement. New York: AMACOM.

Farrell, J. P., & Robbins, M. M. (1993, July/Aug). Leadership competencies for physicians. *Healthcare Forum Journal*, pp. 39–41.

Gurvis, J. P., & Grey, M. T. (1995). The anatomy of a competency. *Journal of Nursing Staff Development, 11*(5), 247–252.

Jeska, S. (1996). Applying leadership competencies for nurse executives. In Disch, J. (Ed.). *The managed care challenge for nurse executives*, pp. 55–61. Chicago: American Hospital Publishing, Inc.

Jeska, S. B. (1994). Luminous leadership: A qualitative study of nursing administration practice (Doctoral dissertation, University of St. Thomas). *Dissertation Abstracts International, 55*(9):9503514.

Jeska, S., Anderson, L., & Bach, M. (1995). *Blueprint for competence: The University of Minnesota Model*. Pensacola, FL: National Nursing Staff Development Organization.

Joint Commission on Accreditation of Healthcare Organizations. (1996). *Comprehensive accreditation manual for hospitals: The official handbook*. Oakbrook Terrace, IL: Author.

McGregor, R. J. (1990). Advancing staff nurse competencies: From novice to expert. *Journal of Nursing Staff Development, 6*(6), 287–290.

Parry, S. B. (1996, July). The quest for competencies. *Training*, pp. 48–56.

Pollock, M. B. (1981, Jan/Feb). Speaking of competencies. *Health Education*, pp. 9–13.

Scott, B. (1982). Competency-based learning: A literature review. *International Journal of Nursing Studies, 19*(3), 119–124.

7

Managing the Mandatories: Back to Basics

REBECCA KATZ

This chapter addresses the concept of mandatory training and the unwritten purpose of mandatory training, discusses competence with mandatories, and offers suggestions about realistic ways to manage mandatories. Throughout the chapter, there are diagrams, tables, and samples of policies and procedures to augment the written text.

WHAT ARE MANDATORIES?

"Mandatory" is a word bandied about by many in the health care arena. Often, in an effort to satisfy mandates from the Joint Commission on Accreditation of Healthcare Organizations (JCAHO), educators and managers implement fragments of a competency program without fully understanding its potential. They may not realize that mandatories provide an opportunity for staff to demonstrate basic competencies.

On hearing the term "mandatory education," many educators envision JCAHO and Occupational Safety and Health Administration (OSHA) requirements such as fire and safety, utility outage, and bloodborne pathogen education, to name just a few. Definitions for mandatories abound, but it is more difficult to translate this information into reasonable programs for everyday practice.

However, mandatories are not always related to a regulatory body that requires the organization to do something. In fact, it is a good idea for the educator to question the directive, "this is mandatory" or "this agency says we must do this." Request a copy of the standards. A standard can be interpreted many different ways. For example, there can be several interpretations of OSHA fire and safety standards in the same institution. One person can interpret this standard to mean that everyone in the system must pass a test; another may construe this standard to mean that only persons providing patient care need to meet the standard. The regulatory agencies offer consultative services for help in interpreting the standards, but they do not prescribe a process for meeting the standard.

It will be helpful to reiterate four key terms used here and throughout the text: standards, competence, competency, and competency assessment.

> **STANDARDS** "Authoritative statements, promulgated by the profession, by which the quality of practice, service, or education can be judged" (ANA, 1994, p. 14)
>
> **COMPETENCE** A person's or group's capacity to perform job functions. Competence is concerned with whether or not the person has the required knowledge, skills, behaviors, and personal characteristics necessary to function well in a given situation. The word "competence" is often applied to the overall capacity of people and groups to perform global behaviors and activities, such as "provides care to oncology inpatients."

COMPETENCY A person's actual performance in a particular situation. It describes how well a person demonstrates his or her knowledge, attitudes, skills, and behaviors according to expectations for specific situations. Competency focuses on the person's ability to put knowledge to work. Within the workplace, knowledge is expected; however, there may be people who have the knowledge but cannot do the job.

COMPETENCE ASSESSMENT An organized staff development activity that systematically ascertains if the person actually has the knowledge and skills and can put them into action. Just as we assess patients, plan for their care, and then evaluate their care, competence assessment allows the educator to assess the knowledge and skills of employees. These assessments provide baseline data about knowledge and skills before implementing patient- and family-centered care models or new clinical skills or procedures. Many managers assume that the institution's current evaluation process will assess these competencies, but often the system is not set up to provide adequate data to conduct an adequate evaluation. Staff development specialists and managers work together to develop relevant competence assessment activities based on the populations served and the scope of services provided. Staff development specialists and managers also work together to conduct these activities as they plan the overall staff development program for the specified unit or service. Unit or department competence assessment activities help people and teams identify opportunities for learning.

COMPETENCIES A new word developed through popular use; the identified essential skills considered necessary to perform a specific job.

A summary of definitions is found in Chapter 4, Table 4-1. These definitions are the guiding operations for the competency framework in Figure 7-1. A corresponding institution-wide policy and procedure is found in Display 7-1. The diagram identifies core hospital-wide competencies specified by regulatory agencies or strategic initiatives ("mandatory competencies") as one dimension of competency needed in an ongoing program of competence assessment.

Mandatories, for purposes of this discussion, refer to the organized and systematic competence assessment activities usually identified by the organization to illustrate the competence of groups and persons to the public and selected regulatory and accrediting bodies. Data are aggregated to reflect the overall capacity of the organization to perform the identified skills. The educator is assessing the competence of mandatory or essential job skills of employees, contract workers, volunteers, or anyone the organization deems must demonstrate a skill to ensure safe, quality patient care.

When referring to demonstrable skills, an institution must meet all regulatory agency requirements. Other sources must also be reviewed to ensure that employees are competent in providing safe care. In the next section, various sources of standards will be reviewed. Mandatory competencies usually make no distinction between the new and the experienced employee. The literature is replete with references about developing competency programs for both the new employee and the experienced one.

WHO SAYS THEY'RE MANDATORY?

The regulatory agencies that fuel mandatory education include, but are not limited to, JCAHO, OSHA, and state health departments. The Clinical Laboratory Information Act of 1987 and the Health Care Financing Agency have also set forth required competencies

Grant/Riverside Methodist Hospitals
Organization-Wide Framework for Competency Assessment

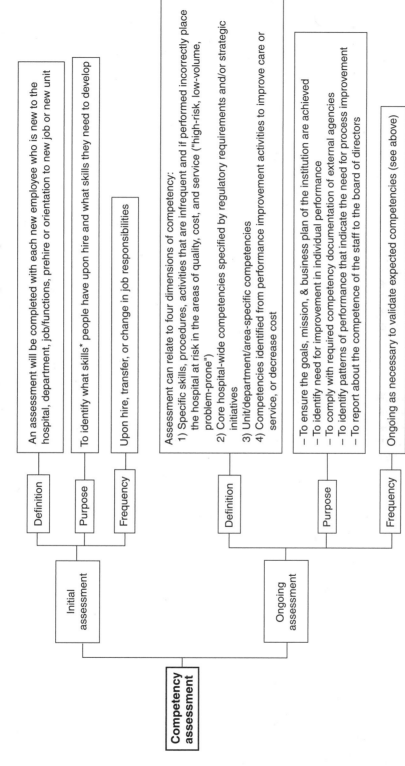

* "Skills" may include process (*e.g.*, critical thinking, interpersonal) and technical skills

Final - Adopted by G/RMH Competency Assessment Group 5/10/96

FIGURE 7-1. Organization-wide framework for competency assessment.

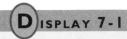

Institution-Wide Policy and Procedure, Competency Assessment

Grant/Riverside Methodist Hospitals
Columbus, Ohio
Standard Policy and/or Procedures

Date Effective: August 6, 1996
Title: COMPETENCY ASSESSMENT
Distribution: All SPP Policy Holders
Approval: Office of the President

Purpose:

To establish a process that will:

- ensure that the goals, mission, and business plan of the institution are achieved
- identify need for improvement in individual performance
- comply with required competency documentation of external agencies
- identify patterns of performance that indicate the need for process improvement
- report about the competence of the staff to the Board of Directors

Policy

Department leaders provide staff with appropriate authority and responsibility to perform their work processes, to have a sense of ownership of work, and to be held accountable for their performance. In addition, department leaders support and encourage staff to continuously improve their performance, thereby improving the organization's performance.

Hospital leaders are responsible for defining the competencies needed for the provision of patient care and other organizational processes. Through recruitment, retention, retraining, and other activities, the hospital department leaders ensure that the appropriate number of qualified staff are available to carry out the individual and collective responsibilities in service to the hospital's mission.

An assessment will be completed with each new employee who is new to the hospital, department, or job/functions, prehire or as part of orientation to new job or new unit. The attached flowchart visually presents the organization's framework for competency assessment.

The Education staff or designated persons will assess competency after training to validate that an employee can perform the process and/or skill. Skills may include process (*e.g.*, critical thinking, interpersonal) and technical skills. Staff development needs are addressed on the organizational, departmental, and individual levels, and such needs are used in planning continuing staff education activities.

Definitions

Competence is defined as an individual's **capacity** to perform his or her job functions. Competence is concerned with whether or not the individual possesses the knowledge, skills, and attitudes required to function at the level expected in specific role/job category.

Competency, on the other hand, is defined as an individual's **actual performance** in a particular situation. It describes how well an individual demonstrates his or her knowledge, skills, attitudes, and behaviors in accordance with expectations. Competency focuses on the individual's ability to use knowledge and skills on the job.

Competencies are the identified **essential knowledge and skills (technical and process)** and other characteristics such as critical thinking that are considered necessary to the performance in a specific role/job/category.

Competency assessment is the process of identifying and validating a person's ability to perform as expected. *High-risk* refers to a process or skill that if not correctly performed affects the hospital's quality, cost, or service. *Low-volume* refers to a process or skill that is not done frequently enough to be observed by a peer or customer, and, therefore, competency or demonstrated performance is not known. *Problem-prone* relates to a process or skill that, by virtue of the number of steps or difficulty, is inclined to mistakes.

DISPLAY 7-1 (Continued)

Procedures to Implement Policy

A. INITIAL ASSESSMENT

Each job incumbent needs to have an orientation to the specific job. To plan the orientation and build on the knowledge/skills that the new employee brings to the job, a *competency assessment* is conducted prehire and/or upon hire. The initial competency assessment is not performed again if the employee remains on the hiring unit, unless the employee changes job titles or transfers to another unit/area.

All prehire, orientation, or focused assessments are performed by the staff development instructors or by a department-identified trainer.

B. ONGOING ASSESSMENT

Each unit/department identifies skills that are considered high-risk, low-volume, and problem-prone.

Ongoing competency assessments are performed at least annually. These competency assessments can be done at any time during the course of the year, or more frequently, as designated in the clinical area.

If a change in the level of an employee's performance is noted, a focused assessment of competence may be requested.

C. FOCUSED ASSESSMENT

Competence needs to be validated for the individual(s) who has demonstrated inconsistent performance or who has been involved in a critical incident. Knowledge and skills related to his/her job functions are explicitly assessed. Outcome of the assessment is correlated with the individual's performance and serves to focus a work improvement plan.

---

and require evidence of training or assessment. These organizations and their regulations or guidelines provide numerous standards and recommendations that discuss the types of behaviors needed to:

- Manage patients in high-risk environments
- Manage patients of various ages and developmental stages
- Manage bloodborne pathogens
- Implement emergency and fire prevention plans
- Initiate CPR
- Prevent workplace hazards and communicate hazardous situations
- Implement action plans in the event of hazardous situations
- Use identified training for care of patients in special settings such as long-term care, maternal care, and psychiatry.

These standards, guidelines, or recommendations often define the intent of training but leave the process of the training up to the institution. It is the responsibility of the professional staff of the health care organization to define to whom each standard applies, how to implement it, and how to maintain it.

Professional organizations also provide standards and guidelines that address expected competencies for care providers. The following are but a few of the professional associations and societies that promulgate standards and guidelines for health care providers:

- American Heart Association
- ANA
- American Physical Therapy Association
- American Association of Critical Care Nurses

- Licensed Practical Nurses Association
- American Occupational Therapy Association
- American Association of Neuroscience Nurses
- Association of Women's Health, Obstetric and Neonatal Nurses.

It is productive for the novice staff development specialist to ask health care providers about their associations and societies. A wealth of information about standards, guidelines, and competence is available from many of them. In addition, many of the clinical nursing specialty organizations are members of the Nursing Organization Liaison Forum, an organization of associations sponsored by the ANA that discusses common issues across specialties. The American Hospital Association serves a similar purpose for issues and workers in hospital settings.

A SAMPLING OF STANDARDS

The following standards illustrate the vagueness of many standards. Clear, precise informa-tion is not always available from the regulatory agencies, but most regulatory and accredit-ing bodies have staff who can answer questions and interpret standards. The novice staff development specialist will find these citations useful to understand why the processes for compliance vary from institution to institution.

OSHA standard 29 CFR, 1910.38, Employee Emergency Plans and Fire Prevention Plans, states:

(5). "Training."

(i) Before implementing the emergency action plan, the employer shall designate and train a sufficient number of persons to assist in the safe and orderly emergency evacuation of employees.

(ii) The employer shall review the plan with each employee covered by the plan at the following times:

(A) Initially when the plan is developed,

(B) Whenever the employee's responsibilities or designated actions under the plan change, and

(C) Whenever the plan is changed.

(iii) The employer shall review with each employee upon initial assignment those parts of the plan which the employer must know to protect the employee in the event of an emergency. The written plan shall be kept at the workplace and made available for employee review. For those employers with 10 or fewer employees the plan may be communicated orally to employees and the employer need not maintain a written plan.

OSHA expects the employer to define the type of training, to whom the standards apply, and the process for training.

Similar language is found in the OSHA regulations for hazard communication and bloodborne pathogen education. Standard 29 CFR 1910.1200 states:

(iii) Employers shall ensure that employees are provided with information and training in accordance with paragraph (h) of this section (except for the location and availability of the written hazard communication program under paragraph (h)(2)(iii) of this section), to the extent necessary to protect them in the event of a spill or leak of a hazardous chemical from a sealed container.

(h) "Employee information and training."

(1) Employers shall provide employees with effective information and training on hazardous chemicals in their work area at the time of their initial assignment, and whenever a new physical or health hazard the employees have not previously been trained about is introduced into their work area. Information and training may be designed to cover categories of hazards (e.g. flammability, carcinogenicity) or specific chemicals. Chemical-specific information must always be available through labels and material safety data sheets.

The standard further defines what the training should include.

Standard 29 CFR 1910.1030 refers to bloodborne pathogens; the parts of the standard referring to training are:

(2) Information and Training.

(i) Employers shall ensure that all employees with occupational exposure participate in a training program which must be provided at no cost to the employee and during working hours.

(ii) Training shall be provided as follows:

(A) At the time of initial assignment to tasks where occupational exposure may take place;

(B) Within 90 days after the effective date of the standard; and

(c) At least annually thereafter.

(iii) For employees who have received training on bloodborne pathogens in the year preceding the effective date of the standard, only training with respect to the provisions of the standard which were not included need to be provided.

(iv) Annual training for all employees shall be provided within one year of their previous training.

(v) Employers shall provide additional training when changes such as modification of tasks or procedures or institution of new tasks or procedures affect the employee's occupational exposure. The additional training may be limited to addressing the new exposures created.

This standard continues to define the minimum elements needed in a training program.

The Clinical Laboratory Information Act of 1987, as well as JCAHO (1996) defines "waived testing" as those tests performed at the bedside by patient care staff. One of the most common waived tests is for blood glucose. The organization must define which job titles can perform this test and the competence standards for them. In accordance with the previous definition, competency in the skills used at the bedside must be demonstrated in any laboratory testing such as blood glucose testing.

JCAHO's *Accreditation Manual for Hospitals* (1997) addresses what has become known as mandatory education in Chapter 6, "Management of Human Resources," and Chapter 7, "Management of the Environment of Care." Because JCAHO surveyors review employees' files for compliance with competence in safety management, security management, hazardous materials waste management, emergency preparedness management, life safety management, medical equipment management, and utility management programs, these programs have informally become known as "mandatory." The intent of the JCAHO standards is for all persons who have contact with patients to be knowledgeable about fire safety, for example, and to demonstrate competence in case of a fire. The educator responsible for the mandatory fire and safety education should work with the hospital's appointed safety officer to define competence. Competence in fire and safety involves more than answering knowledge questions on a test; the employee needs to demonstrate knowledge about what to do if a fire occurs or how to shut off an oxygen valve.

To help decide what global competence is related to job performance, such quality measures as the following can be used:

- High risk to patient or care provider
- Low volume of procedures by providers for patients
- Problem-prone issue or concerns related to volume or the system of care expressed by providers or patients.

Del Bueno (1993) said there were two opportunities to assess competence: at the beginning of employment and throughout employment. With the publication of the 1995 edition of the *Accreditation Manual for Hospitals*, JCAHO emphasized not only the assessment of competence but also the maintenance and improvement of competence on an ongoing basis. This standard indicates that competence should be assessed at periodic intervals, rather than just at the beginning of employment. Also, JCAHO emphasizes the "trending" of competence information, or the demonstration of data change over time. The intent of the standard is not to review numbers of employees who have attended a certain program, but to develop a program that identifies trends in competence. For example, if an initial problem is identified with staff in the quality of 12-lead EKG tracings, JCAHO would be interested not only in the program that was instituted to correct this problem, but also in the improvement and trend over time in changing the competence of the staff.

Thus, many organizations have implemented "mandatory" performance reviews or education days during which the staff perform, for example, a 12-lead EKG. Before setting up an education day or a series of mandatory stations, the educator should ask whether performing an EKG in the simulated environment, usually on a mannequin or in a classroom, really simulates the conditions of performing a 12-lead EKG on a patient who is diaphoretic or obese or has a hairy chest.

Standards for practice are found in the literature of many professional organizations, as noted above, and can be used to define components of basic competencies. Reference to those documents will strengthen the criteria used to assess competence. However, these standards do not define the competencies unique to an institution.

RETHINKING THE TERM

A better way of defining education and what should be mandatory is to think about what is necessary for any employee to demonstrate and meet the standards of the department. To define what regulatory agencies require and to review employee competencies requires a organized process and a systematic approach—a staff development strategy.

Another common myth is, "We have to do it annually." In many cases, but not all, the interval between training and reassessment of competency for those areas defined as mandatory is left up to the institution. As seen previously, however, OSHA defines blood-borne pathogen education as an annual requirement. Also, the conflicting standards of the regulatory agencies can be confusing. For example, for some standards OSHA requires education at the time of hire, but JCAHO may state annual education requirements. Because compliance by all employees is difficult to ensure, annual assessment of competencies identified by the organization as core or "central to the mission" has often been established in an effort to achieve a satisfactory figure of compliance, such as 70% or 80%. However, for the most part, the institution should decide how often mandatory competencies need to be reassessed. When developing a system to demonstrate compliance with mandatory training, the staff development specialist should bear in mind that if the institution states in a policy that the training should be completed annually, then the regulatory agency will expect compliance annually.

DETERMINING A FRAMEWORK
FOR ASSESSING MANDATORIES

There are many approaches to defining competencies. However, there are probably at least two times when competency should be measured: once during orientation and once during the course of the year to assess skills that are high-risk, low-volume, and problem-prone (Table 7-1) (JCAHO, 1997).

Unit: 9E/W

Indicator	Epidural Analgesia	12-Lead EKG	Peritoneal Dialysis	Identification Stage I, II, III, IV for Skin Staging	Identification Arterial/Venous Circulation	Phlebotomy	Orders in HBOC	ABG's Direct Sticks	Turbo Infuser
High risk	x	x	NA	x	NA	NA	x	NA	NA
Low volume	x	x	NA	x	NA	NA	x	NA	NA
Problem prone	x	x	NA	x	NA	NA	x	NA	NA

Unit: 8E/W

Indicator	Epidural Analgesia	12-Lead EKG	Peritoneal Dialysis	Identification Stage I, II, III, IV for Skin Staging	Identification Arterial/Venous Circulation	Phlebotomy	Orders in HBOC	ABG's Direct Sticks	Turbo Infuser
High risk	x	x	X	x	NA	NA	x	NA	NA
Low volume	x	x	X	x	NA	NA	x	NA	NA
Problem prone	x	x	X	x	NA	NA	x	NA	NA

Unit: 7W

Indicator	Epidural Analgesia	12-Lead EKG	Peritoneal Dialysis	Identification Stage I, II, III, IV for Skin Staging	Identification Arterial/Venous Circulation	Phlebotomy	Orders in HBOC	ABG's Direct Sticks	Turbo Infuser
High risk	x	x	NA	x	NA	x	x	x	NA
Low volume	x	x	NA	x	NA	x	x	x	NA
Problem prone	x	x	NA	x	NA	x	x	x	NA

Problem-prone refers to the complexity of the function or criteria; often it is not performed well. It could be a procedure for which some type of monitoring or quality check is already performed and problems have been identified. *High risk* usually relates to the potential for adverse outcomes to the patient. *Low volume* is critical because if a procedure is not performed frequently enough by the employee, competence will not be maintained. Let's review some examples of how a matrix can help the educator determine what education or competency is mandatory.

Table 7-2 shows an example of a grid developed for procedures by unit. This type of grid could be also developed for job titles on a particular unit or for departments. As illustrated, peritoneal dialysis is marked as being high-risk, problem-prone, and low-volume for only two units. Some units are marked "NA" because no patients requiring peritoneal dialysis are cared for on these units. It was determined that the RNs on these units have very little exposure to peritoneal dialysis during the year from which to maintain competence. However, it would be high risk to the patient if the RN did not know or demonstrate competence, because failure to be competent could result in an adverse outcome to the patient. Peritoneal dialysis is also marked as a low-volume procedure because only about 70 of 4,000 patients per year who require this procedure are admitted to the nursing units.

To determine the competencies that should be incorporated into the matrix, the educator should review not only the mandatories from regulatory agencies but also the data from quality improvement efforts, risk management programs, or stated needs from management staff. There may be identified areas where employee competence needs to be assessed. These areas could be added to the matrix. In the preceding example, peritoneal dialysis had originally been defined by physicians as a function requiring attention.

The specialist should solicit the assistance of staff and managers in developing grids of the basic and unit-based skills to assess for mandatory competencies. This process can be accomplished through committee or staff meetings. If staffing and budget do not support taking staff away from direct patient care, use staff meetings to educate. It is imperative to seek staff nurse input.

Several skills may be identified as high-risk, low-volume, or problem-prone. The educator should attempt to limit the number defined: remember, once these mandatories are defined, educational opportunities must be offered. Some points to remember about high-risk, low-volume, and problem-prone mandatories are:

- These competencies or mandatories are dynamic and can change as the job changes. For example, as an institution decentralizes phlebotomy, phlebotomy competency might be mandatory for employees on units where this skill is not performed frequently enough (low volume) to maintain competence. However, this phlebotomy competency might not be mandatory when blood draws are performed frequently (high volume), even though they are considered problem-prone and high-risk.
- An ongoing competency assessment can be performed at any time during the year. For some clinical areas, certain skill assessments may need to be more frequent. For example, if environmental service duties have been decentralized to a job class of service associates, the skills of buffing floors might need to be assessed on a monthly schedule until this new skill is learned.
- Competency needs to be assessed by someone who knows the skill or has the knowledge, such as case managers, case coordinators, staff development instructors, clinical care managers, or peers. Usually, peers are staff peers and are not budgeted to have off-unit time (Chap. 14 addresses competence assessment budget strategies). Initially, peer review may sound like the most practical way of

TABLE 7-2

Matrix for Skills by Unit, by Shift: High-Risk, Low-Volume, Problem-Prone

Skills	9E/W	8E/W	7W	6E/W	SNF	MIU	5E	LD	NICU	ICU	CCU	ER	GS3	TP	OSC	OOMS	MOR/PACU/ASC
Epidural analgesia	X	X	X	X	NA	NA	NA	NA	NA	X	X	NA		NA		NA	PACU
12-lead EKG	X	X	X	X 7P-7A only	X	NA	NA	NA	NA	X	X		X	X	NA	NA	NA
Peritoneal dialysis	NA	X	NA	NA	X	NA	NA	NA	NA	X	X	NA	NA	NA	NA	NA	NA
Identification Stage I, II, III, IV for skin	X	X	X	X	X	X	X	NA	X	X	X		X	X	X	X	X
Identification arterial/venous circulation	NA		NA	X	NA	NA	NA	NA	NA	X	X	X	NA	NA	NA	X	
Phlebotomy	NA	NA	X	X	X	X	NA	NA	NA	X	X	X	X	NA	NA	X	NA
Orders in HBOC	X	X	X	X	X	X	X	X	X	X	X	X	X	X	X	X	X
ABG's direct sticks	NA	NA	X	NA	NA	NA	NA	NA	NA	X	X	X	NA	NA	NA	NA	NA
Turbo infuser	NA	NA	NA	NA	NA	NA	NA	NA	NA	NA	NA	X	NA	NA	NA	NA	NA

NA = not applicable to unit; applicable to both 7A–7P and 7P–7A shifts unless otherwise noted evaluating mandatory competencies. However, time needs to be built into the schedule for initial training as well as for revalidating the skills of peers. In addition, content regarding the mandatory competency may change. For example, if peers are assessing the competency of staff about the proper method of restraining patients, the trainer will want to reinstruct the peers about any revisions in standards or guidelines about restraints. Usually, an annual review and validation of peer competency is needed if the organization chooses department- or unit-based "train-the-trainer" or peer-to-peer programs for competence assessment.

TIPS FOR ASSESSING COMPETENCE

The process of competence assessment is more defined than most performance review methods. Data from competence assessment activities should be included in summary comments made on annual reviews about individual employees. This symbiotic relation between competence assessment and performance review by managers generates challenges and opportunities. Many skills and procedures that organizations assume staff know how to accomplish are identified as problems during the assessment process. In some cases, this is due to the competence assessment framework or assessment strategies used in the organization. The staff development specialist must clearly recognize that performance in simulated scenarios may be markedly different because of the simulation equipment, the experience of the care provider, and the experience of the assessor. It is certainly possible, and in many cases preferable, to conduct competence assessment activities during the actual performance of tasks. However, competence assessment conducted during actual care must be stopped immediately if the patient or provider is placed at risk. Intervention at that point changes the competence assessment activity to a coaching or counseling activity.

Once the major functions and the specific units to which these functions apply have been identified, the competency criteria can be constructed. Table 7-3 shows a sample competency statement, along with the corresponding criteria, that was developed for an orthopedic unit. There are various methods of constructing criteria, but this is one of the easiest to explain to staff. It also streamlines the tracking and reporting of data.

Even though the manager hires the best-qualified person for the position, there is no real opportunity to assess the knowledge and skills that are needed to do the job. The process of verifying credentials, checking references, and interviewing the candidate does not allow the manager to observe the candidate's skills or knowledge. The orientation period can be used to assess the new employee's skills and knowledge and customize his or her orientation.

Each job title requires orientation to the specific job. To plan the orientation and build on the knowledge the new employee already brings to the job, a competence assessment program for new employees provides a baseline for what is needed. This process is lengthy but needs to be accomplished only once during the tenure of the employee in a specific job title. The manager might request another competency assessment if there is a significant change in job performance.

TRACKING DATA

A reliable tracking system, preferably computerized, should be developed to provide cumulative data, charts, and graphs for reports. The system should be easily accessible for routine reporting and during scheduled or unannounced regulatory agency visits. Once competency statements and criteria are developed, the educator, collaborating with

TABLE 7-3

SAMPLE COMPETENCY STATEMENT, ALONG WITH CORRESPONDING CRITERIA

Unit-Specific Competency: GS3

Evaluator: _____ Date: _____

Note to the evaluator: no prompting of the employee is permitted; if prompting is needed for any of the criteria, criteria is then marked as "not met."

Competency: **Applies Jones dressing according to policy and procedure**

Criteria	Met	Not Met
1. Cleanses the incision with soap and water and dries prior to applying the dressing		
2. Applies Adaptic to incision and covers with 4×4 or ABD		
3. Applies Webril to hold dressings in place		
4. Applies pound cotton wrapping from foot to thigh, including the foot		
5. Wets down casting splints one at a time and applies 1st splint over the knee • Second splint to one side of knee overlapping the initial splint • Third splint to the other side of knee overlapping splint number one		
6. Wraps the entire dressing with webril to help conform splints to leg		
7. Wraps entire leg from foot to thigh with Ace bandage including foot		

the information system department, can create a data base system. Today's software will track not only attendance but also the delinquencies—those not maintaining current competence as defined by the organization. Although some type of oversight procedure is necessary, it is not realistic to expect 100% compliance. Sample policies and procedures are shown in Displays 7-2 and 7-3. The former applies to all departments, contract workers, and volunteers, the latter only to patient care services.

These policies provide managers with a disciplinary process to use when employees are not compliant. In most cases, only one verbal warning is needed when word gets around that the policies are expected to be followed.

To support the policies and procedures, reports must be generated from the data base. Also, JCAHO standards require the institution to review trends. Several reports can be set up to run from data base applications; examples are shown in Tables 7-4, 7-5 and 7-6. Table 7-4 reports the actual attendance at a program. Table 7-5 is a delinquency report, developed to assist the manager in determining compliance with mandatory education. Table 7-6 compares organization-wide compliance with actual and targeted partici-

(*text continues on page 161*)

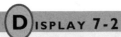

DISPLAY 7-2

Hospital-Wide Policy and Procedure, Annual Requirements: Educational, Safety, and Employee Health

Standard Policy and/or Procedure

Date Effective: September 1, 1994
Title: ANNUAL REQUIREMENTS: EDUCATIONAL, SAFETY, AND EMPLOYEE HEALTH
Distribution: All SPP Manual Holders
Approval: Office of the President

Statement of Purpose

To establish requirements for mandatory attendance at training programs to meet applicable regulatory standards.

Policy

Grant Medical Center provides for education and training designed to maintain and improve the knowledge and skills of all personnel via orientation classes, inservice programs, and continuing education offerings. Grant Medical Center adheres to guidelines from the Centers for Disease Control and Prevention (CDC) and Occupational Safety and Health Administration (OSHA). These guidelines apply to employee health testing and training of employees. Each department determines if employee training in cardiopulmonary resuscitation and other lifesaving measures is appropriate. If appropriate, divisional policies will be contained within the manual concerning performance criteria for annual evaluations.

Procedure

A. All employees are required to attend a Fire and Safety training program annually.
B. All employees who have exposure or potential exposure to blood-borne diseases are required to attend the OSHA blood-borne pathogen/TB training program annually.
C. All employees who have exposure to hazardous materials are required to attend the OSHA hazardous materials training program annually.
D. Additional mandatory programs may be required on an as-needed basis; employees are required to attend these as determined by the department director.
E. All employees are required to report to Employee Health annually for the Mantoux TB test.
F. Failure to attend programs or to report to Employee Health results in progressive disciplinary action in the form of a verbal counseling, written counseling, and written reprimand. Discharge will result on the third Class III reprimand within a 12-month period. Disciplinary action will be administered by the manager/supervisor and occur on at least a monthly basis until the requirement has been met or failure to participate in mandatory programs has resulted in termination.
G. Tracking of attendance is the responsibility of the employee's department director.

REVIEWED/REVISED BY:

Mike Heys / Rebecca Katz   5/11/94

APPROVED BY:

Executive Staff   9/19/94
Medical Executive Committee   N/A
Board of Directors   N/A

Any previous edition of this Standard Policy and Procedure becomes null and void with the enactment and announcement of this edition, now numbered SPP 82-94.

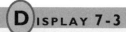

DISPLAY 7-3

Policy and Procedure, Requirements for Annual Acquisition of Educational Credit and Participating in Departmental Staff Meetings

Grant Medical Center
Columbus, Ohio

Patient Care Services Policy and Procedure

SUBJECT

Requirements for Annual Acquisition of Educational Credit and Participation in Departmental Staff Meetings

PURPOSE/OBJECTIVE

To define the expectations of nursing personnel associated with attending and participating in required educational programs and staff meetings.

E 01
———————————
Number

E 01   11/22/93
———————————
Replaces

03/01/96
———————————
Date Effective

Suzanne De Woody
———————————
Authorization

Suzanne DeWoody
Vice President
Patient Care Services

2/16/96
———————————
Date Signed

Policy Statements

1. Grant Medical Center believes that the ongoing education of its staff is vital to the provision of high-quality, individualized patient care. Formal and informal education programs are designed to improve each nursing staff member's competence. Ongoing education programming is based on findings from quality assessment and improvement activities, new or changing technology, therapeutic or pharmacological interventions, and identified or stated learning needs of nursing staff members.

2. Staff participation and attendance at either formal or informal educational programs and committee meetings is planned for, scheduled, and documented on the unit schedule. Educational time and attendance at committee meetings may be reflected on an employee's schedule via the Automated Nurse Staffing Office System (ANSOS). ANSOS permits the user to enter two (2) scheduling codes per day in the SCHEDULER module.

3. Divisional and unit staff meetings are conducted on at least a monthly basis and afford staff members the occasion to exchange information and to seek out, and act on, opportunities to improve care and resolve identified problems in the provision of nursing care. Staff members are expected to attend seventy-five (75) percent of the total staff meetings conducted per year. Discussions at unit meetings are based upon (but are not limited to) findings from quality assessment and improvement activities and divisional/unit operational issues. Staff meeting minutes will be made available for staff review following each meeting. The manager makes the decision for paying the employee for attending the staff meeting on own time based upon the unit's budget allocations.

4. Meetings or activities that assist with the improvement of the unit may be paid. Examples are Quality Improvement Team meetings, cluster group meetings, meetings for Patient-Family–Centered Care and various unit task force groups. The manager makes the decision based upon the budgeted allocation for orientation and educational time.

5. Attendance records that document each staff member's participation in required education programs are maintained in the Education Department's database. Attendance will be documented and maintained for all participants for each educational activity for which an OBN (Ohio Board of Nursing) number has been assigned.

(continued)

DISPLAY 7-3 (Continued)

6. Each classification of nursing personnel is required to attain a minimum number of educational credits annually as an opportunity to improve competence. These requirements are outlined as follows:

Position/Title	Hours Required
Registered Nurse	12 OBN contact hours
Licensed Practical Nurse	12 OBN contact hours
Patient Care Assistant	10 GMC class hours
Health Unit Coordinator	8 GMC class hours
Clinical Assistant	10 GMC class hours
Patient Care Technician	10 GMC class hours or proof of nursing school enrollment for PCTs who are student nurses
Technicians	10 GMC class hours

7. During the first year of employment, mandatory programs and any program selected by the manager with substantial rationale will be paid at the hourly base rate. All Patient Care Services' employees are required to attend a Fire and Utility Safety, Hazardous Communication, and Blood-Borne Pathogen training program annually. RNs, LPNs, and PCT/CCTs are also required to complete Accu-chek competency performance verification annually. CPR recertification is required annually for all Patient Care Services' employees, with the exception of the Health Unit Coordinators, for whom it is optional. (Refer to Patient Care Services' Policy on CPR recertification, C 16.)

   RNs are to demonstrate competency with defibrillator checks annually. Failure to attend these programs will result in progressive disciplinary action in the form of verbal counseling, written counseling, and written reprimand. Discharge will result on the third Class III reprimand within a twelve (12) month period. Disciplinary action will be administered by the manager/supervisor and occur on at least a monthly basis until the requirement has been met or failure to attend mandatory programs has resulted in termination.

8. After the first year, 16 hours of paid workshop time will be allowed for full-time employees (regularly scheduled 72 and 80 hours per pay period), while part-time employees will be allowed 8 hours. Contingent employees are not paid for workshop time over and above any class hours that are required (e.g., CPR, etc.). This workshop time may be paid and includes workshops held either at Grant Medical Center or outside of it.

9. Employees may select workshops of their choice and present to their manager for approval. If the manager approves the workshop time to be paid, it is expected that the employee attending GMC-sponsored workshops will clock in and out appropriately.

10. Workshop hours will be tracked by the manager and are based on the fiscal year from July 1st to June 30th.

11. No time will be paid for workshop attendance unless pre-approved by the manager.

12. Grant Medical Center class hours are awarded by Grant Medical Center for participation in inservice education that consists of planned instruction or training programs provided by the employer in the work setting. Inservice education is designed to promote compliance with institutional policies and procedures, the demonstration of new equipment, the explanation of revised procedures, and the practice of previously learned skills. Cardiopulmonary resuscitation certification/recertification is classified as inservice education.

13. OBN contact hours are awarded through the ONA Provider program for continuing nursing education offerings, independent studies, and programs. OBN contact hours may be obtained through attendance at internal or external continuing nursing education programs.

DISPLAY 7-3 (Continued)

PROCEDURE

1. EXPECTED OUTCOMES
   Employees participate in educational activities to improve competence; attendance is documented.
2. EQUIPMENT
   ANSOS SCHEDULER module
   Staff meeting minutes
   Attendance records

Implementation Steps	Rationale/Amplification
Scheduling Committee Participation in ANSOS With Other Duty Code	
1. Select unit from the **SCHEDULER** menu.	
2. Select **View/Alter Skeletons**.	2a. Scheduled workshops and conferences may be scheduled as a request in ANSOS using the appropriate scheduling code.
3. Select employee.	
4. Tab to desired date and enter duty code (*e.g.,* D, A, etc.).	
5. Tab to the second line of the employee's schedule using the right, left, up, and down arrow keys and enter one of the following codes: **I = PMtg** (committee or meeting scheduled after 1200 hours); **m = AMtg** (committee or meeting scheduled before 1200 hours)	5a. The printed schedule will indicate the scheduled duty as well as the meeting. The meeting length, however, will not be deducted from the length of the shift because I and m are generic codes and do not differentiate the specific meeting or the length of the meeting. The duty code and meeting will be noted on the schedule, which should hlep in planning. 5b. As needed, update the "**note fields**" in Controller (Alt U) and record the date of committee meetings for your employees (*e.g.,* P&P Committee, 2nd Friday). Four note fields are available which should be sufficient for most staff. The notes can be helpful when entering requests, because they will be a reminder of staff committee responsibilities.

pants. A trend report would show if there were similar competency issues on units throughout the institution.

Another method of ensuring compliance with mandatory competencies is to use the performance evaluation system. An example is shown in Table 7-7. This evaluation is a pilot one using a skills-based pay system for an orthopedic unit. The employee must give the documentation to the manager, as outlined in "criteria for achievement of rating of 2." The person cannot proceed with the evaluation if the documentation is not received by the manager. An additional positive outcome related to mandatory activities was noted as a result of this approach. The manager said that before 1995, when this evaluation was implemented, she never had staff approach her to find out where the independent studies for fire and safety were kept or how they could facilitate others' attendance at the mandatory competencies.

TABLE 7-4

REPORT FROM DATA BASE SHOWING ATTENDANCE AT ONE PROGRAM

Program Participation

Program Code: GMC-1826
Program Title: OSHA Bloodborne Pathogen Update
Speaker: Bernie Deed
Time Span: Since the beginning of the program

Unit	Clock No.	Last Name	First Name	Prof. Title	Job Title	DNA Hours	GMC Hours	LPNAO Hours	SW Hours	Date
5E	2249	Edwards	Irene		Clinical Assistant		1.0			4/30/96
5E	2327	Mobley	Marjorie A.	RN	Registered Nurse		1.0			4/14/96
5E	7587	Fisher	Nancy	LPN	Licensed Practical Nurse		1.0			7/11/96
5E	15373	Madden	Arlene	RN	Registered Nurse		1.0			7/11/96
5E	15651	Cornell	Theresa	LPN	Licensed Practical Nurse		1.0			2/02/96
5E	17035	Thomas	Ava		Clinical Assistant		1.0			1/24/96
5E	20213	Ridenour	Lisa Marie	RN	Registered Nurse		1.0			3/26/96
6E	10773	Blount	Anna		Secretary II		1.0			2/05/96
6E	11867	Waters	Terri		Patient Care Assistant		1.0			5/04/96
6E	12687	Schwenk	Justine		Patient Care Technician		1.0			5/25/96
6E	12825	Fitzgerald	Judy	LPN	Licensed Practical Nurse		1.0			5/05/96
6E	13341	Williams	Mercedes		Patient Care Assistant		1.0			5/24/96
6E	16388	Anderson	Barbara	RN	Registered Nurse		1.0			6/12/96
6E	16836	Brown	Deborah	RN	Registered Nurse		1.0			5/05/96
6E	18813	Smegal	Tracy	RN	Registered Nurse		1.0			4/03/96
6E	19052	Carney	Sue	RN	Registered Nurse		1.0			5/20/96
6E	19122	Brooks	Sheila Elyse	RN	Registered Nurse		1.0			5/14/96
6E	19471	York	LaVerne	LPN	Licensed Practical Nurse		1.0			5/02/96

TABLE 7-5

REPORT FROM DATA BASE SHOWING EMPLOYEES WHO ARE EITHER DELINQUENT IN ONE OF THE MANDATORIES OR ABOUT TO BE DELINQUENT

No.	Last Name	First Name	Prof. Title	Job Title	Program Code*	Title*	Exp. Date
Unit: 5E							
20176	Bourne	Ruby		CA	GMC-1826	OSHA Bloodborne Pathogen Update	8/30/96
20476	Woods	Toni Lynn	RN	RN	GMC-1826	OSHA Bloodborne Pathogen Update	6/08/96
20635	Miller	Julia	RN	RN	GMC-1826	OSHA Bloodborne Pathogen Update	8/29/96

* These two fields are blank if there is no record of prior OSHA training on file

USING A SYSTEMATIC APPROACH

Once the educator, along with the designated safety director, has defined the content, competencies, and criteria that employees need to demonstrate competence, he or she must determine the number of hours required to demonstrate mandatory employee competencies. Then the educator should determine if the current staff have enough knowledge and skills or if training is needed. A competency checklist should be developed.

Competency checklists should include the critical steps. The educator, manager, and staff need to collaborate to determine these critical steps. Lengthy competency checklists are unnecessary (Table 7-8).

After the initial process for determining the competency assessment of mandatories is developed, a method of budgeting time for employees to accomplish these competencies should be selected. One large hospital system in central Ohio uses a process for budgeting that includes allocating time for mandatory requirements (Display 7-4). The mandatories included in determining this formula are CPR, hazard communication, fire safety and utility loss, and bloodborne pathogen education. The actual number of employees, not just the number of budgeted full-time equivalents (FTEs), is multiplied by the number of hours each employee will need to attend or complete mandatory education. This figure is equated to FTEs and added to the overall budget.

(*text continues on page 168*)

TABLE 7-6

REPORT FROM DATA BASE COMPARING ACTUAL PARTICIPANTS WITH TARGET AUDIENCE

Primary Course #	Course Title	Contact Hours	Target Participants	Actual Participants	Percent of Target Audience Reached
GMC-1826	Bloodborne training/TB training	1.2	2253	957	42%

TABLE 7-7

PILOT EVALUATION USING SKILLS-BASED PAY MODEL

Performance Evaluation Addendum #1 Team Player Evaluation

Your Name: _____

Instructions: Complete a self-evaluation; this will be used for feedback to your immediate supervisor. Choose 2 peers to complete this; your immediate supervisor will choose 2 peers also. You can duplicate these forms, but they must be returned to your immediate supervisor by 6/1/96. The manager will also complete this form.

Competency	Rating		
1. Promotes teamwork and cooperation with others on same unit/department and with other departments; assists coworkers with assignments. Comments:	3	2	1
2. Sets appropriate priorities; takes responsibility for effective communication with team members; assists in identification of problems and effective methods of solving problems. Comments:	3	2	1
3. Maintains confidentiality; displays positive relationship with patients, families, physicians, other departments; demonstrates behaviors that constitute positive customer service as identified by department goals. Comments:	3	2	1
4. Practices effective communication skills by listening respectfully, giving feedback directly and honestly, and talking with others to clarify differences. Comments:	3	2	1
5. Assists with developing change and creative approaches to problem-solving; reacts positively to creativity and innovation and demonstrates a willingness to accept change. Comments:	3	2	1

Reviewer: _____ Date: _____

Rating scale
3 = consistently exceeds expectations
2 = meets expectations
1 = does not meet expectations

TABLE 7-7 (Continued)

PILOT EVALUATION USING SKILLS-BASED PAY MODEL

Performance Evaluation Addendum #2
Technical Evaluation Form and Direct Patient Care (Completed by immediate supervisor)

Complete this form with dates and appropriate documentation; this form is to be given to immediate supervisor by 6/1/96.

All documentation is to be handed to supervisor; evaluation cannot be scheduled until documentation is completed.

Competency	Criteria for Achievement of Rating of 3	Criteria for Achievement of Rating of 2	Rating		
1. Initiates and performs Basic Life Support skills according to the Emergency Cardiac Care guidelines of the American Heart Association	• Asks for "delinquent CPR list" and assists 5 team members in successfully completing CPR in interactive video lab	• CPR Course C card • Mock code blue QI monitor	3	2	1
2. Initiates and maintains competency with Accuchek II blood glucose monitoring	• Asks for "delinquent Accuchek list" and checks 5 team members in successfully completing Accu-chek competency checklist after attending an Accu-chek training class	• GMC certificate for Accuchek blood glucose monitoring	3	2	1
3. Demonstrates knowledge and integration of bloodborne pathogen regulations/TB into practice	• Asks for "delinquent bloodborne pathogen/TB list" and facilitates 5 team members in successfully completing independent studies	• GMC certificate for completion of bloodborne pathogen/TB education • Documentation of TB test on education report	3	2	1
4. Demonstrates knowledge and integration of fire/safety practices	• Asks for "delinquent fire/safety list" and facilitates 5 team members in successfully completing independent studies	• GMC certificate for completion of fire/safety	3	2	1
5. Demonstrates knowledge and integration of hazardous materials practices	• Asks for "delinquent hazard materials lists" and facilitates 5 team members in successfully completing independent studies	• GMC certificate for completion of hazardous materials	3	2	1

COMMENTS:

(continued)

TABLE 7-7 (Continued)

PILOT EVALUATION USING SKILLS-BASED PAY MODEL

Competency	Criteria for Achievement of Rating of 3	Criteria for Achievement of Rating of 2	Rating		
6. Demonstrates knowledge and integration of utility outage and life safety practices	• Asks for "delinquent life safety and utility outages list" and facilitates 5 team members in successfully completing independent studies	• GMC certificate for completion of utility outage and life safety	3	2	1
7. Demonstrates knowledge and skill for age-specific patients	• Provides formal appropriate educational activity as documented on educational summary report	• Competency checkoff list for age-specific patients completed	3	2	1
8. Demonstrates knowledge and skill in caring for patient populations of all activity levels commonly seen on patient care unit	• Teaches POP classes • Provides formal appropriate educational activity specific to orthopedic patients as documented on educational summary report	• Anecdotal notes • Customer letters • Physician comments	3	2	1
9. Demonstrates safe practice during the following: • Dysrhythmia interpretation and documentation • Obtaining blood samples by venipuncture • Obtaining 12-lead EKG • Assisting with physical therapy skills		• 80% on EKG QI monitor • Absence of negative reports from lab about venipuncture or contamination on blood cultures • Absence of abnormal 12-lead EKGs • Feedback from physician therapist		2 2 2	1 1 1
10. Demonstrates training with new equipment		• Documentation on education report sent to immediate supervisor		2	1
11. Demonstrates training/education regarding new documentation forms, policies/procedures, quality issues	• Assists training on unit, becoming a trainer for equipment after attending formalized class	• Documentation on education report sent to immediate supervisor	3	2	1

TABLE 7-7 (Continued)

PILOT EVALUATION USING SKILLS-BASED PAY MODEL

Competency	Criteria for Achievement of Rating of 3	Criteria for Achievement of Rating of 2	Rating		
Unit-specific Competency 12. Demonstrates application of Jones dressing	• Precepts team members on proper application of Jones dressing	• Completion of competency check-off list	3	2	1
Unit-specific Competency 13. Demonstrates Shantz application	• Precepts team members on proper application of Shantz dressing	• Completion of competency check-off list	3	2	1
Unit-specific Competency 14. Demonstrates setup for double traction	• Precepts team members on proper setup for double traction	• Completion of competency check-off list	3	2	1

PROFESSIONAL DEVELOPMENT PLAN:

Scoring Sheet for GS3

	Indicator	Weight	Score	Numeric Wt.
T	Press Ganey goal	30%		
E	Physician Satisfaction	10%		
A	Expense	35%		
M	Unit or department goals	25%		
40%				
			×0.4 (40%)	
I	Team Player	30%		
N D	Technical competencies	30%		
60%				
			×0.6 (60%)	

TABLE 7-8

COMPETENCY STATEMENT ALONG WITH CRITERIA FOR ONE PROCEDURE CONSIDERED TO BE PROBLEM-PRONE, HIGH-RISK; HOSPITAL-BASED

••

Hospital-Specific Competency: Age-Specific

Employee name: _____ Clock number: _____

Evaluator: _____ Date: _____

> Note to the evaluator: no prompting of the employee is permitted; if prompting is needed for any of the criteria, the criteria is then marked as "not met."

Competency: **Modified care for pediatric and/or elderly patients as appropriate**

Criteria	Met	Not Met
Applies principles of growth and development in caring for pediatric and/or elderly patients		
Adjusts plan of care and interventions to meet individual psychological needs for pediatric and/or elderly patients		
Anticipates need for adjustment in medication dosing based on pediatric and/or elderly patient's needs		

In the past, some staffing plans included only FTEs needed to care for patients. Time needed for staff to attend meetings and mandatory and optional educational offerings had to be carved out of existing FTEs. Using the method described above has provided concrete support for off-unit activities by budgeting replacement staff for direct patient care.

Administrative support is essential before starting the process of defining and evaluating competencies. Standards or competencies should be defined for all employees, including any nonemployees who are working in the institution. For example, from an administrative approach, anyone who is in an institution must know the procedure to follow if a fire occurs. So when defining competencies, the process must address not only employees, but also contract workers, physicians, and physicians' staff.

PROCESS FOR EDUCATING FOR THE MANDATORIES
••

Next, the educator needs to determine the best method of educating staff. Because many institutions are downsizing and the traditional approach of educating staff in a classroom has disappeared, a self-learning package may help an institution to educate a critical mass of employees (Display 7-5). Self-learning packages are relatively simple to develop and maintain. They can be placed on the units, in lobbies, or in areas for easy access. A paper-and-pencil test can assess cognitive knowledge but does not assess if the employee can demonstrate the skills. For example, completing the exercises shown in Display 7-5 would not ensure that the employee could locate fire extinguishers on the unit. To ensure this skill, use questions like those shown in Display 7-6. This requires the employee to find the fire extinguishers and the shut-off valves.

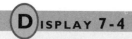
Budgeting for Mandatory Education

Grant/Riverside Methodist Hospitals—Grant Campus FY97 Budget For: 569—Skilled Nursing Facility

Patient days	9,833
O/P Obs patients	0
Budget ADC	26.9
Budget HPPD	5.7
Variable staff	55,689
Variable FTE's	26.8
Hours per shift:	12
Patient days/week:	188.6
Total shifts/week:	89
Variable hours/week:	1,068
Calculated HPPD:	5.7

Skill mix:		
	1	37.08%
	2	19.10%
	3	43.82%

Sample Staffing:

	Sun	Mon	Tues	Weds	Thur	Fri	Sat	Totals
1	2	2	3	3	2	3	2	17
2	2	2	1	1	2	2	2	12
3	3	3	3	3	3	3	3	21
1	2	3	2	2	2	3	2	16
2	1	0	1	1	1	0	1	5
3	2	3	2	3	2	3	3	18
1	0	0	0	0	0	0	0	0
2	0	0	0	0	0	0	0	0
3	0	0	0	0	0	0	0	0

Replacement Staff

ORIENTATION STAFF:

No. of Staff	Hours/ Staff		Total Hours
1	5.0	240	1,200
2	2.0	120	240
3	5.0	80	400
			1,840

FIE's: 0.9

Calculated % to variable hours: 3.30%

ETO/SICK HOURS:

	Total
Estimated ETO/sick hours:	6,348
FIE's	3.1
Calculated % to variable hours:	11.40%

NON-PRODUCTIVE HOURS:

Factor	Stat		Total
1	0.14	9,833	1,377
2	0.00	9,833	0
3	0.00	9,833	0
			1,377

FIE's: 0.7

Calculated % to variable hours: 2.47%

FIXED PERSONNEL:

1.0	Manager
1.0	Other (specify) Admission/discharge coordinator
2.0	Total

MANDATORY EDUCATION:

No. of Staff	Hours/ Staff		Total Hours
1	13.0	12	156
2	6.0	12	72
3	14.0	12	168
			396

FIE's: 0.2

Calculated % to variable hours: 0.71%

SUMMARY:

	Fixed	1	2	3	Total	Check
Variable		9.9	5.1	11.7	26.7	26.8
Orientation		0.6	0.1	0.2	0.9	0.9
Non-productive		0.7	0.0	0.0	0.7	0.7
ETO/Sick		1.1	0.6	1.3	3.0	3.1
Mandatory Ed		0.1	0.0	0.1	0.2	0.2
Fixed	2.0	0.0	0.0	0.0	2.0	2.0
Total FTE's	2.0	12.4	5.8	13.3	33.5	33.6

Legend:	1-RN	2-LPN	3-PCT/PCA

DISPLAY 7-5

Fire and Safety Independent Study

Life Safety
Fire Safety & Utility Loss
Independent Study

This program was designed for staff in direct patient care departments. Portions of this program are not applicable for staff working in other areas. Contact Safety Management at extension #3671 if you have questions.

INSTRUCTIONS

1. Obtain a copy of the fire & safety videotape from your nursing unit/department. View the videotape and read all of the enclosed information.
2. Complete the attendance roster on the back of this page.
3. Complete the post-test and program evaluation form.
4. Return the attendance roster, post-test, and evaluation form to Safety Management.

NAME: (PLEASE PRINT) _____ CLOCK # _____

UNIT: _____ TITLE: _____ DATE: _____

1. What is the <u>first</u> action you should take upon discovering a fire in a patient room?
   Circle <u>all</u> correct answers

   a. Report the fire.   c. Run to an exit.
   b. Get a fire extinguisher.   d. Remove the patient(s) from the room.

2. To alert other staff to the fire you should yell:
   Circle <u>one</u> correct answer

   a. "Condition X."   c. "Condition frank."
   b. "Condition Red."   d. "Help Fire."

3. In case of a fire that involved oxygen, you should attempt to shut off the oxygen at the flowmeter on the wall in the patient room where the fire is occurring. If this is not possible, your next action to stop the oxygen should be to:
   Circle <u>one</u> correct answer

   a. Page the plant operation engineer.   c. Call Security STAT!
   b. Shut off the oxygen at the valve located in   d. Wait for the fire department.
      the corridor.

4. In case of a loss of electrical power to the hospital, the only patient care equipment that will work is equipment that is plugged into:
   Circle <u>all</u> correct answers

   a. Green-colored outlets.   c. Black-colored outlets.
   b. Outlets that are red in color. d. Blue-colored outlets.

5. In case of a water, medical gas, or electrical outage in the hospital, the telephone operator will make the following announcement:
   Circle <u>one</u> correct answer

   a. "Code Brown."   c. "Code White."
   b. "Code Yellow."   d. "Utility Alert."

Display 7-6

Independent Study, Fire and Safety Test

For the next three questions you will need to examine the equipment in your work area.

10. On top of each fire alarm pull station is a number. Walk around your work area and locate at least four fire alarm pull stations.

Station #	Location
#1 _____	_____
#2 _____	_____
#3 _____	_____
#4 _____	_____

11. Identify the type and location of at least three fire extinguishers in your work area.

Type	Location
#1 _____	_____
#2 _____	_____
#3 _____	_____

12. List the location of the oxygen shut-off valves in your department. A typical unit in the main hospital will have four valves, Grant South three valves. *Note: If you do not have wall outlets for oxygen in your area, mark this question "NA."*

    #1 _____

    #2 _____

    #3 _____

    #4 _____

13. A patient who is receiving oxygen is not permitted to:
    Circle all correct answers

    a. Use a toothbrush.   d. Use a hair dryer or curling iron.
    b. Use an electric shaver.   e. Place the television closer than 1 foot from the face.
    c. Smoke.

Please complete the Security and Safety program evaluation on the back of this page.
   Mail your completed test, attendance roster, and safety program evaluation to Safety Management.

EVALUATING SUCCESS

How do you know if you've been successful in your approach to mandatory education? Obviously, a successful JCAHO visit is a positive indicator. If the management team perceives that employees can achieve the mandatories, the process is not cumbersome, and the managers understand the process and participate in implementation, the process will be deemed successful. Employees will appreciate it if the self-learning studies are available 24 hours a day, 7 days a week. Cost is not a useful measure: the cost of not maintaining JCAHO accreditation, or a fine by OSHA, would outweigh any amount of money needed to educate employees. However, cost can be calculated and used as a measure of changing from classroom-based education for mandatories to self-learning packages.

SUMMARY

Some react to the word "mandatory" as if chalk had just scraped the blackboard. However, if the educator assesses what is needed by reviewing the standards, planning the education in an efficient, cost-effective manner, and providing an oversight procedure, the outcome will enhance quality in patient care. Then, the term "mandatory" will come to mean something positive: a process that contributes to the quality of care provided to patients in the facility.

Managing Mandatories

DENISE PETRAS

The word "mandatories" typically conjures up images of programs on fire and safety, infection control, body mechanics, and CPR, and historically members of staff development departments have provided these programs. Over the years, educators have explored a variety of ways to ensure that health care professionals and support staff receive the relevant information contained in these programs to complete their annual requirements.

Paradoxically, mandatory in-services are both static and dynamic in nature. Like death and taxes, mandatories have a stable presence in health care organizations because of regulatory and accrediting agencies' requirements, as well as organizational policies. The standard programs of fire, safety, infection control, bloodborne pathogens, and body mechanics make up what are usually called mandatories, with CPR and point-of-care testing added for patient care providers. On the flip side, mandatory program content needs to be updated or expanded and new content needs to be added on a regular basis. Hospitals and other health care facilities also may add their own requirements for mandatory education based on their mission and values, specific population, or other regulatory guidelines.

At Shadyside Hospital, a 450-plus-bed acute care institution in Pittsburgh, Pennsylvania, managing mandatories and other required programs for the nursing and related staff always has been a function of the nursing education (staff development) department. Like all staff development specialists, the challenge is how best to provide any educational program, given the available resources.

In the mid-1980s, the department was staffed with five full-time educators and two coordinators who worked in a centralized department under a director. Each had specific and what may be considered traditional staff development roles; providing mandatory programming took up much of their time. Centralized programming, using a basic lecture format, was common practice. Staff compliance was adequate but could have been better. As organizational and staff development department changes occurred, alternative modes of program delivery began to evolve. Through attrition of department members and subsequent collapse of positions, followed by position eliminations in 1993, the department evolved in a variety of ways and now is made up of two professional staff and one secretary.

To be able to manage the essential functions of the department and provide a higher level of service, it was essential to redesign the work of staff development. Four themes emerged from the organizational changes that were occurring, involving the traditional belief that staff development educators must "do it all."

The first theme was, and continues to be, sensitivity to available resources. With fewer people to do the same amount of work, the educators explored innovative ways to provide services.

Shift of accountability to staff was the second theme. The concepts of decentralization, participative leadership, and accountability are core values within Shadyside Hospital's Nursing Division and have been influential in having the staff take "ownership" of specific educational programs.

The next theme was that traditional modes of learning became less acceptable and feasible.

Gone were the days of conducting multiple all-day programs for basic topics. Staffing mix changes, shorter lengths of stay, and more acute patients made it difficult for staff to complete annual program requirements.

The last theme was the changing role and work of staff development educators. Instead of providing the required programs, the educators created an environment in which staff would be accountable for completing the annual mandatory programs. Mandatories and other required programs were targeted as areas that staff could independently manage because staff had knowledge of the content.

The CPR program was the first to be decentralized, and support was obtained from the unit managers to implement the program. What once was an all-day program with educators lecturing and certifying staff became a unit-based program using a videotape and unit-based CPR instructors. Unit managers provided one or more staff from their units to be trained as CPR instructors. The nursing education department provided CPR instructor training, supplies, materials, and recordkeeping; the task of cleaning the CPR equipment was redirected to the sterile processing department. Today, all nursing units continue to be fully accountable for completing the biannual CPR requirement. Skill competency programs and point-of-care testing programs are managed in the same way.

Mandatories, which originally were offered as a full-day and then half-day lecture program, first were converted to the mandatory "box" self-learning format. Because staff and managers alike complained that leaving the patient care unit to attend the program was too difficult, this alternative learning mechanism was developed to meet the learners' needs and facilitate compliance. These brightly covered paper boxes (one per unit) included a videotape of all required subjects, an in-service record (sign-in sheet), instructions for use, and learning evaluations. Each unit manager was given a box and was instructed on its use.

It worked perfectly—for a while, anyway. It wasn't too long, however, before the film became outdated and incomplete. The expense of developing or purchasing a new film and the increased frequency with which new programs needed to be added to the mandatory repertoire made it necessary to develop another mechanism for teaching

this information. Also, this format, although more convenient and efficient than a day-long program, had its own limitations, such as access to a VCR, inflexibility for group viewing, inability to complete the program at any location, and the need to complete the program in one sitting.

Subsequently, a written self-learning instructional exercise was developed for the staff in the Nursing Division. The nursing education department worked collaboratively with a variety of departments (rehabilitation services, clinical engineering, infection control, safety and security, quality, customer relations) to obtain information relevant to their areas of expertise. Additional writing, final editing, and compilation, as well as development of the learning evaluation tool, were completed by the nursing education department. The evaluation tool, which consisted of multiple-choice, true-or-false, and fill-in-the-blank questions, was included at the back of the material. Employees were asked to complete this form and submit it to their supervisors. Supervisors were to ask the employees if they had any questions about the material they read, then sign the form to say it had been properly completed. When returned to the department of nursing education, this page served as the documentation for the completion of mandatories. Bimonthly compliance reports were generated for the unit managers. Most staff complete their mandatories self-learning material during their CPR/competency day to fulfill their requirements.

In light of the JCAHO requirement that all hospital employees complete mandatory in-services, a team had been established to develop an all-day lecture format program to teach the required content. The program was offered twice monthly to accommodate as many employees as possible. Realizing that this method was not the most cost-effective mechanism for completing mandatories, the nursing education department encouraged the use of the self-learning booklet and made it available to all employees. A great deal of positive feedback was received from many department managers because of its convenience and lower time requirements; employees liked working at their own pace and having a reference tool to keep.

The self-learning module for mandatory in-services is still not the sole tool for meeting mandatory in-service requirements at Shadyside Hospi-

	Instructor Cost	Employee Cost*	Non-prod. Hours	Total Cost	FTEs
8-hr. program	$2208	$255,040	16,000	$257,248	7.8
SLP	0	$63,760	4,000**	$63,760	1.9

Total annual cost savings: $193,488
*Based on 2,000 employees
**2 Hour estimated completion time

tal, but more employees are taking advantage of the tool and fewer are attending the all-day program. The tool is a cost-effective strategy for meeting the mandatory in-service requirements and has the potential to save a substantial amount of money annually (see calculations above).

The self-learning material also has many other advantages over a lecture-type format. The material can be completed at the employee's own pace. It requires active participation, which is likely to result in better retention of information. When employees finish the material, they have a reference booklet for future use. The material is also much easier to update as needed.

Managing the mandatories usually is a challenge for staff development educators, but it also can be an opportunity to stretch thinking and become more innovative. Decentralizing required programs helps to foster staff nurse accountability and independence and allows the staff development department to focus on other aspects of the role that truly help to develop staff and promote professional practice. A process of letting go occurs when any responsibility is relinquished. But it's only letting go of the task, not the assurance that requirements are being fulfilled. The staff development department must continue to oversee the process and provide leadership, direction, support, and expertise to achieve the best outcome.

REFERENCES

American Nurses Association. (1994). *Standards for nursing professional development: Continuing education and staff development.* Washington, DC: Author.

Cosolo, N., Hicks, A., & Tietsort, J. (1995). *The competency primer: The building of a competency-focused system from the ground up.* Los Angeles: Academy Medical Systems.

Del Bueno, D. J. (1993). Competence, criteria, and credentialing. *Journal of Nursing Administration, 23*(5), 7–8.

Joint Commission of Accreditation of Healthcare Organizations. (1997). *Accreditation manual for hospitals.* Oakbrook Terrace, IL: Author.

Occupational Safety and Health Administration. (1996). *Employee emergency plans and fire prevention plans* (Standard 29 CFR 1910.38, 1996); *Hazard communication standard* (Standard 29 CFR 1910.1200, 1996); *Bloodborne pathogen training* (Standard 29 CFR 1910.1030, 1996).

8

Outcome Measurement in Clinical Staff Development

SUZANNE K. SIKMA

Outcome measurement is an important concern and function in clinical staff development. The staff development specialist is expected to be accountable for positive outcomes from the resources invested by an organization in the staff development program. He or she must demonstrate value, merit, effectiveness, goal attainment, and positive output or results. Evaluation of staff development outcomes may result in information that demonstrates how competent the staff are and how well the staff development interventions are working, and gives input for planning, policy-making, and accreditation. Measuring staff development outcomes will help demonstrate that staff development makes a difference and will provide insight into how interventions can be improved to make staff development programs even better for the people being served.

MULTIDISCIPLINARY PERSPECTIVES ON OUTCOMES

Educational Outcome Evaluation

Goals, objectives, intents, judgments, contexts, inputs, processes, and products are terms that have been defined and discussed as they relate to the evaluation of educational outcomes. Several models and conceptions from the education literature are relevant to measuring outcomes in staff development.

OBJECTIVE-BASED MODEL

In Tyler's (1967) objective-based evaluation model, the learner's behavioral objectives are the desired performance outcomes measured before, during, and after a program. In this model, learner behaviors are the ultimate criteria. This model focuses primarily on the classroom and the teacher and does not take into consideration structural, contextual, or procedural factors that might affect student performance (Stufflebeam & Shinkfield, 1985).

COUNTENANCE MODEL

Stake's (1967) countenance evaluation model, built on Tyler's, expands the concept of educational goal or outcome to include the results of the education process, which can take many forms. He used the term "intents" to reflect these educational goals or outcomes. He defined intents as including the environmental conditions, demonstrations, subject matter to be covered, and student behavior. Intents need to include the goals and plans that others have, particularly the students. Thus, intents includes a list of all that may happen as a result of the educational effort, not just narrowly defined student behavioral outcomes. He encouraged educators not to focus narrowly on a few variables in a program (such as outcomes associated with objectives) but to pay attention to the full countenance of evaluation. This full-countenance approach includes description and judgment of the program, using a variety of data sources, and multiple analyses to describe the program fully (Stufflebeam & Shinkfield, 1985).

RESPONSIVE EVALUATION MODEL

Stake expanded his philosophy of evaluation to include the necessity of "responsive evaluation" (Stufflebeam & Shinkfield, 1985). Responsive evaluation's dominant theme is providing a service to specific clients, making comprehensive statements about what the program is observed to be and about the satisfaction and dissatisfaction that appropriately selected people feel toward the program. Stake emphasized that evaluations are not useful if evaluators do not know the language and interests of their audience and if they do not couch their reports in this language.

CONSUMER-ORIENTED EVALUATION

Scriven (1967) emphasized that the goal of evaluation is to judge value, but that the roles of evaluation are varied. He defined two main roles of evaluation: formative (to assist in developing programs) and summative (to assess the value of the program once it has been developed and put into use). Formative evaluation helps the educational staff improve what they are developing; summative evaluation is more consumer-oriented, providing assessments that compare the costs, merits, and worth of competing programs or products and judgments about the extent to which the goals validly reflect the assessed needs of the consumer (Stufflebeam & Shinkfield, 1985).

IMPROVEMENT-ORIENTED EVALUATION

Stufflebeam (1971) characterized his "CIPP" model as improvement-oriented evaluation (Stufflebeam & Shinkfield, 1985). This model includes four types of evaluation:

1. Context: the environment in which the program takes place (including institutional conditions, target population and needs, opportunities and problems underlying the needs)
2. Input: the system capabilities (internal and external resources, alternate strategies and procedural designs)
3. Process: the implementation (identification, predicting and monitoring for potential problems, recording and judging the procedural events and activities)
4. Product: interpreting the worth and merit of the outcomes (descriptions and judgments of outcomes related to objectives and context, input and process information).

Stufflebeam (1971) claimed that this model is more in line with a systems view of education and human services, concentrating not so much on an individual study but rather on providing ongoing evaluation services to the decision-makers in an institution. It is based on the view that evaluation is not merely an instrument of accountability and that the purpose of evaluation is not to prove but to improve. Evaluation is seen as a tool by which to make programs better for the people they are intended to serve.

Human Resources and Staff Development Outcome Evaluation

Concepts from the educational outcome literature are strongly reflected in the literature on evaluation in human resources development and staff development. Literature in this field of practice addresses the multiple levels of evaluation required when education is

DISPLAY 8-1

Sample of Reaction-Level Questions to Measure Critical Thinking Indices

1. At what moment during this course were you most engaged with what was happening?
2. At what moment were you most disconnected with what was happening?
3. What action taken (by anyone) did you find most helpful or affirming?
4. What action taken (by anyone) did you find most puzzling or unhelpful?
5. What, if anything, surprised you the most?
6. How would you rate your ability to apply your learning in practice?
   diminished ability   no change   enhanced ability

Developed by Susan Jeska, Fairview Hospital and Healthcare Services. Based on the work of Stephen Brookfield. Used with permission.

practiced in organizations whose primary purpose is something other than education. The staff development specialist in these contexts must look at outcomes beyond the level of the individual learner.

Kirkpatrick (1994) described a four-level model of evaluation for professionals in education, training, and human resources development that included the evaluation levels of reaction, learning, behavior, and results:

1. Reaction evaluation measures "the reaction or satisfaction of the participants in the program" (p. 21). Two application samples of reaction-level questions are shown in Displays 8-1 and 8-2.
2. Evaluation of learning is defined as "the extent to which participants change attitudes, improve knowledge, and/or increase skill" (p. 22).
3. Evaluation of behavior is defined as "the extent to which change in behavior occurs as a result of participation in training" (p. 22).
4. Evaluation of results is defined as "final results that occur because participants attended the program" (p. 25), such as increased production, improved quality, decreased costs, reduced frequency or severity of accidents, increased sales, decreased turnover, and higher profits.

Puetz (1985) discussed program evaluation in nursing staff development and differentiated between approaches to individual evaluation and program evaluation. She reviewed both qualitative and quantitative methodologies and instruments for program evaluation

DISPLAY 8-2

Sample of Reaction-Level Questions Related to Appreciative Inquiry Indices

1. What was your peak experience during this conference?
2. What did you value most about this conference?
3. If you could imagine that you have fully integrated your learning into practice, what would be different from your present practice?
4. If you had three wishes for next year's conference, what would they be?

Developed by Susan Jeska, Fairview Hospital and Healthcare Services. Based on the work of David Cooperrider. Used with permission.

and delineated four stages of evaluation: needs assessment, program planning, formative evaluation, and summative evaluation. She also presented a variety of approaches to program evaluation, including judicial, transactional, discretionary, and cost analysis, as well as the quality assurance process.

In nursing staff development, Alspach (1995) proposed a comparable evaluation model that included four levels of evaluation output or results:

1. Satisfaction: the learner's satisfaction or happiness in reaction to content, teaching methods, instructors, materials, and so forth
2. Learning: whether learning has occurred, as measured by changes in cognitive, affective, and psychomotor behaviors
3. Application: the learner's application of learning in the work setting, such as increased clinical competence and improvements in nursing practice
4. Impact: the impact of the program on the organization and its patients or customers; includes elements such as length of stay, incidence of negative outcomes, patient satisfaction, productivity, cost of care, and quality of care.

Abruzzese's evaluation model (1996) in nursing staff development is similar to Kirkpatrick's but adds a fifth level:

1. Process evaluation: general happiness with the learning experience
2. Content evaluation: change in knowledge, affect, or skill on completion of a learning experience
3. Outcome evaluation: changes in practice on a clinical unit after a learning experience
4. Impact evaluation: organizational results attributable in part to learning experiences
5. Total program evaluation: congruence of program goals and accomplishments.

Patient and Health Outcome Evaluation

In health care organizations, clinical results, referred to as patient outcomes, are a priority concern. The clinical staff development specialist must consider patient outcomes in needs assessment and planning and evaluation of educational offerings. The patient and health outcome literature defines the staff development outcomes relevant in broader clinical, multidisciplinary, and organizational contexts.

Lang and Marek (1992) reviewed the past and present use of outcome measures in the evaluation of the effectiveness of nursing practice. They described the construct of outcome as highly complex and defined it as "an end result of a treatment or outcome" (p. 27). They described and grouped outcomes reflected in the nursing literature in several areas:

- Physiologic status measures
- Psychosocial status measures
- Functional measures related to activities of daily living
- Behavioral measures
- Knowledge and cognitive understanding
- Quality of life
- Safety
- Home functioning
- Family strain

- Goal attainment
- Patient satisfaction
- Caring achievement
- Nursing diagnosis resolution
- Use of services.

They pointed out several key issues and questions that need to be asked when evaluating outcomes:

- What is the population for which the treatment is done and to which the outcomes are related?
- What is the treatment or intervention?
- When is the end point?
- Are multiple measures needed?
- Does the outcome measure represent the end result desired?

Hegyvary (1992) acknowledged the variety of perspectives involved in outcomes research and proposed that practitioners, providers, and researchers need to broaden their conceptual horizons, approaching problems not only from the point of view of their own discipline in parallel with others, but also in an integrated way across disciplines, organizations, and communities. She pointed out the need to assess and define the various assumptions and perspectives being used in the current and desired positions and also to be clear about the nature of the questions being asked. For example, what conditions and actions produce what outcomes? How are the conditions, actions, and outcomes defined?

Lohr (1988) described how the definition of medical outcomes has shifted over time. The classic definition of the five "D's" was rather negative (death, disease, disability, discomfort, dissatisfaction) and reflected outcomes to avoid. The shift she described has been to more positive aspects of health, including survival rates, states of physiologic, physical, and emotional health, and satisfaction with health care services. These more positive indicators are also best measured using an integrated, multidisciplinary view.

Eddy (1992) also defined health outcomes from a medical practice point of view, asserting that the identification of health outcomes is a crucial step in the assessment of a health practice and the design of a practice policy. He defined health outcomes as those "that people can experience (feel physically or mentally) and care about. They relate to the length and quality of life, including death, functional disability, appearance, pain, anxiety, reassurance, and peace of mind" (pp. 24–25).

Crane (1992) proposed a multidisciplinary definition of outcomes research as "any inquiry that is designed to measure—and ultimately improve—the outcome of treatment and thereby the health status of individuals and communities" (p. 56). He claimed that this definition would encompass efficacy, effectiveness, and appropriateness research. He described three distinguishing characteristics of outcomes research:

1. A focus on conditions and alternative treatments for conditions
2. A concern not just with clinical or physiologic outcomes, but also with measures of health-related quality of life
3. A recognition that the outcomes of any treatment process are affected by both nonclinical factors (*e.g.*, patient sociodemographic characteristics, organization and delivery of care, financial incentives) and clinical intervention factors. Thus, he argued that a multidisciplinary approach to outcome research is necessary.

The Joint Commission on Accreditation of Healthcare Organizations has defined an outcome as "the result of a process" (1994, p. 22). A good outcome is a result that achieves the goal of the process. Goals that relate to patient health include avoiding adverse effects of care, improved physiologic status, decreased signs and symptoms, and increased functional status and well-being. Non–health-related but still relevant outcomes include patient satisfaction, minimizing the cost of care, and maximizing revenues.

Program Outcome Evaluation

Staff development outcomes are often articulated in the broader context of clinical program implementation and evaluation. The field of program evaluation is developing as a strong multidisciplinary practice area. Literature in this area is strongly influenced by research theories; program evaluators have described research models applied in the real world of evaluating programs in dynamic, complex organizational environments.

Ingersoll (1996) defined evaluation as research and described approaches to developing theory-driven evaluations. She argued that theory can help guide the selection of outcome indicators, clarify what actually occurred as opposed to what was intended, and identify, describe, and understand both intended and unintended outcomes. She reviewed several evaluation theories and elaborated how they might be applied in guiding evaluation research. She argued that the intent of evaluation is to determine whether something makes a difference or not. In an input–process–outcome model of evaluation theory, the outcome component would include the unique characteristics of the intervention and would describe what should be seen as a result of the intervention. It may be subdivided into early and late outcomes. Ingersoll wrote that although this model provides some guidance about what influences intervention, implementation, and outcome, it does not give much information about how or why.

Ingersoll also discussed McClintock's model, in which a concept map is used to define relations among intervention components and anticipated outcomes. The guiding philosophy and the service components are noted at the top of the model. Next are the causal processes by which these are expected to benefit patients in relation to the measurable outcomes of each component. This type of model or map allows for operationalizing the concepts and facilitates monitoring of implementation and the extent of outcomes.

Chen defined program theory as "a specification of what must be done to achieve the desired goals, what other important impacts may also be anticipated, and how these goals and impacts would be generated" (1990, p. 43). He divided program theory into two parts:

1. Normative (prescriptive) theory deals with what the structure of a program should be, including such things as treatments, outcomes, and implementation processes that are related to the values of the program. Normative theory can come from experience, assumptions, customary practices, or prior knowledge and theory. It guides program planning, formulation, and implementation. A program is created for the purpose of providing services or solving problems. These purposes are formally called goals or intended outcomes. The outcome domain of normative theory addresses the goals or intended outcomes that the program strives to achieve. The outcome domain concerns both intended and unintended outcomes. Normative outcome evaluation (often referred to as summative or outcome evaluation) is defined as "an attempt to assist stakeholders in identifying, clarifying, or developing the goals or outcomes of a program for program improvement" (p. 91).

2. Causative (descriptive) theory specifies how the program works by identifying conditions under which certain processes arise and what their likely consequences will be. Causative theory represents empirical knowledge about

causal relations between treatments and outcomes. It specifies the underlying causal mechanisms that link, mediate, or condition the causal relation between treatment variables and outcome variables. This is referred to as the impact domain—assessing the impact of treatment on the outcome.

Patton defined evaluation as "the systematic collection of information about the activities, characteristics, and outcomes of programs for use by specific people to reduce uncertainties, improve effectiveness, and make decisions with regard to what those programs are doing and affecting" (1987, p. 15). Patton argued that "there is no one best way to conduct an evaluation" (p. 19). Every evaluation situation is unique; a successful evaluation emerges from the special characteristics of a particular situation. He stated that evaluation decision criteria must be multiple, flexible, creative, and diverse. This suggests that it is important to understand the scope and nature of clinical staff development practice and the complex contexts in which it is practiced.

WHO IS THE STAFF DEVELOPMENT CLIENT?

The staff development specialist provides services in the context of often complex and rapidly changing organizational environments. Thus, evaluation of staff development outcomes requires consideration of the multiple levels of clients we serve. Staff development clients may be conceptualized at the individual, group, or community level.

The primary clients served by the staff development specialist are the health care providers to whom the specialist provides instruction. The goal is to build their capacity and competence for providing care to health care consumers. Staff development interventions at the individual level are grounded in an understanding of individual learning needs, style, goals, and capacity. Competence (the capability or possession of knowledge, skills, and attitudes to function) may be seen as a primary desired outcome of individual-level staff development interventions.

Staff development interventions are also sometimes geared toward groups—for instance, all the staff on a particular nursing unit, or a particular group of staff with a common role, such as nurse case managers from multiple units. The goal is to develop capacity and competence of a group with a common relationship such as function, program or specialty, or clientele. Staff development interventions at this level might be geared toward supporting a group or departmental goal, program, or care delivery model.

An organization is a type of community, a group of persons with a common affiliation and some level of interdependence in the larger whole of the organizational environment. The organizational environment may also be the target of staff development interventions. For example, organization-wide interventions designed to promote collaboration, cooperation, and involvement of care providers might be designed with organizational needs, goals, and outcomes in mind. Staff development interventions can create and influence the environment, not just develop a person's capacity to respond to it.

DEFINITION AND CHARACTERISTICS OF STAFF DEVELOPMENT OUTCOMES

The previous discussion has illustrated the broad range of contexts and definitions used to describe the term "outcome" in related disciplines. For the rest of this chapter, "staff development outcome" will be defined as an end result of a staff development intervention.

This broad definition is proposed so that it may be applied to the multiple levels of clients that staff development specialists serve in a wide range of clinical disciplines and health care organizations.

The following are characteristics of staff development outcomes:

- People can experience them. Staff development outcomes are changes in human capacity, competence, and behavior that individually or collectively are experienced and can be measured, described, or observed.
- People care about them. Staff development interventions are designed with stakeholders in mind; thus, the outcomes of the interventions (or lack of them) are also important. A key issue in defining outcomes is determining the purposes and desired outcomes of the various stakeholders in the process.
- Multiple levels of clients create multiple levels of expectations. Defining and measuring staff development outcomes involve considering the needs and goals of the multiple clients served on the three levels mentioned. Outcomes are defined differently based on the intentions, needs, and desires of the various clients or groups. Describing unexpected as well as expected outcomes is important in reporting results.
- Outcomes occur in the context of organizational conditions. It is important to clarify and describe the conditions in which staff development interventions and outcomes occur. Attention must be devoted to the context as well as to the processes of staff development interventions to understand their relation to outcomes of staff development efforts.

A MODEL FOR CONCEPTUALIZING STAFF DEVELOPMENT OUTCOMES

Relation Between Level of Client and Outcomes

In planning an evaluation of staff development outcomes, the staff development specialist must consider both the level of the targeted client and the goal of the intervention to select appropriate types of outcomes and measures of those outcomes. Table 8-1 shows how staff development interventions might target four types of staff development outcomes at each level of intervention (individual, group, or organizational levels). The four types of outcomes are:

1. Well-being and satisfaction (or reaction) of the client
2. New competence or capacity of the client
3. Enactment of learning through performance or application of learning by the client
4. Direct and indirect impacts on the well-being and health of patients, the organization as a whole, or the community.

This model might be applied by the staff development specialist in planning small- or large-scale outcome evaluations. With the goals of the intervention in mind, the intervention and targeted level of implementation are selected. The staff development specialist can then select or negotiate with other stakeholders the desired outcomes of different types to include in the evaluation.

TABLE 8-1

EXAMPLES OF LEVELS AND TYPES OF STAFF DEVELOPMENT (SD) OUTCOMES

Level of Client	Type of SD Outcome			
	Well-being (satisfaction and reaction) of SD Client	New Capacity and Competence of SD Client	Enactment of Learning (performance/application of SD client)	Well-being (direct/indirect impacts) of SD Client
Individual	Individual satisfaction measures	Individual changes in knowledge, skill, attitude (KSA)	Individual enactment and application of new KSA	Individual patient outcomes: positive, avoid negative. Customer satisfaction.
Group	Aggregate satisfaction measures	Group competence. Readiness for program change. Shared meanings.	Collective enactment of learning: knowledge, skill, attitudes, teamwork.	Cost-effectiveness at unit level. Group retention and satisfaction. Unit changes managed successfully.
Organization	Aggregate satisfaction measures. Measures of organizational learning climate.	Shared vision/goals/attitudes. Organizational level expertise.	Care standards met. Information processed efficiently. Efficient process adaptation.	Profit or fiscal viability. Reputation. Goal accomplishment on multiple levels.

Application of the Staff Development Outcome Model in a Clinical Organization

Consider the example of a long-term care facility that implements a clinical program through a special care unit for older adult residents with advanced cognitive impairment due to Alzheimer's disease and related disorders (ADRD). The organization has determined that there is a strong community need for such a program, with a good potential for maintaining high census. The program is not without risks, however. The population is extremely vulnerable, and without well-trained, competent staff, the potential for adverse outcomes is high. People will need to be prepared at several levels (individual, group, and organizational) to provide respectful, individualized care for this challenging population while maintaining a balance of freedom and safety for their residents in a home-like environment.

INDIVIDUAL-LEVEL INTERVENTIONS

The staff development specialist might develop and implement an workshop to prepare caregivers to work with residents with ADRD and manage common behavioral manifestations. He or she might develop a reaction evaluation tool to give to learners at the end of the workshop to measure their satisfaction with the offering. He or she might also prepare tests of knowledge, skills, and attitudes about dementia care to learners at the beginning and end of the workshop to evaluate if their individual capacity or competence in ADRD care had changed as a result of the workshop. To measure outcomes at the performance level, the staff development specialist might pick a high-risk, high-volume behavioral issue such as wandering, observe the unit during high-risk sundown hours, and validate and quantify the interventions being used by trained staff to minimize and manage wandering behaviors. This would also be an opportunity for additional one-on-one coaching; staff development evaluation does not need to be a controlled experiment with detached, uninvolved observers. Finally, the staff development specialist might use the quality assessment data already being routinely gathered. Examples might include routine data collected on door alarms or elopement attempts by residents, review of unusual incident reports to determine any negative client outcomes related to wandering, or review for possible correlation between such quality assessment indicators and the staff on duty.

GROUP-LEVEL INTERVENTIONS

An example of a group-level staff development intervention is a special care unit team session facilitated by the staff development specialist. The goal is to minimize and manage effectively agitated behavior on the unit. The intervention would include an overview of the progressively lowered stress threshold (PLST) model (Hall & Buckwalter, 1987) of caregiving. A discussion would follow about each team member's roles in managing the level of stimulus and stress in the unit environment and how they as a team could work together to manage both environmental stressors on the unit and internal stressors within residents that might make people with ADRD become more agitated.

A simple way of measuring group satisfaction outcome would be to ask each group member to rate on a scale of 1 to 5 how satisfied he or she is with the process of the meeting and to report on their responses in aggregate. Competence change might be evaluated by having the group members reflect on what they have learned from the discussion; this discussion is facilitated by the staff development specialist and summarized into a team plan of the strategies they will use to manage the unit environment. An observation tool that measures environmental stressors as well as the team-designated approaches might be used during various times of the day to validate performance application of the PLST model by the staff in managing the unit environment. Residents' health and well-being outcomes might be demonstrated by measuring the incidence and persistence of agitation in the population.

ORGANIZATION-LEVEL INTERVENTIONS

An example of an organization-level intervention would be educating the total facility on the importance of security when entering and leaving the special care unit. The goals of the intervention are to promote security awareness, to prevent negative resident outcomes due to elopement, and to promote family satisfaction with the unit and security. An organization-level well-being or satisfaction indicator might be that the staff buy into and express satisfaction with the security consciousness philosophy. Competence and capacity would be demonstrated by all staff being able to use the alarm system properly in the learning activity. Performance application and enactment of learning could be monitored through quality assurance monitoring of alarms set off by staff or resident elopements that occur after staff enter or exit the unit. Impact outcomes on the organizational community might include quality assurance measures of resident and staff safety or overall congruence between the intervention's goals and accomplishments—for instance, no adverse events due to resident elopement, or family satisfaction with the safety and security of the unit.

SELECTING METHODS AND MEASUREMENTS FOR STAFF DEVELOPMENT OUTCOMES

There is no one best way to conduct an evaluation; what constitutes the best in a given situation depends on the criteria chosen. A variety of factors and alternatives must be taken into account to match the evaluation to the situation. Patton (1987) states that creative evaluation is a "paradigm of choices" involving a broad range of viable methods and approaches, including situation responsiveness, methodologic flexibility, conscious matching of evaluation approaches to the needs and interests of stakeholders, and sensitivity to the unique constraints and possibilities of particular circumstances. The following are questions to ask and issues to consider when planning an outcome evaluation:

1. What is the problem or need that is the basis for the educational intervention? Clarify the nature of the problem to be addressed through the educational intervention. What assumptions have been made about the problem and the educational interventions chosen to address the problem? Clarify the utilitarian as well as political needs being addressed by the educational intervention. The staff development specialist should reflect on his or her understanding of the original problem and educational need to provide perspective on where the outcome evaluation priority should be placed.

2. Who are the other stakeholders in the staff development intervention? What will they need to know and be interested in knowing about the outcome? Stakeholders may include the learners, decision- or policy-makers, program managers or administrators, or other persons or interest groups who sponsor the program or benefit from or use the results. It is important in planning an outcome evaluation to understand who the key stakeholders are and what their values, issues, and expectations are. What are their assumptions and expectations regarding program resources, activities, and intended outcomes? What are the crucial evaluation issues to them? How will they want to use the evaluation results in the future?

   Identifying and understanding stakeholder needs and expectations is a key consideration in the political aspect of outcome evaluation. In complex organizational environments, stakeholders are looking not only for observable, measurable "truth tests" of staff development outcomes but also for relevance tests that emphasize political values and utility tests, such as plausible results that offer new perspectives or support the status quo (Chen, 1990).

   Evaluations can be shaped to enfranchise or disenfranchise stakeholder groups in a variety of ways. Selectively involving stakeholders in the design and implementation of the evaluation and negotiating courses of action on which most stakeholders can agree makes it possible for persons to find a reason to support it, work at it, and feel good about it (Guba & Lincoln, 1989).

3. What is the nature of the outcome to be measured? The staff development specialist must clarify the type of outcomes most important to measure in the situation (as outlined in Table 8-1). Is the main concern demonstrating learner well-being and satisfaction, competency and capacity, performance and application of learning, or organizational impact? Or does this situation call for evaluating several or all of these types of outcomes? Also consider the client

level (individual, group, or organization) as it relates to the desired outcomes. Ranking the types and levels of outcomes desired and most important to the situation will help in selecting measurement methods and tools.

4. What or who are potential data sources? Obviously, the targeted learners of the intervention are a potential and an important data source. Other potential data sources to consider include the patients of the learners or other stakeholders who have interest and involvement in the situation. Finally, other data sources, if available, should not be overlooked, such as quality improvement or quality of care measurements, clinical documentation, financial and cost reports, customer satisfaction and quality of life measurements, staff satisfaction and retention data, and reports from external accreditation or review bodies.

5. What are the potential measurement methods and data collection tools available? Once the desired outcome and potential data sources have been clarified, the appropriate measurement methods will become more apparent. Does the desired outcome lend itself best to objective measures of adaptation and change? Or is the desired outcome better addressed by more subjective description, such as discovery of insights, learning, and change? Is the goal to measure incremental or widespread change?

Table 8-2 provides examples of measurement approaches or methods appropriate to a continuum of subjective to objective perspectives. Depending on the nature and scope of the evaluation, one or several methods to measure

TABLE 8-2

METHODOLOGIC APPROACHES TO OUTCOME MEASUREMENT

Subjective	Objective
Methods that involve discovery or disclosure of perceptions, descriptions of insights, learning, or other qualitative changes.	Methods that involve objective, quantitative measurements of adaptation/change from incremental to revolutionary change
• Interviews	• Pretests and posttests of knowledge, skill, or attitudes
• Participant observation	• Return demonstration
• Focus groups	• Discrepancy evaluation
• Advisory boards	• Goal accomplishment appraisal
• Critique	• Simulation testing
• Dialogue	• Rating scales of indicators such as quality of life, quality of care
• Games/experiential exercises	• Record audits
• Disclosure of unintended outcomes	• Document audits
• Picture or story thinking	• Competency measurement
• Satisfaction measures	• Cost-effectiveness measures
• Open-ended surveys	• Surveys with quantitative measures
• Case study—qualitative in-depth	• Case study—quantitative in-depth
• Critical incident analysis	• Critical incident analysis

the desired outcomes of the intervention may be selected. The more complex the nature of the client and the broader the scope of the intervention, the more important it may be to consider multiple methods from different points of view (both subjective and objective). Some of the measurement approaches in Table 8-2 may be adapted to either end of the continuum; others, by their nature, are better suited to one end of the continuum or the other. The key is to match the method selected with the evaluation question, purpose, and audience need.

6. What is practical and appropriate in this situation? In the world of practice, resources for evaluation are limited, so an outcome evaluation must be shaped by matters of practicality. The staff development specialist should consider resource limitations, the nature and scope of the intervention, the interests and priorities of the client and other stakeholders, and the specifics and risks of the particular situation to determine what is the most practical. The goal is to find the most appropriate approach with the most potential for accomplishing the desired goals within the context of the situation and the resources available.

REPORTING AND USING THE RESULTS OF OUTCOME MEASUREMENT

Once the outcome evaluation is complete, the challenge is to report and use the results effectively. The following areas should be addressed in developing the outcome evaluation report:

1. Consider audience needs. Who is the audience for this report? Is there one audience or several? Is only one report needed, or are several needed for different audiences? Thinking about audience needs will help determine how much information and detail to include in the report and what results to highlight. What format will be most effective? Will a written report, a presentation, or a combination be used to present the result to a single or different audiences?

2. Describe the context of the need for the staff development intervention and outcome evaluation. Summarize how the intervention and evaluation relate to the overall mission and goals of the organization, unit, or program. Remind the audience of the need behind the intervention. If the intervention was related to a clinical program change, consider summarizing the relevant clinical factors related to the program before the intervention, as well as the desired clinical program changes. Consider including a description of learner characteristics and competencies as they were before the intervention. Also describe noneducational and nonclinical contextual factors that may have influenced the perception of the need for the intervention—for instance, personal attributes and preferences of the staff, the way service is organized and delivered, and financial incentives.

3. Describe the intervention process and desired outcomes. Describe the needs assessment, the plan for the intervention, and the desired outcomes. What actions were taken to implement the intervention? Once again, when describing the intervention process, consider the effect of context. What, if any, contextual events (*e.g.*, unanticipated events, occupancy changes, change in leadership or staff, budget cuts, regulatory changes) occurred during the course of the intervention that may have affected it?

4. Describe the evaluation. Summarize the evaluation methods selected and the rationale for choosing them. Describe data sources used in terms of type, number, and characteristics. Describe the data collection methods used and provide examples of relevant data collection tools as appropriate to the audience's needs. Describe any efforts made to ensure credibility and trustworthiness or validity and reliability of the results. Also describe any efforts made to protect confidentiality and the rights of humans participating in the evaluation.

5. Describe the outcome evaluation results. Descriptions of the evaluation results will vary based on the type of measurement strategies chosen for the evaluation. For more subjective evaluation methodologies such as interviews, focus group discussions, or advisory board critiques, descriptions of themes, issues, and insights emerging from the discussions may be presented. Commonalties and disparities among themes from different stakeholder groups might be highlighted. If a strategy such as "picture thinking" or story-telling (Patton, 1987) has been used, a series of pictures or excerpts from stories may be used to highlight themes from the evaluation. If more traditional objective measures have been used, tables and figures summarizing ratings, quantitative performance measures, and statistics may be effective in illustrating the results. For evaluations that have used multiple and diverse methods, a combination of reporting types may be used to illustrate the results in ways that would appeal to a wide and diverse audience. It is important to know the audience members so that they are not either overwhelmed with detail or underwhelmed with inadequate evidence to convince them of the significance of the results.

Sometimes the staff development specialist is asked for progress data on outcome evaluations in process. Deciding whether or not to provide preview results is an important decision. There are scientific and political risks in revealing preliminary results that may not be substantiated when the total evaluation is completed. Some stakeholders may be looking for preliminary information to support or refute a particular point of view to subvert the implementation and change process. On the other hand, stakeholders providing resources for the intervention may expect accountability from the staff development specialist in terms of interim reports or accounts of ongoing progress in an extended project. Once again, the staff development specialist must consider the circumstances, risks, and requirements of the situation to determine whether this is appropriate. If the decision is made to offer preliminary data, the nature of the interim results most appropriate to share must be determined.

6. List and discuss conclusions and recommendations. This is the staff development specialist's opportunity to interpret and summarize significant results. Highlight the most significant conclusions from the evaluation. Interpret the strengths and weaknesses of the intervention and evaluation. Suggest what needs to be continued, changed, or discarded. Tie the recommendations to unit or organizational goals, needs, and priorities. Emphasize how value has been added through staff development interventions. Make suggestions for continuing evolution of the program.

Outcome evaluation may be used in single interventions or projects or in a total staff development program. In looking at a total program, it is useful to identify where resources will be expended on outcome evaluations. A department may routinely collect satisfaction or reaction data on most offerings or measure competencies routinely on identified groups of staff at designated points in time (*e.g.*, orientation). This type of routine outcome data summary can be combined with the results of one or two high-priority organizational change projects and staff development utilization and productivity statistics to illustrate the effectiveness of the staff development program or department as a whole. Taking the time to consolidate and summarize a wide range of evaluation data in an annual or other periodic report is a good investment of time and energy before a new budget or departmental planning cycle.

SUMMARY

This chapter has reviewed multiple perspectives on outcome evaluation and has presented a model that may be used to guide outcome evaluation of staff development interventions at several levels. Selecting salient outcome measures and reporting and presenting them in a meaningful way to interested stakeholders not only demonstrates accountability but also helps clinical staff development specialists demonstrate that their programs make a difference to individual learners, groups of learners, patients, organizational decision-makers, organizations, and systems.

Comparison of Outcomes Assessment of Teaching Strategies of the Foundations of Intensive Care Course

DONNA GLOE

Each of us is concerned about how the changes in health care are going to affect us and the quality of the care we provide. When hiring practices changed, it affected St. John's Department of Continuing Education, and we had to search for effective ways to deliver education in a more cost-effective manner. It was the concern for quality that led us to devise the following study to compare outcomes.

St. John's Regional Health Center is a tertiary health care facility with 866 licensed beds. It offers an array of medical and surgical services, including intensive care nursing. About 500 nurses are employed in the seven adult intensive care units. Nurses who practice in an intensive care nursing area need a certain body of knowledge to assess, monitor, and provide nursing care to critically ill patients. St. John's Department of Continuing Education offers a Foundations of Intensive Care (FIC) course. All RNs employed in the adult intensive care units must take the FIC course or successfully complete challenge testing.

The didactic course was fairly typical of other courses used to prepare nurses for specialized

practice. It consisted of body systems and disease review, dysrhythmia recognition, Code Blue protocol, pharmacology, patient care interventions, and patient education. The original course was 80 hours long and was given Monday through Friday for 2 consecutive weeks.

Early in 1994, it became necessary to integrate nurses employed on a merged medical nursing unit into other areas in the health center. Two nurses chose to transfer to critical care areas. Because those two nurses needed the course immediately, a vice president requested the development of a self-directed learning version of the FIC course. Also, due to changing health center needs, fewer nurses were being hired, which made the original didactic course impractical. June 1994 was the last time the 80-hour didactic course was held.

Instead, a self-directed learning (SDL) FIC course was developed. This course was presented as a pilot for the two nurses who were moving into critical care employment and then was revised based on their experiences and feedback. The SDL course covered the same topics as the didactic course. The course materials consisted of reading modules, videotapes, and some discussion between the participants, the course facilitator, and members of the department of continuing education who had critical care background and expertise. The course was held Monday through Wednesday for 3 consecutive weeks.

The quality and cost-effectiveness of the SDL course were evaluated. Several questions were posed concerning the comparison of the two courses. International (via the Internet) and regional trends in critical care courses were solicited via a questionnaire, the scores of three tests (dysrhythmia, Code Blue, and comprehensive) were statistically compared (two-tailed t-test with Bonferroni technique), the cost of each course was calculated, the performance evaluations written at the end of the nurses' probationary period were obtained and statistically compared (two-tailed t-test), and level 1 (reaction) evaluations from both groups were also statistically compared (two-tailed t-test with Bonferroni technique). A search of the literature revealed that no study of this kind had been published.

The results of this study were very interesting. The response to the trends questionnaire posted on the Internet bulletin board NURSENET yielded nine responses out of total membership of 1,886, which was not a large enough sampling from which to draw conclusions. The regional trends questionnaire was mailed to similar hospitals in the geographical region surrounding southwest Missouri and yielded an 81% response rate. The analysis showed that St. John's fit into the regional trends related to critical care courses, course content, testing procedures, and so forth. St. John's expectations in test completion (90% in a total of three attempts) was a higher standard than that used in the surrounding hospitals.

The didactic FIC held in June 1994 had 32 participants. A comparative sample of 32 was gathered from the SDL course held in the fall and winter, 1995 into 1996. The test comparison

(level 2) yielded no results that were statistically significant, but the mean SDL score was slightly higher than the mean didactic score (due to space limitations, the statistics are not reported). The performance evaluation results were the same; the two groups were not statistically significantly different.

However, the cost calculations for the two courses were very different. The initial didactic course was estimated to cost $114,689, the initial SDL course $86,562. The costs of subsequent courses were estimated at didactic, $106,122 and SDL, $41,916. The SDL course was significantly less costly than the didactic course.

Also very different were the level 1 (reaction) evaluation comparisons between the two courses. Participants' reactions to the didactic course were much more positive than to the SDL course. The reasons for this preference could be as varied as the participants. Participants may be accustomed to the didactic format and feel comfortable with it; many people feel threatened and uncomfortable with the unfamiliar. Another factor may be the motivation of the participants. It is much less work to sit in a lecture than to be self-directed in learning. SDL requires more responsibility and diligence toward the learning goals on the part of the participant than does a didactic format. Except for cost calculations, level 3 and 4 strategies were not done.

These analyses led to several conclusions. First, there were no significant differences in knowledge assessment or performance evaluation between the didactic course and the SDL course; the major differences were cost and student learning preferences. Therefore, the cost was weighed against student preferences. The cost savings of providing the SDL course was significant over a year's time. Continuing the more cost-effective course was a logical choice, while helping the participants make the transition from didactic learning to SDL.

REFERENCES

Abruzzese, R. S. (1996). *Nursing staff development: Strategies for success*, 2nd ed. St. Louis, MO: Mosby.
Alspach, J. G. (1995). *The educational process in nursing staff development*. St. Louis, MO: Mosby.
Chen, H. T. (1990). *Theory-driven evaluations*. Newbury Park, CA: Sage.

Crane, S. C. (1992). A research agenda for outcomes research. In National Center for Nursing Research (Ed.). *Patient outcomes research: Examining the effectiveness of nursing practice. Proceedings of the State of the Science Conference* (NIH Publication No. 93-3411, pp. 54–62). Washington DC: Department of Health and Human Services, Public Health Service, National Institutes of Health.

Eddy, D. M. (1992). *A manual for assessing health practices and designing practice policies.* Philadelphia: American College of Physicians.

Guba, E., & Lincoln, Y. (1989). *Fourth-generation evaluation.* Newbury Park, CA: Sage.

Hall, G. R., & Buckwalter, K. C. (1987). Progressively lowered stress threshold: A conceptual model for care of adults with Alzheimer's disease. *Archives of Psychiatric Nursing, 1,* 399–406.

Hegyvary, S. T. (1992). Outcomes research: Integrating nursing practice into the world view. In National Center for Nursing Research (Ed.). *Patient outcomes research: Examining the effectiveness of nursing practice. Proceedings of the State of the Science Conference* (NIH Publication No. 93-3411, pp. 17–24). Washington DC: Department of Health and Human Services, Public Health Service, National Institutes of Health.

Ingersoll, G. L. (1996). Evaluation research. *Nursing Administration Quarterly, 20*(4), 28–40.

Joint Commission on Accreditation of Healthcare Organizations. (1994). *A guide to establishing programs for assessing outcomes in clinical settings.* Oakbrook Terrace, IL: JCAHO.

Kirkpatrick, D. L. (1994). *Evaluating training programs: The four levels.* San Francisco: Berrett-Koehler.

Lang, N. M., & Marek, K. D. (1992). Outcomes that reflect clinical practice. In National Center for Nursing Research (Ed.). *Patient outcomes research: Examining the effectiveness of nursing practice. Proceedings of the State of the Science Conference* (NIH Publication No. 93-3411, pp. 27–38). Washington DC: Department of Health and Human Services, Public Health Service, National Institutes of Health.

Lohr, K. N. (1988). Outcome measurement: Concepts and questions. *Inquiry, 25*(1), 37–50.

Patton, M. Q. (1987). *Creative evaluation,* 2d ed. Newbury Park, CA: Sage.

Puetz, B. E. (1985). Evaluation in nursing staff development. Rockville, MD: Aspen.

Scriven, M. (1967). The methodology of evaluation. In Tyler, R. (Ed.). *Perspectives of curriculum evaluation.* Chicago: Rand McNally.

Stake, R. E. (1967). The countenance of educational evaluation. *Teachers College Record, 68*(7), 523–540.

Stufflebeam, D. L. (1971). *Educational evaluation and decision making.* Itasca, IL: F. E. Peacock.

Stufflebeam, D. L., & Shinkfield, A. J. (1985). *Systematic evaluation: A self-instructional guide to theory and practice.* Boston: Kluwer-Nijhoff.

Tyler, R. (1967). *Perspectives of curriculum evaluation.* Chicago: Rand McNally.

9

Staff Development Programs: Strategic Thinking Applied

LORRY SCHOENLY

This chapter discusses application of curriculum design and strategic thinking principles to the planning of an overall staff development program. For the purposes of this discussion, the term "staff development program" will be used to mean the overall plan of staff development activities performed in an organization. This program is likely to involve multiple courses, individual programs, offerings, in-services, and orientation and seeks to meet the learning needs of a diverse group of health care providers. Curriculum design elements will be discussed and applied to clinical and nursing staff development. Common staff development programs will be discussed as they relate to curriculum design.

STRATEGIC THINKING IN STAFF DEVELOPMENT

Staff development in health care institutions encompasses a wide scope of content. Staff development specialists are being asked to manage the staff development and continuing education needs of professional and support staff, along with continuing responsibilities for nursing staff education. In most situations, these new responsibilities are not met with increases in the number of educators on staff—indeed, sometimes departments that have been reduced in size are assigned added responsibilities.

Strategic thinking and creative planning are necessary to meet the educational needs of a larger group of health care staff. Strategic planning is no longer a luxury; it has become a necessity. A well-designed program of offerings in orientation, in-service, and continuing education can move the health care organization and its staff to higher levels of expertise, enhancing both patient care, the product of the organization, and effective, efficient operations, the process of the organization.

Planning is future thinking (Bolan, 1974) and action laid out in advance (Sawyer, 1983). Schwendiman (1976) defined planning as the fitting together of ongoing activities into a meaningful whole. It is this aspect of the meaningful whole that leads to strategic thinking and curriculum design in nursing staff development. Rather than relying on individual units of educational activity created to meet needs as they arise, strategic thinking allows for future thinking and action laid out in advance, thereby creating a meaningful whole.

A well-thought-out total program of staff development allows for the productive educational activities and the ability to move the organization forward. Coordinating common themes in individual developmental needs allows for an integrated and comprehensive approach to erasing learning deficits.

TOTAL PROGRAM PLANNING

To design well-constructed staff development programs, staff development specialists can use many elements of a curriculum planning model. Curriculum design is a format for total program planning in staff development.

Several authors have documented the need for curriculum design in nursing staff development (Leroux & Cody, 1996, Schoenly, 1994, Alspach, 1995, O'Connor, 1986). Total program planning through curriculum design provides a proactive approach, focusing on the critical needs of staff (Leroux & Cody, 1996). It provides a basis for ranking programming options for staff education (O'Connor, 1986). This means that programming is done in response to strategic organizational needs rather than on the demands of short-term crises or budget allocations. A well-designed curriculum is more likely to involve all levels of organizational staff rather than just the immediate needs of beginning staff, such as survival and entry-level skills.

CURRICULUM DESIGN MODEL

Alspach (1995) described curriculum development as the determination and arrangement of the educational components such that there is "optimal facilitation" of learning. To reach this goal, she identified five aspects of curriculum design (Display 9-1). Traditional academic models of curriculum design identify four elements of curriculum design (Display 9-2). The design elements of conceptual framework, objectives, curricular threads, and process elements make up O'Connor's model (1986) (Display 9-3).

Using concepts from all three models, a nursing staff development curriculum design model for total program planning was created (Display 9-4). This design model was created specifically for this text to help staff development specialists and is a continuation of the author's model development (Schoenly, 1994).

As shown in Figure 9-1, this curriculum design model is thematic rather than linear. Although curriculum design can follow a general sequence, planning involves the continual re-evaluation of elements in relation to one another. Therefore, the designer may choose to begin at any one topic in the framework and move to other areas as he or she continues to re-evaluate the design for consistency and fit among the elements. Instructional design and evaluation are not included as major themes in this curriculum design model; rather, instructional design and evaluation of individual programs and classes within the curriculum are considered as they relate to the elements of the total staff development program.

The entire curriculum design revolves around the organizational and individual developmental needs of the target audience. The curriculum's conceptual framework and the curricular threads support the design.

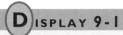

DISPLAY 9-1

Elements of Curriculum Design According to Alspach (1995)

1. Selection of content or subject matter
2. Planning the order and timing of instruction
3. Selecting instructional media
4. Designating and managing faculty
5. Preparing instructional schedules

DISPLAY 9-2

Elements of Curriculum Design According to Ornstein and Hunkins (1988)

1. Aims, goals, and objectives
2. Subject matter
3. Learning experiences
4. Evaluation approaches

DISPLAY 9-3

Elements of Curriculum Design According to O'Connor (1986)

1. Conceptual framework
2. Objectives
3. Curricular threads
4. Process elements

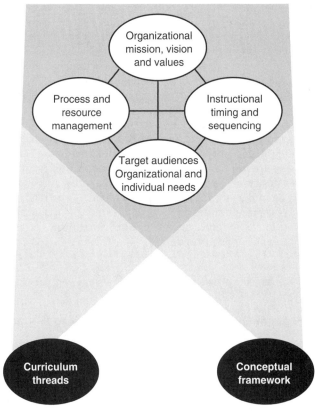

FIGURE 9-1. Nursing staff development curriculum design model.

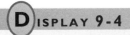

ISPLAY 9-4

Nursing Staff Development Curriculum Design Model

Organizational mission, vision, and values
Conceptual framework
Target audiences
Organization and individual developmental needs
Curriculum threads
Process and resource management
Instructional timing and sequencing

Organizational Mission, Vision, and Values

Understanding the organization's mission, vision, and values is the vital first step in total program planning. Strategic thinking is based on an understanding of the organizational culture in which the staff development department operates. An organization's mission is, in effect, the definition of who it is and what it does. The vision is who it hopes to be and where it is going. Finally, every organization works from an underlying set of values, whether implicit or explicit. These values drive strategic decision making at the senior management level.

Staff development specialists must align the department's mission, vision, and values with those of the organization. Inconsistency between these will hinder total program outcomes. Should educators find that the organization's mission, vision, or values are incompatible with sound educational principles, steps should be taken to influence organizational change toward embracing these principles.

Cues in the work environment, usually linked to money and time allocation, can show the organization's and management's values about educational planning. Examples include budgetary allocations for off-site continuing education, leadership support of release time for management development, policies for staffing coverage during times of heavy orientation, or level of support for trying new and innovative educational technology.

Information regarding the organization's mission, vision, and values can be used to plan the overall staff development program. The inclusion of values in the latest Joint Commission for the Accreditation of Healthcare Organizations (JCAHO) standards for health care (1996) has led many institutions to analyze the values that underlie patient care and operational decision making. Staff development specialists can take advantage of this new interest in values identification when developing the total program.

Conceptual Framework

A conceptual framework provides a frame of reference in which staff development specialists may order their educational activities. Conceptual frameworks provide an organization for thinking, making observations, and interpreting the phenomena in the learning environment (Fawcett, 1989).

The discipline of nursing staff development has evolved to include several conceptual frameworks common to most practice settings. Of course, each staff development department is unique and may choose to diverge from commonly held concepts to try new "ways of knowing." The following conceptual frameworks are popular with staff development specialists and can be used in curriculum design.

ADULT LEARNING PRINCIPLES

The unique characteristics of adult learners (Knowles, 1980) can be used as a conceptual framework to guide staff development specialist practice. The target audience for all staff development activity is the adult learner. Knowles postulated that as adults, learners are self-directed and internally motivated. They need to know "what's in it for me." Adult learning must have immediate application and incorporate each participant's life experiences. New information must be linked to previous information and experience and must be applicable in the immediate work environment. An underlying tenet of an adult learning conceptual framework is that adults develop a readiness to learn based on their current needs, so educational experiences must be based on current work requirements.

Adult learning principles provide an excellent choice as a staff development curriculum conceptual framework. These tenets can guide curriculum choices regarding timing, sequencing, flexibility, and content elements. Using adult learning principles as a curriculum guide, staff development specialists would time in-service education to coincide with new equipment implementation and sequence the "roll-out" first to meet staff's immediate needs and later to provide more in-depth information and mastery. Flexible educational options would be planned for self-directed adults needing immediate applicability. Classroom learning would make reference to life situations and would include immediate application of learning to the current work situation.

BENNER'S NOVICE-TO-EXPERT FRAMEWORK

Benner (1984) analyzed the development of nursing skill and developed a model based on Dreyfus's work with pilots. She posited that nurses move through five levels of career and skill development on their way to becoming expert practitioners. Those levels—novice, advanced beginner, competent, proficient, and expert—provide a conceptual framework for developing the sequencing of nursing staff development curricula.

This conceptual framework could be used to determine the depth of content for continuing education programs. Evaluations of orientees can be developed using these levels of skill. The framework can be useful in programs geared toward developing an understanding of orientee needs by new preceptors.

REALITY SHOCK

Kramer (1974) described "reality shock," a process of entry into professional nursing practice. Kramer postulated that graduate nurses proceed through a series of phases as they socialize into the role of practicing RN. This process of entry into practice corresponds to the phases of socialization of employees into any new job situation. Therefore, the reality shock conceptual framework provides guidance in preparing health care practitioners for new and changing roles within an organization, whether due to unit consolidation, unit closure, or delivery of care changes.

The nursing staff development department using a reality shock conceptual framework would take into account important socialization issues in its orientation and education activities. A curriculum so framed would acknowledge the affective needs of the reality shock period and would seek to move the new employee to "biculturalism."

LEARNING STYLE MODELS

Learning style concepts can be an effective conceptual framework for a nursing staff development curriculum. Several learning style models have emerged:

- Kolb's learning styles (1976)
- Brain dominance (Hermann, 1988)
- Mind mediation channel theory (Gregorc, 1982).

Each of these provides perspective regarding methods for presenting information to meet the many ways that people learn.

A learning style conceptual model allows for diverse presentation methods in determining educational process. Diversity in presentation, including audio, video, artistic representation, and role playing, provide multiples channels for learning.

CHANGE THEORY

Change theory is an appealing theoretical framework for staff development specialists working in our current health care delivery environment. Although always in a state of change, institutions today are undergoing a major industry reorganization that could extend into the 21st century. Each shift of course in the larger industry creates shock waves of change in each health care organization. Staff development specialists are in the forefront of implementation for any change within an institution. They may readily see themselves as "change makers" and would therefore benefit from viewing their organizational role through a change theory conceptual framework.

Several change theorists have published models of the change process (Havelock, 1973, Lewin, 1951, Lippitt et al., 1958, Rogers & Shoemaker, 1971, Spradley, 1980). An excellent overview of these and other change theorists was published by Gloe and Stefanik (1995). Two recent entries into the body of work regarding change management deserve discussion as they relate to a nursing staff development conceptual framework. Bridges (1991, 1994) and Noer (1993) developed change models emphasizing the human side of change, which is of particular interest to health care institutions in transition.

Framing organizational change as a transition, Bridges postulated that both the person within an organization and the organization itself move through the three phases:

- Endings
- Neutral zone
- Beginnings.

Using this model as a conceptual framework for a staff development department, curriculum elements would focus on moving people and the organization successfully through these three phases. Each phase requires attention to the feelings and emotions generated by the transition state. Table 9-1 reviews the phases and corresponding characteristics.

Noer's healing model also focuses on the human toll of organizational change. Bridges' model is linear and moves through a time line of activity, but Noer's model is topical, focusing on four key elements of organizational change:

- Downsizing
- Grieving
- Breaking the old employment contract
- Accommodating the new employment contract.

Table 9-2 depicts the four elements of Noer's model with corresponding characteristics. Staff development specialists using this conceptual framework to guide curriculum design would focus on helping staff members in the grieving process while developing a new employee paradigm focusing on career and skill development.

Target Audiences

The target audience for staff development activities has expanded greatly in recent years. Not long ago, staff development specialists in health care facilities planned and implemented education only for nurses. Many managed the orientation and in-service programs

TABLE 9-1

BRIDGES' TRANSITION MODEL

Phases	Characteristics
Phase 1: Endings	• The end of what used to be • Letting go of the old identity • Feelings of loss
Phase 2: Neutral zone	• Interval between the old and the new • Low stability • Increased conflict • Feelings of overload, polarization
Phase 3: Beginnings	• New ways become familiar • New goals are articulated • Feelings of purpose

for ancillary nursing staff (*e.g.*, unit secretaries, nursing assistants). Mandated regulatory in-services might have been under the purview of the nursing educators in an institution as well. However, the movement toward multidisciplinary care, cost containment, and patient-focused activities has led to the need for nursing staff development specialists to redefine their target audience to include all hospital employees.

The target audience for specific curricular activities must be identified to develop appropriate content. Different target audiences bring different amounts of preparation and experience to the orientation, in-service, or continuing education program being provided. For example, the anatomy and physiology background an RN brings to a class on 12-lead EKG interpretation is much broader than that brought by an EKG technician. The technician may require a preliminary class or self-directed learning component before entering the 12-lead EKG class, but the RN can enter it immediately.

The heterogeneous nature of the current employee base can create significant challenges

TABLE 9-2

NOER'S HEALING MODEL

Concept	Characteristics
Downsizing	• Principles of equity and fairness required • Consideration of the impact on survivors
Grieving	• Symbolic acknowledgment of organizational grieving required
Breaking the old employment contract	• Letting go of organizational codependency • Embracing ''good work''
Accommodating the new employment contract	• Empowering the workforce • Increasing autonomy

TABLE 9-3

SUGGESTED PERSONNEL DIFFERENTIALS FOR ESTABLISHING TARGET AUDIENCES

Category	Personnel	Commonalities
Administrative	Financial Managerial Secretarial	Not involved in patient care Generally well educated Focus is operational vs. service issues.
Professional care providers	Nurses Technologists Therapists Social workers	Strongly involved in patient care Usually degreed and licensed Well-defined professional discipline Focus is on service more than operations issues.
Support staff	Dietary services Environmental services Unlicensed assistive personnel Patient care–based clerical workers	Interact with patients Could have minimal education Could have problems with literacy and verbal skills Focus is service more than operations.

to be surmounted. One challenge is determining how best to group people for educational activities. Table 9-3 shows three suggested categories of employee groups within a health care facility:

- Administrative personnel
- Professional care providers
- Support staff.

The administrative category includes financial, managerial, and secretarial positions. These workers are generally removed from patient care activities but provide the operational infrastructure to allow patient care services to take place. These employees are generally well educated and typically have in-service and continuing education needs in the areas of information technology, communication skills, human resources management, and decision making. Often, they need a more in-depth understanding of the services provided by the health care institution and would benefit from programming on basic patient care principles.

The professional care providers, on the other hand, are strongly involved in the services provided by the institution and have less understanding of operational activities such as budgeting and management. They are usually well educated in their chosen profession and often must hold a license to provide their services. Many have a well-defined professional discipline and must continue in education to maintain licensure. Most understand medical terminology and prepare or work with plans of care or individualized programs of interventions for their patients.

Support staff are those who have regular contact with patients. Although their focus is on service, rather than operations, they typically have an unclear understanding of their role in patient care or the institution as a whole. These employees are more likely to have minimal education and to suffer from literacy and language difficulties. They are a challenge for staff development specialists because as adult learners, they are likely to be adept at masking their shortcomings.

Individual and Organizational Developmental Needs

The developmental needs of the organization and individual staff members guide curriculum design. Meeting the learning needs of these two entities contributes to the mission of the organization and increases the likelihood that organizational goals will be attained.

NEEDS OF THE PRACTITIONER

Each employee is on a learning continuum throughout his or her employment. Some employees come to the institution with a wealth of experience and education; for others, it is their first job, and they have little education. The staff development curriculum should take into consideration the developmental needs of each person that specifically affect the fulfillment of the organization's mission and vision.

The initial evaluation of individual developmental needs occurs in the interview process. Here, the candidate learns about the job performance requirements and presents his or her experience and education. Often people are hired with the understanding that they will require job training to meet performance requirements. The staff development curriculum should include mechanisms for communicating the needs of new employees and a plan for meeting their common educational needs.

Individual developmental needs are ranked according to the job description. Writing a clear, concise job description for each type of employee is a priority for quality curriculum development. An ambiguous or unclear job description will create difficulties in developing educational outcomes for individual development activities.

Performance standards are used to evaluate workers' performance of their duties. Written in an objective format, performance standards are often identical to the primary responsibility statements found in a job description. Performance standards are most often used to evaluate the employee's performance. Performance standards can assist staff development specialists in determining trends in individual developmental needs for the institution.

Trends noted in individual performance evaluations can guide curriculum design. For example, a trend of below-standard performance in correct medication administration across a general medical unit may lead to a curriculum plan for medication review classes. If, however, below-standard performance is found in only one or two persons, the intervention may be a self-directed learning plan for correcting the deficit.

State boards of nursing may mandate continuing education requirements for RNs, licensed practical nurses, or nursing assistants that require attention in the curriculum design. Some boards of nursing require specific content elements; others require a specific amount of contact hours. The staff development curriculum should reflect these requirements, or adequate funding to attend outside programming to meet licensing needs should be provided.

Other professional staff members may require continuing education to maintain licensure. The staff development specialist should consult with the state boards overseeing the licensed practices of radiology technology, physical therapy, pharmacy, and occupational therapy, to name a few. These licensing bodies may require specific amounts and areas of continuing education to meet relicensure needs. Once again, curriculum design should accommodate these licensure needs or provide the employees with the needed funding to attend outside programs.

NEEDS OF THE ORGANIZATION

The larger organization has educational requirements related to its operational and cultural developmental needs. It could be said that the accumulation of individual needs within an organization constitutes the organization's developmental needs. However, outside agencies often require organizations to develop in ways they did not expect.

Federal and state regulatory agencies force health care agencies to comply with a wide variety of standards. These can include infectious disease standards from the Centers for Disease Control and Prevention and hazardous waste standards through the Occupational Safety and Health Administration. Federal laws such as the Americans with Disabilities Act and the Patient Self-Determination Act have led to organizational developmental needs that must be considered in curriculum design. Of course, the JCAHO frequently challenges health care organizations to meet quality standards, and these may create developmental needs. An in-depth review of these regulatory requirements is found in Chapter 7.

Changes in the larger profession of health care management also lead to organizational needs. Methods such as total quality management, continuous quality improvement, and outcomes management have required major education efforts throughout health care organizations. These quality activities have evolved into the development of clinical pathways and the case management process.

The national movement to reform health care and major changes in reimbursement created another group of organizational development needs as health care institutions began embracing re-engineering, work redesign, and restructuring. These organization-wide changes produce massive developmental needs requiring a coordinated staff development effort for success.

Curriculum Threads

Curriculum threads are recurring themes that emerge throughout the total program of staff development. Curriculum threads can be described as vertical or horizontal and together produce a rich educational tapestry. Horizontal threads are the levels of course content; vertical threads are the concepts covered in all courses (Leroux & Cody, 1996, O'Connor, 1986).

The horizontal threads of course content come from the identified needs of the target audiences and the organizational and individual developmental needs. Many of the programming standards discussed later in this chapter are excellent examples of horizontal threads. There are many potential vertical curriculum threads important to health care. These curriculum threads define the emphasis of the content of individual programs within the larger educational plan of the organization. The following curriculum threads can be considered by nursing staff development specialists planning a total educational program. They were chosen as representative of common themes that would encompass learning experiences planned for any of the three categories of target audiences.

CARE ACROSS THE LIFE SPAN

Although growth and development has always been a significant component of nursing education, the recent emphasis placed on age-related competency requirements by the JCAHO (1996) makes this a strong candidate for a horizontal curriculum thread. Used as a horizontal thread, any program to any target audience would include age-specific criteria. The JCAHO (1996) has identified several age groups that must be considered: neonate, infant, child, adolescent, adult, geriatric.

Using "care across the life span" as a horizontal thread would require that an in-service program for radiology technologists regarding new radiographic equipment would include implications for diagnostic testing for pediatric and geriatric clients. Mental health technician continuing education would include care of the adolescent; pharmacist continuing education would include the geriatric implications of medication absorption.

CUSTOMER SERVICE AND VALUES ORIENTATION

The competitive nature of the health care arena has led to increased focus on customer service. Continuous quality improvement programs identify customers as patients, physicians, vendors, other institutional departments, and other employees. Customer service as a horizontal thread in a staff development curriculum design would guarantee that this important theme was a part of all in-service and continuing education programs. This would suggest that customer service elements would be a natural part of telephone skills workshops or new employee orientations.

Likewise, a greater emphasis on applied institutional values can lead to the use of values orientation as a horizontal curricular thread. Many health care institutions are promoting the organizational values embedded in their mission and vision statements. Reinforcing explicit organizational values is an appropriate part of employee orientation, in-service, and continuing education content.

CRITICAL THINKING SKILLS

More than ever, the fast-paced and high-acuity health care setting requires all care providers to think critically. Educators have found it difficult to teach critical thinking skills in preparing professional care providers (Brookfield, 1993, Schank, 1990, Snyder, 1993). An even greater challenge may be the preparation of support and administrative staff members in critical thinking and problem-solving skills.

A critical thinking horizontal curriculum thread would allow for application of critical thinking skills in all content areas. Emphasis would be placed on applying the educational content in ways that allow for critical thinking. Teaching methods such as case studies and role playing would allow for critical thinking episodes during the educational program. Evaluation of educational programs could include outcome in the patient care setting, such as appropriate response to crises and effective communication of changes in patient status.

SELF-DIRECTED LEARNING PRINCIPLES

Self-directed learning principles provide a timely horizontal thread for today's staff development curriculum design. Health care employees need to be skilled at seeking and obtaining necessary information. Staff development specialists must maximize their time and increase productivity by teaching care providers how to acquire the information they need to provide quality care. Dependency is no longer an acceptable educational practice.

Using self-directed learning principles as a horizontal curricular thread provides many opportunities for educators to coach staff members in literature review, on-line searching, policy and procedure locations, and peer consultation. Teaching methods can be adapted to correspond to self-directed learning. Self-learning modules in a written or computer-assisted instruction format can be created and made available to staff at any time. A flexible lending library of audiocassettes and videotapes allow staff to acquire knowledge when they need it or have time available for it. A staff education channel on the in-hospital network can also encourage self-directed learning.

These four potential themes for vertical curricular threads are just a few of the options available. Staff development specialists should spend time assessing the learning environment and learning needs when deciding on horizontal threads.

Process and Resource Management Elements

Nursing staff development curriculum design must involve the application of education in a continuous around-the-clock setting with, by necessity, very little time allocated for educational experiences. This environment must be considered when designing a strategic staff development plan. Process elements under consideration in curriculum design include flexible learning options, 24-hour, 7-day-a-week educational accountability, and the use of information technology.

FLEXIBILITY

Staff development specialists can best meet the needs of their target audiences when they allow flexibility in the means by which they accomplish educational goals. The unpredictability of patient care requires a serious look at flexibility in the overall curriculum. Flexibility is unique to curriculum design in nursing staff development: the focus is on providing education around patient care priorities.

A flexible curriculum design takes into account the frequency of educational programming and includes innovative formats such as poster presentations, self-learning packages, learning "suitcases," flyer in-services, educational newsletters, and E-mail "sound bites." A concerted effort is made to take the education to the person and package it in a format to accommodate the work situation.

AROUND-THE-CLOCK ACCOUNTABILITY

Most health care-based staff development departments are required to meet the educational needs of staff working on all shifts. Providing programming on all shifts is a challenge to a primarily day-shift development staff. Total program planning must accommodate the needs of staff who work evenings, nights, and weekends. Timing of direct delivery education must be evaluated related to the ebb and flow of patient care activity on the various shifts. A balance between the times most convenient for the educators and the times most likely to meet the needs of the patient care staff must be struck. Popular in-service times include midshift and meal break times (particularly when food is provided at the educational event!).

USE OF TECHNOLOGY

Advances in computer technology and the computerization of medical records have led to increased availability of personal computers in patient care areas. Curriculum designers can look to new and innovative methods to provide "just-in-time" in-service programming. Institution-based home pages can provide information to employees when they need it. Computer-assisted instruction for regulatory and mandated education is now available, allowing employees to obtain instruction and information on any shift and at any time. Institution-based E-mail systems can allow communication between participants and educators regarding registration, course changes, or course locations.

PRODUCTIVITY

Consideration should be given to the productivity of activities that contribute to the total staff development program. In particular, staff development specialists should attempt to maximize the time consumed by literature review and content formatting. Once developed, educational content can be used for multiple programs targeted to multiple audiences, so the return on the invested time is significantly increased.

Likewise, productivity is enhanced by reviewing duplicate offerings. Consideration should be given to the frequency of orientation sessions and mandated programming. If class size is not a factor in the choice of instructional strategy, it may be advantageous to replace frequent small-group offerings with less frequent large-group offerings. This multiplies the effectiveness of instructor time: when weekly orientations are changed to biweekly or even monthly programs, the effective use of instructor time is doubled or quadrupled.

Finally, a staff development specialist's productivity is enhanced when programs are modulated so that various categories of staff can enter and leave at appropriate times. Participants thereby receive the information needed without the instructor's duplicating efforts with segregated programs. For example, a modulated dysrhythmia interpretation course would allow experienced coronary care nurses to attend only the modules needed for review after unsuccessful competency evaluation; beginning critical care nurses, however, would attend all the modules. Mandatory education can be modulated so that all employees attend some sections while professional patient care staff attend all sections. These considerations during curriculum design will increase the overall productivity of the staff development specialist.

REALITY-BASED EXPECTED OUTCOME

Although 100% attendance at new-product in-services and continuing education programs is ideal, strategic education planning must incorporate realistic outcome expectations: ideal attendance is thwarted by staffing, budgetary, and acuity factors.

The concept of critical mass can have an intriguing application to issues of educational outcome in curriculum design. Critical mass is defined in *The American Heritage College Dictionary* (1993) as "the smallest mass of a fissionable material that will sustain a nuclear chain reaction." This term has come into common use to mean reaching a large enough number within a population to allow for diffusion of new information throughout the population. Rogers (1995) identified diffusion as a social process among peers. This concept, applied to staff development education, allows for the sharing of new information throughout an organization once enough people have attended the educational session. Although it requires more research, the application of critical mass principles and Rogers' diffusion theory could prove effective in increasing the productivity of a staff development department.

Instructional Timing and Sequencing

The final element of this nursing staff development curriculum design model is instructional timing and sequencing. This component refers to the timing of program elements and their relation to each other.

Instructional timing takes into consideration the time of year, season, cycle, or time of day the educational program is implemented. Annual periods of peak vacation leave such as summer and winter holidays may reduce staff availability. Cyclic institutional periods such as annual budget preparation or triannual JCAHO review should also be avoided when possible. Organizations may have weekly patterns that must be taken into account in total program planning. Many staff development planners schedule programs during midweek, when staffing is most plentiful. Conflicts with organizational meetings such as monthly staff meetings also must be considered.

The ordering of instructional elements is important to learner outcomes. People cannot learn everything at once; they must have information arranged so as to build on previous

---

DISPLAY 9-5

Instructional Design Sequencing Options

General to specific
Known to unknown
Concrete to abstract
Simple to complex
Facts to principles
Principles to application
Most to least important
Most to least interesting
Part to whole (or whole to part)
Chronologic order
Inherent logic of the subject matter
Established order of steps in a procedure
Customary or traditional way of teaching the content

From Alspach, J. G. (1995). *The educational process in nursing staff development* (p. 34). St. Louis: Mosby.

information. Several design choices are available to staff development specialists. The sequencing format may be altered to match the type and complexity of the educational content. Sequencing options, as identified by Alspach (1995), are presented in Display 9-5.

COMMON PROGRAM STANDARDS

Staff development in health care institutions consists of a common group of program expectations. These standard programs make up the greatest part of a nursing staff development curriculum. The needs of each organization, of course, dictate the priority placed on each of these program entities.

Orientation

The orientation of new employees to the organization and their new job responsibilities is a major staff development activity. No matter what the new employee's position, orientation consists of three core areas: organizational orientation, departmental orientation, and position orientation.

Organizational orientation can be completed with all new employees in a large group. The major theme of organizational orientation is an understanding of the mission, vision, and values of the organization. Other elements include organizational systems and processes (*e.g.*, quality processes and communication mechanisms), human resources issues (*e.g.*, compensation, benefits, job transfer, and promotion), and general safety information (*e.g.*, infection control, hazardous waste disposal, and back safety). Frequently, senior management officials speak at organizational orientation programs to meet new employees and to explain their goals for the organization and the new employee's role in accomplishing these goals.

Departmental orientation typically follows organizational orientation. A large department with many similar processes such as nursing may have departmental orientations in large groups. Smaller departments such as radiology or physical therapy may accomplish departmental orientation in a one-on-one fashion or incorporate this with position orientation.

Departmental orientation involves sharing information regarding the environment and facilities, department-specific standards, and departmental application of organization-wide systems and processes. This could take the form of the application of safety principles in the specific department, human resources policy application, and department-specific standards, policies, and procedures. During department-specific nursing orientation, for instance, time is typically spent reviewing the safe use of department-wide equipment such as IV pumps, skin care products, and respiratory care equipment. Department orientation in a dietary department may include general food preparation and handling policies and a review of the scheduling policy.

Another important element of departmental orientation is the integration of the new employee into the work team. This could take the form of a unit tour and introduction to staff members. Departments may wish to arrange a welcome lunch or arrange for staff members to accompany orientees during break periods.

Finally, new employees are oriented to their position and specific job description in the organization. This orientation often involves a precepted experience and competency evaluation. Many positions also require credentialing. Age-specific criteria and equipment-specific competencies may also be applicable.

In-Service Education

The ever-changing practice of health care requires continual updates. In-service education provides learning experiences intended to help staff members acquire, maintain, or increase competence in fulfilling expectations of employers regarding the application of technology, equipment, medications, procedures, and techniques in the specific work setting (ANA, 1994).

The staff development specialist may accomplish this through direct delivery or the organization of materials presented by other specialists or educators provided by the product vendor. Planning the content, timing, process, and implementation of the in-service education is the responsibility of the staff development specialist, regardless of who delivers the content. Even if vendor-sponsored educators provide the in-service education, the staff development specialist should preview the material for appropriateness and monitor the initial delivery of the education. Quality of material and delivery varies widely, and some vendor-initiated education is little more than marketing material. Vendor educators are often less intent on meeting the needs of the organization's employees and more intent on meeting their own organization's marketing and sales goals. That aside, vendors can be an excellent source of in-service education materials. Establishing good relationships with the companies doing business with the organization can prove very helpful.

Continuing Education

Continuing education consists of professional learning experiences designed to enrich the employee's health care practice and contribute to quality health care (ANA, 1994). Unlike in-service education, continuing education builds on the learner's current knowledge with information that is applicable to care provision in a wide variety of practice settings.

All employees working in a health care setting have continuing educational needs. These needs are of varying degree and priority. The goal in nursing staff development curriculum development is to meet the continuing education needs of employees that will also move the organization toward its intended goals. Examples are:

- Courses in triage for emergency nurses seeing an increase in major trauma
- Programs on premature infant assessment for nursery personnel faced with more high-risk deliveries
- Updates on invasive radiology therapy for radiology technologists
- Updates on the outcomes of speech therapy in stroke clients for occupational therapists
- Courses on medical terminology for patient care clerical support staff
- Programs on current trends in budget analysis for financial administrative staff.

The savvy staff development specialist will use information prepared for one group of employees to educate other employees. For example, a medical terminology class or self-study module to meet the organizational need of upgrading the knowledge of patient care clerical staff might also be offered to unlicensed assistive personnel desiring greater health care knowledge, even though this information does not directly tie into an organizational need. RNs might also desire information regarding speech therapy, so the program intended for occupational therapists could be made available to a multidisciplinary group, thereby increasing the educational outcome of the efforts. When preparing continuing education programming, the staff development specialist should always ask, "Who else could benefit from this information?"

Mandatory or Regulated Training

Great amounts of educator time and efforts are directed toward meeting mandated education programming. As identified earlier in this chapter, health care organizations are required to provide employees with periodic education to meet the requirements of JCAHO, the Occupational Safety and Health Administration, the Centers for Disease Control and Prevention, state departments of health, and the federal government. The staff development specialist responsible for providing mandated and regulated training must develop methods for remaining abreast of changes and additions to these requirements. Suggestions include:

- Regular monitoring of agency publications (make sure you are on their mailing lists)
- Review of health care education publications
- Involvement in local staff development consortiums.

Close, continuous monitoring of these requirements will allow time for planning and avoid crisis education as new laws and regulations are enacted.

Some state boards of nursing have specific mandatory content required for relicensure; examples include New York's abuse education requirement and Florida's IV therapy requirement. Other professional licensure boards, such as physical therapy and radiology technology, may have mandated education. Staff development specialists responsible for other professional staff must develop information pipelines to remain updated on licensure board needs.

The regulatory education needs for support staff must be considered as well. Unlicensed assistive personnel may be required to receive mandated education to maintain state certification.

The challenge in providing mandated or regulatory education lies in the delivery. The content of mandated programs is often prescribed by the agency and allows for little deviation. Staff development specialists must struggle with motivating staff to attend annual and biannual programs with unchanging information. Keys to success involve flexible delivery and creative teaching methods. Curriculum designs featuring alternative delivery methods such as poster presentations, self-directed learning packages, and computer-assisted instruction are recommended. Light, humorous teaching styles add an entertainment quality to the perceived monotony of content, offering motivation for attendance. Staff development specialists have successfully used games, education fairs, and raffles to entice reluctant staff members to annual reviews of mandated and regulatory materials.

Leadership Development

Most health care organizations require some form of leadership development as part of the staff development curriculum. Supervisory and management staff who are promoted from within due to their clinical expertise will need development in employee management, communication, budgeting, and strategic planning. In addition, leadership principles such as motivation, change management, delegation, and meeting management are necessary elements of successful manager development. Large nursing departments may have specialized nursing management courses, but more often staff development specialists provide leadership development for a broad range of novice health care managers.

Leadership courses are an excellent training ground for the development of multidisciplinary efforts in the health care organization. Attention to the socialization of leaders is necessary. Courses should promote the development of problem-solving and critical thinking skills in the real-life framework of actual institutional challenges.

Organizational Transitions

The nursing staff development curriculum most likely will include programming related to organizational transitions. Most health care organizations are in some form of transition as the industry moves through a major reorganization. Transitions may include the closing of units, combining of units, changing of target patient populations, or the opening of new patient care "product lines." Staff and management may be required to change their practice focus or career path with little input on their part.

The staff development professional has an opportunity to improve the outcomes in these transition periods through educational programming regarding the human impact of organizational transition. Content can include the emotional impact of loss, "survivor sickness," motivational theory, career planning, and "meaning-making" activities. Curriculum conceptual frameworks such as those proposed by Bridges and Noer, reviewed earlier in this chapter, provide assistance in structuring these important programs.

Preceptor Development

Preceptor programs have gained popularity as a major part of most nursing orientations. As staff development specialists expand their practice to encompass professional and support employee orientations, preceptor programs have been adjusted to encompass all organizational orientees. Preceptors are experienced and competent staff members who serve as clinical role models and resource persons for new employees. They orient new staff to their roles and responsibilities and introduce them to the formal and informal rules, customs, culture, and norms of their coworkers and the workplace.

The development of a group of mature employees who understand the preceptor role is an important function of the staff development department. Preceptor development programs involve the identification, recruitment, and initial and ongoing education of chosen staff members. Major content elements of initial preceptor training include:

- Preceptor roles and responsibilities
- Reality shock theory
- Adult education principles
- Socialization principles
- Education and teaching approaches
- Problem solving
- Case study or role playing
- Evaluation and documentation.

Train-the-Trainer

Due to ever-increasing productivity demands, many staff development departments have started using "train-the-trainer" education delivery. In this process, staff development specialists teach other staff members the educational content and how to teach it. These newly trained "content experts" then provide in-service education to a large target audience. Train-the-trainer activities are most often used when the content is specific, the target audience is large, and the time frame is short. This method frees the staff development specialist from having to provide large amounts of direct delivery and allows for more education coordination and facilitation.

It is important to analyze the expected outcome of the educational activity before initiating the train-the-trainer method. If this method were used to present large amounts of complex content requiring unfamiliar education delivery methods, it would be inappropriate and probably unsuccessful. Examples of appropriate uses of train-the-trainer programs in staff development curricula include the house-wide implementation of new intravenous equipment and the preparation of staff for an upcoming JCAHO survey.

When developing the train-the-trainer program, the needs of the training assistant and the target audience must be carefully analyzed. The staff development specialist should spend ample time preparing the material so that it is already formatted for easy delivery by the training assistant. A training kit should be prepared with all the information, equipment, and teaching materials he or she will need. Educators should be available to the training assistants during their first few in-services to provide support and assistance as necessary.

Informatics

The increased use of computer technology for the provision of clinical services and the operations of health care institutions requires curriculum design efforts in the area of informatics. Basic, intermediate, and advanced programming is likely to be required for the use of clinical computers. Attention to informatics in the organizational, departmental, and position orientation of new staff is warranted. Ongoing improvements in the clinical application of information technology requires continuing education.

The direct delivery of informatics education can often be delegated to information services personnel. Once again, the staff development specialist must review the content, format, and delivery of the information to ensure it is appropriate for the large audience. As education experts in the institution, staff development specialists may find themselves acting as consultants to information services regarding the dissemination of computer application information and manual creation.

SUMMARY

This chapter presented an overview of strategic thinking and curriculum design concepts. A suggested model for nursing staff development curriculum design was created and each of its seven elements discussed, and its application to nursing staff development in present health care organizations was explained. Common staff development program standards were described.

The future of staff development in health care organizations will be enhanced by the use of a curriculum design that allows for the incorporation of the organization's mission and vision. Careful application of realistic and flexible teaching strategies to a content based on targeted individual and organizational learning needs is warranted in today's cost-conscious, quality-driven industry.

Strategic Targeting for Oncology Education

DONNA K. WRIGHT

Part of my staff development role has been to oversee the orientation and education for oncology nurses. The goal was to equip caregivers with the knowledge and skills to provide sound, consistent, safe care for cancer patients throughout the organization. In designing a program to achieve this outcome, I first identified the potential learners. These included nurses from the oncology units, med/surg units, float pool, clinics, and ER, as well as other health care professionals assigned to oncology populations, such as social workers, chaplains, and dietitians. Because of the diverse needs of the target groups identified, the program had to be designed to meet the needs identified by the various groups involved.

I began my program design by talking with managers from the groups identified above. Some managers knew exactly what they wanted; others didn't even recognize that they had oncology education needs until I called. After talking with the various managers, I divided the potential learners into four categories:

- Nurses who needed in-depth knowledge to carry out all aspects of oncology care, including chemo administration (mostly oncology unit, med/surg unit, and clinic nurses)
- Nurses who needed basic knowledge to carry out safe care for oncology patients, not including chemo administration (mostly float pool and some med/surg unit nurses)

- Employees who worked around chemotherapeutic agents who needed a basic understanding of safe handling of cytotoxic agents (all employees who work in areas where cytotoxic agents are used)
- Employees who needed a basic overview of the oncology patient experience to understand the disease process and treatments (social workers, chaplains, dietitians, some nurses from other areas).

My next step was to review information established by oncology associations that articulated outlines for an oncology curriculum, as well as safety requirements. I divided the curriculum ideas I found into categories that reflected our needs: basic cancer overview, chemo administration, chemo safety, and the response of the patient to the disease process and treatment.

I put this content into a 1-day workshop format but kept each of the four sections as a free-standing 1- to 2-hour class. This made it possible for learners to attend one or several sections without feeling like they were coming into the middle of something. For example, new oncology unit nurses came to all four sessions, social workers came to the basic cancer overview and the session on patient response to the disease process and treatment, and the chaplains attended only the basic cancer overview.

I also took the class content and developed

other learning methodologies to meet the individual learner's preference and style of learning. Each class section was put into a self-learning video packet available to employees through the check-out library in the organization. I developed an oncology challenge examination to provide a way for learners with extensive knowledge to verify their competency, thus avoiding the cost of orientation for those who already had the knowledge.

Because so many staff needed chemo safety education, I developed a variety of learning methods—fact sheets, videos, classes, posters, self-learning packets, and even a fairy tale entitled *The Princess and the Chemo Spill* (Wright, 1993).

After the curriculum was identified and methodologies were created, I developed guidelines to help managers identify which learners needed what part of the curriculum. These guidelines mapped out what part of the curriculum each person needed, as well as the options they could choose from to meet their needs.

I also advertised each part of the curriculum as educational opportunities in our education newsletter. This allowed any staff member to take the class or use the self-learning packets on their own time, free of charge. This was a great option for people seeking continuing education and ongoing learning opportunities.

The content of the classes, self-learning packets, and videos addressed more than just oncology objectives. Job descriptions and expectations were clarified for the employees, as well the roles of others with whom they would be working as they provided service to the oncology population. Competency expectations were articulated, and options for verification of these competencies were discussed. Organizational philosophies were frequently associated with the various concepts of oncology care. This strategy helped bring the organizational philosophies out of the policy book and into the real world. Safety concepts were reinforced, and many real-life examples were used to challenge the learner to think about the intent behind OSHA and JCAHO safety standards. This promoted the use of critical thinking skills.

The education described above was followed by mentoring sessions in the actual work area to which the employees were assigned. The mentors designated for each area were oriented to the oncology program curriculum and given periodic updates. To reinforce this process, some mentors were asked to audit the classes periodically to help review content and evaluate teaching methods, instructor approach, and overall class flow. Other mentors were asked to review or help develop self-learning packets and videos. This strategy was great for addressing many needs. It helped keep the material fresh and up to date. It also spread the work out and helped promote team building among oncology employees. This was a great opportunity to bring together outpatient and inpatient services, as well as nursing and other disciplines. A sense of ownership was created for oncology education that went far beyond the educator. This approach helped keep the program responsive to the ever-changing needs of the organization and health care.

In more than 5 years of providing and maintaining this program, we had many voluntary repeat customers. Their response was, "I just wanted to participate in another part of the education to make sure my skills and knowledge are up to date." We also had several quality improvement monitors in place that reflected that our education was hitting the mark.

I am glad I took the time to use strategic thinking in my program development. I feel confident that we have cost-effective strategies in place for meeting our goals, and the energy and resources we use to carry out this program are worth it for our organization and quality patient care. Taking the time to do it right does pay off.

REFERENCES

Alspach, J. G. (1995). *The educational process in nursing staff development.* St. Louis: Mosby.

The American Heritage college dictionary, 3rd ed. (1993). Costello, R. B., et al. (Eds.). Boston: Houghton Mifflin.

American Nurses Association. (1994). *Standards for nursing professional development: Continuing education and staff development.* Washington DC: Author.

Benner, P. (1984). *From novice to expert: Excellence and power in clinical practice.* Menlo Park, CA: Addison-Wesley.

Bolan, R. S. (1974). Mapping the planning theory terrain. In Godschalk, D. R. (Ed.). *Planning in America: Learning from turbulence.* Boston: American Institute of Planners.

Bridges, W. (1991). *Managing transitions.* New York: Addison-Wesley.

Bridges, W. (1994). *Job shift: How to prosper in a workplace without jobs.* New York: Addison-Wesley.

Brookfield, S. (1993). On impostership, cultural suicide, and other dangers: How nurses learn critical thinking. *Journal of Continuing Education in Nursing, 24*(5), 197–205.

Fawcett, J. (1989). *Analysis and evaluation of conceptual models on nursing,* 2nd ed. Philadelphia: F. A. Davis.

Gloe, D., & Stefanik, R. (1995). Change. In Avillion, A. E. (Ed.). *Core curriculum for nursing staff development.* Pensacola, FL: National Nursing Staff Development Organization.

Gregorc, A. F. (1982). *An adult's guide to style.* Maynard, MA: Gabriel Systems.

Havelock, R. G. (1973). *The change agent's guide to innovation in education.* Englewood Cliffs, NJ: Education Technology Publication.

Hermann, N. (1988). *The creative brain.* Lake Lure, NC: Brain Books.

Joint Commission on Accreditation of Healthcare Organizations. (1996). *1996 Comprehensive accreditation manual for hospitals.* Oakbrook Terrace, IL: Author.

Knowles, M. S. (1980). *The practice of adult education: From pedagogy to androgogy.* Chicago: Follett.

Kolb, D. A. (1976). *Learning style inventory.* Boston: McBer and Company.

Kramer, M. (1974). *Reality shock: Why nurses leave nursing.* St. Louis: Mosby.

Leroux, D. S., & Cody, B. (1996). Curriculum planning and development. In Abruzzese, R. (Ed.). *Nursing staff development: Strategies for success.* St. Louis: Mosby.

Lewin, K. (1951). *Field theory in social science.* New York: Harper & Row.

Lippitt, R., Watson, J., & Westley, B. (1958). *The dynamics of planned change.* New York: Harcourt, Brace & World.

Noer, D. M. (1993). *Healing the wounds: Overcoming the trauma of layoffs and revitalizing downsized organizations.* San Francisco: Jossey-Bass.

O'Connor, A. B. (1986). *Nursing staff development and continuing education.* Boston: Little, Brown.

Ornstein, S., & Hunkins, F. (1988). *Curriculum: Foundations, principles, and issues.* Boston: Allyn & Bacon.

Rogers, E. (1995). Lessons for guidelines from the diffusion of innovations. *Journal of Quality Improvement, 21*(7), 324–328.

Rogers, E., & Shoemaker, F. (1971). *Communication of innovations: A cross-cultural approach.* New York: Free Press.

Sawyer, G. C. (1983). *Corporate planning as a creative process.* Oxford, OH: Planning Executives Institute.

Schank, M. J. (1990). Wanted: Nurses with critical thinking skills. *Journal of Continuing Education in Nursing, 21*(2), 86–89.

Schoenly, L. (1994). Curriculum design in nursing staff development. *Journal of Nursing Staff Development, 10*(4), 187–190.

Schwendiman, J. S. (1973). *Strategic and long-range planning for the multinational corporation.* New York: Praeger.

Snyder, M. (1993). Critical thinking: A foundation for consumer-focused care. *Journal of Continuing Education in Nursing, 24*(5), 206–210.

Spradley, B. W. (1980). Managing change creatively. *Journal of Nursing Administration, 5*(2), 32–37.

Wright, D. (1993). The princess and the chemo spill: A policy magically turned into a fairy tale. *Journal of Continuing Education in Nursing, 24*(1), 37–38.

10

Program Planning: Solving the Problem

JULIA W. AUCOIN

Program planning is the responsibility of the staff development specialist (SDS) in collaboration with content experts, managers, and learners. The content expert knows what should be taught; the manager directs what the learners should know; the learner should be able to identify what is needed to be effective on the job; and the SDS brings it all together. Comprehensive program planning is the first step to providing cost-effective staff development and ensuring success for the SDS. As always, alignment with administrative philosophy and mission are required for success. For the purposes of this chapter, a program is defined as any educational activity designed to meet a particular learning need. These educational activities are components of the total staff development program plan, which is not intended or implied in this chapter; it is discussed in Chapters 4, 5, and 6.

NEEDS ASSESSMENT STRATEGIES

The SDS may employ a variety of needs assessment strategies to plan the program. More often than not, more than one approach is used at a given time. The purpose of assessing learning needs is to discover what must be taught. Needs assessment is also used to determine the instruction, if necessary, and the extent of instruction needed. Assessment is used to prioritize the identified needs and interests of the learners. The information is then used to set objectives and plan appropriate and effective teaching methodologies. The following steps are useful in performing a needs assessment (Bastable, 1997):

1. Identify the learners. Will the audience include everyone that you or others think needs this information?
2. Choose the right setting. Is the environment conducive to getting accurate information, which the learner may think is confidential?
3. Collect data on the learner. Is this learner typical of a larger group?
4. Include the learner as a source of information. Actively engaging learners in defining their learning needs motivates learning because there is already an investment in the process.
5. Involve members of the health care team. As our work becomes more multidisciplinary, it is important to get the perspective of the rest of the team.
6. Prioritize needs. Using needs theory as an organizing framework, needs can be prioritized so that basic needs necessary for survival are accommodated first, with higher stages of development reserved for the more experienced learners.

Needs assessment is commonly thought of as a printed survey given annually to the staff, who rank the choices listed. This method can be useful for generating ideas in a large organization but can also imply to staff that all the topics listed will be covered at

TABLE 10-1	
NEEDS ASSESSMENT STRATEGIES	
Advisory groups	Meeting minutes
Brainstorming	Nominal group technique
Critical incident review	Observation
Delphi technique	Participant feedback
Exit interviews	Performance appraisal
Focus groups	Qualitative research
Incident reports	Questionnaire/survey
Interviews	Records review/quality improvement activities
Introduction of new policies, procedures, or products	Satisfaction measures

some point, setting the SDS up for failure and the learners up for disappointment. Some effective and frequently used methods for identifying learning needs are interviews, attendance at meetings, and critical incident reviews (Care, 1996, Francke et al., 1996). Table 10-1 lists suggested needs assessment strategies.

Puetz (1992) described a learning needs assessment as an integral part of the staff development program. Without a learning needs assessment to set direction for the staff development program, the SDS essentially is without direction. The assessment serves as the road map, providing direction for the overall staff development effort.

Using Needs Assessment Data in Design

To ensure that programs are on target, the needs assessed early on must be clear. If the problem is resolved or new information becomes available, then the program can be adapted to reflect these latest developments. Basing the program on learning needs will provide a solid foundation for developing objectives, choosing teaching methods, and preparing the evaluation plan.

According to Alspach (1995), the needs assessment process provides the educator with a wealth of data to design specific learning activities and refine the total staff development program. It is the responsibility of the SDS to:

- Solicit needs from all major participants in the education process
- Scrutinize needs to ensure that they can be managed through education
- Categorize needs into orientation, in-service, and continuing education
- Prioritize needs as related to their importance, consequences, and immediacy
- Validate needs with those who identified them.

Based on the data derived from the needs assessment, a learning activity can be designed that is appropriate to the expected outcomes and the level and experience of the learners. Integrating ideas from managers and staff into the design helps build their commitment. A focus of the needs assessment should be on preferred teaching strategies. Attention should also be given to time, cost, and other resources to be invested. The needs assessment data are needed to gain the administrative support necessary for the program.

DOMAINS OF LEARNING

As teaching involves development of the whole person, so should the learning activities. Activities should be planned in diverse ways to match the subject matter. The educational plan begins with a description of what the learner is expected to know, do, or feel at the end of the educational experience. These are the learning or behavioral objectives. A commonly used framework for discussion of objectives within domains of learning is Bloom's taxonomy (Table 10-2), which divides learning into three domains: cognitive, affective, and psychomotor. (Krathwol et al., 1964). The taxonomy provides "guide words" for the SDS to use in developing learning objectives from each domain. They are listed in order of increasing complexity to allow for progressive learning activities.

- Cognitive (ways of knowing): facts and theory. Most commonly used when information is to be delivered, not experienced. Objectives from the cognitive domain often lead to lectures, discussions, readings, and written tests. Guide words include identify, explain, and describe.

TABLE 10-2

DOMAINS OF LEARNING AND SAMPLE LEAD VERBS FOR OBJECTIVES WITH INCREASING COMPLEXITY

Cognitive Domain	Affective Domain	Psychomotor Domain
Recall	Increase awareness	List
Label	Respect	Place in order
Define	Cooperate	Label
Discuss	Accept	Compute
Explain	Value	Arrange
Administer	Defend (beliefs)	Demonstrate
Interpret	Organize (belief system)	Assemble
Examine	Characterize	Construct
Analyze		
Distinguish		
Solve		
Integrate		
Organize		
Modify		
Design		
Diagnose		
Critique		
Appraise		
Prioritize		

From Krathwol, D.R., Bloom, B.S., & Masia, B. (1964). *Taxonomy of educational objectives, Handbook II.* New York: David McKay.

- Affective (ways of feeling): more abstract concepts, such as values and feelings. Programs tend to be on the "touchy-feely" side and may cause the learner some introspection or emotional changes. Guide words include respond and empathize.
- Psychomotor (ways of doing): often the most comfortable to employ. These learning opportunities involve skills development, a common need within health care. Guide words include practice and demonstrate.

Although Bloom's taxonomy may be most familiar, the SDS may choose to use other models developed by Dave (1970), Dyche (1982), House (1972), or Simpson (1966). These differ only in their structure, number of levels, and complexity; the verbs used to guide objectives are the same.

Regardless of the framework's complexity or scope, it is important to address all domains whenever appropriate and to avoid verbs that will not support the program evaluation process or provide good learning activities. For example, verbs to avoid include understand, know, teach, and learn; however, if sound evaluation strategies are part of the program design, these may be the precise verbs needed to describe the anticipated outcome or competency. These are difficult to measure and do not provide enough guidance to the instructor. A little practice will provide the SDS with the expertise to choose the appropriate domain and subsequent objectives to drive the learning experience, using needs assessment data to support the chosen design.

SELECTED TEACHING STRATEGIES

Once the needs assessment has led to the development of instructional objectives, then the appropriate teaching strategy can be selected. The model cited in Figure 10-1 is an example of a classic program-planning process.

Lecture

In this age of entertainment and "sound bites," it is difficult to imagine a group of learners who are eager to sit through a 1- to 3-hour oral presentation of facts and knowledge by an expert without any opportunity for participation. Many novice SDSs begin using this style because it is the one most familiar to them. Many college courses are still taught using this style, although a new university in Florida prohibits its faculty from lecturing, on the grounds that lectures stifle creativity and interest from the learners. However, it remains the most efficient means to ensure that specific information has been conveyed to an audience. Lectures can provide basic information from which discussion and demonstration can stem. To enhance learning, lecture periods should be broken up by small-group discussions, questions to and from the learners, and good audiovisual aids. Lectures should be organized with a clear outline. Movement around the room and good voice modulation by a well-prepared presenter make lecturing a successful means of providing details not commonly available to learners.

Discussion

Providing learners with goals and a clear focus will enable learning to occur from a discussion with peers. "Experiential learning" calls on the breadth and depth of the lives of participants. An effective group discussion draws on the knowledge and styles of the

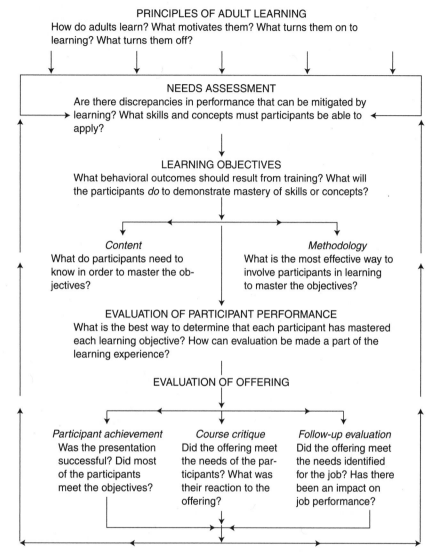

PRINCIPLES OF ADULT LEARNING
How do adults learn? What motivates them? What turns them on to learning? What turns them off?

NEEDS ASSESSMENT
Are there discrepancies in performance that can be mitigated by learning? What skills and concepts must participants be able to apply?

LEARNING OBJECTIVES
What behavioral outcomes should result from training? What will the participants *do* to demonstrate mastery of skills or concepts?

Content
What do participants need to know in order to master the objectives?

Methodology
What is the most effective way to involve participants in learning to master the objectives?

EVALUATION OF PARTICIPANT PERFORMANCE
What is the best way to determine that each participant has mastered each learning objective? How can evaluation be made a part of the learning experience?

EVALUATION OF OFFERING

Participant achievement
Was the presentation successful? Did most of the participants meet the objectives?

Course critique
Did the offering meet the needs of the participants? What was their reaction to the offering?

Follow-up evaluation
Did the offering meet the needs identified for the job? Has there been an impact on job performance?

FIGURE 10-1. Conceptual model for offering development. Holmes, S.A. (1989). Getting started: Educational offering design model. *Journal of Nursing Staff Development, 5*(2), 94.

learners and exponentially increases their learning opportunities. Discussion offers a forum for opposing viewpoints in a safe and accepting environment. Topics and time should be structured so that the objectives can be met and learning maximized. It can be helpful to establish ground rules for discussions (Display 10-1) so that learners will have no doubt that respect and fairness are considered. The SDS should move about and listen, offering support and sharing perspectives as needed.

Questioning learners is an effective way to promote discussion. The presenter will learn what participants bring to the learning experience. It can promote critical thinking and enhance class participation. Everyone may answer the question, although only a few

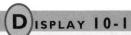

DISPLAY 10-1

Sample Ground Rules for Group Discussion

Everyone has a chance to speak without interruptions.
No one's idea is responded to negatively.
Ideas should be presented briefly.
Participants may seek clarification.
Don't repeat others' ideas; just offer agreement.
The facilitator can close the discussion to keep the group on time.

may speak their responses. Questioning can occur at several levels within Bloom's taxonomy:

1. Recall is the lowest level, with questions beginning with verbs such as state, name, identify, or describe.
2. A higher level of thinking is required to analyze and evaluate information and thus make judgments. Words such as compare, contrast, and differentiate foster critical thinking and decision making.
3. The highest level of questioning may help to invent or create something new or different to the learners. Words to convey this expectation include create, design, invent, predict, or develop.

Skills Training

Repetition of a skill over and over until a learner is comfortable is an ideal that both SDSs and learners would like to achieve. In today's market, we often practice "just-in-time" training: demonstration of a skill, supervised return demonstration of a skill, and then independent performance of the skill within minutes of identifying the learning need. If multiple repetitions are not done, the SDS must identify the person's learning style and adapt the skills demonstration to achieve the most rapid transfer of learning.

Skills fairs are one way to validate multiple skills for a large staff. They do not provide the individual attention of just-in-time training but are efficient strategies to gather a great deal of data about selected competencies.

A well-developed performance checklist will guide skills training sessions. These can be derived from the competence assessment systems described in Chapters 4, 5, and 6 or pulled from journals, procedure manuals, or similar sources. Well-planned skills training sessions require adequate space, simulation aids, equipment, supplies, faculty, and time.

Case Studies

Application of a case study provides the learner with the opportunity to analyze a realistic problem or situation and develop a solution. Adequate information and time must be scheduled for this type of critical thinking exercise. The burden for this strategy lies in the development of the case study: care must be taken to maintain confidentiality, but clinical data must be provided to paint a realistic picture. One strategy for developing a case study is to record facts and events that really happened, but then to disguise them. The case study can be a paragraph or a 100-page document, depending on the learning objectives, the level of the learners, and the amount of time available to achieve the outcome.

Case studies can be used by learners to:

- Identify particular information to be applied later
- Apply models to common situations
- Make decisions regarding care
- Gain more information after successfully satisfying the demands of the current situation.

Computer-assisted instruction commonly uses case studies as the basis for information delivery. Decision trees and algorithms are often applicable to case study analysis. It is important to remain focused on the learning needs because it is easy to digress from the intent of the assignment. The case study is an effective adjunct to delivery of information but should not be considered a substitute.

Self-Learning Packages

Providing an independent environment for learning can meet the needs of staff who cannot leave the work setting to attend to learning. Learners can complete the unit of study in a quiet setting when time allows. Self-learning packages (SLPs) or independent studies are all-inclusive, self-contained packets that allow the student to complete the learning activity without the aid of an instructor. The packet includes the learning objectives, learning activities, and evaluation method for feedback. These forms of learning activities must be accessible to staff. Copies of readings or other media should be a part of the packet or readily available for use with available equipment. A pilot test should be conducted with about five to 10 learners to be sure that the SLP can be accomplished in the allotted time and that it helps the learner achieve the learning objective. Not all learners will achieve learning objectives from an SLP; some learners require a more interactive teaching method or lack the self-discipline to complete the SLP in the allotted time.

Access to independent study materials is easy. Many commercial providers of continuing education have developed this aspect of their business to reach more learners and improve profitability.

Service management and human resources personnel should address how time spent on an SLP is compensated. Professionalism suggests that learning should occur on noncompensated time, but the interpretation of fair wage and salary laws may provide for compensation, especially for mandatory learning activities.

Posters

A consistent and inexpensive method to convey changes in practice or documentation or new programs is the poster. The content of the poster follows the program-planning process, addressing identified learning needs and meeting specified learning objectives. The design of the poster can be simple: paper can be mounted on construction paper or matboard, then mounted on a larger board. Posters are colorful, provide a constant visual reference, and succinctly convey information in a detailed format. A prototype can be developed early for peer and learner review. This strategy allows misconceptions to be identified and corrected before mass production. Volunteer or clerical staff can duplicate the poster as many times as needed to disseminate information efficiently. Topics managed well by posters include:

- Flow charts of new processes
- Examples of the use of new forms
- Photographs of code cart contents
- Reviews of simple procedures.

The poster should not deliver more information than the learner's attention can accommodate; a poster that is too busy or confusing might as well not be displayed. Neatness and good use of color are important to keep the learner's attention.

Others

Many other strategies are available and can be adapted from other settings. Of growing popularity are:

- Storytelling: The use of narrative or oral accounts of actual situations provides learners with an in-depth understanding of issues, concerns, and values of the discipline. It promotes reflective thinking about practice (Rittman & Sella, 1995).
- Nursing rounds: A group of patients, a specific situation, or a challenging case can focus the SDS's discussion with one or more staff members, providing structured "teaching moments" directly in the workplace. Competence validation can occur concurrently with teaching when rounds are the strategy.
- Skits: Having learners play roles in a skit can offer everyone involved an opportunity to experience new or uncomfortable feelings or situations. This is different from traditional role playing, where learners make up their responses to a given situation. Careful and clever scripting is required to help learners have fun while exploring concepts of the affective domain.

PLANNING LEARNING ACTIVITIES

A well-planned activity should provide the SDS with the desired results based on the needs assessment. Often, more time is spent in careful planning than in the actual delivery of the learning event.

Getting Organized

Organization is more than just keeping good records. It involves setting a timetable for activities that will allow enough time for planning. Forms for consistent recording of events also serve as a guide to the steps to be completed before the event. The SDS should set up systems that allow for ready retrieval of information, whether it is a computerized plan, a color-coded file system, a daily to-do list, or an office day focused on planning tasks. Documentation to support the program's organization includes topic, date, time, place, coordinator, faculty, source of learning need, target audience, learning objectives, teaching strategy, evaluation method, and credits awarded. Display 10-2 shows a sample format to record this data.

Brief Activities for a Few

Only one instructor is necessary for planning and teaching when only a few persons need to learn a given topic. An example of this staff development activity is teaching clinical staff how to instill eye drops when a new population with ophthalmic problems is introduced to the agency. Often the steps are critical, and consistency can be achieved if the same faculty teach everyone, without loss of enthusiasm when the audience is small. The program can be quick and to the point and not lengthened to appear to increase its value. An SDS who can offer the staff a new skill in less time than management anticipates has increased value to the organization.

> ## Dispʟᴀʏ 10-2
>
> **Sample Documentation Form for Brief Learning Activity Center for Nursing Education**
>
> | CNE use only |
> | Code _____ |
>
> **Learning Activity Record** _____
>
> **Program Title:**
>
> **Coordinator:**
>
> **Date/Time/Place:**
>
> **Faculty:**
>
> **Source of Need:**
>
> **Learner Objectives:**
>
> **Teaching Strategy:**
>
> **Target Audience:**
>
> **Aids or Equipment:**
>
> **Contact Hours:**
>
> **Evaluation Method:**
>
> **Evaluation:**
> (Completed after activity)
>
> Please attach course outline to this form

Source: Greater Southeast Community Hospital, Washington, DC. Reproduced with permission in Kelly, K.J. (Ed.). (1992). *Nursing Staff Development* (1st ed.). Philadelphia: J.B. Lippincott.

Brief Activities for Many

Occasionally the agency may introduce a new product or policy that requires the majority of employees to participate. New Occupational Safety and Health Administration guidelines may fit this category. This kind of activity can be tedious and redundant for faculty, but the learning curve gets more efficient as more participants complete the training and begin sharing their new skill with peers. To ensure that all learners have received the same content, script the learning activity, provide consistency, and make preparation simple for the faculty. A prop or simple handout is useful to serve as reinforcement. It may be less expensive to develop an amusing video to deliver the information, especially when learners are in several locations. Faculty or facilitators should be scheduled in brief teaching periods so that fatigue does not affect enthusiasm. Learners can be overbooked for these learning activities because distractions, attrition, and shared learning by other staff will influence attendance.

Longer Programs for a Few

When planning 1- to 3-day programs targeted to a very select audience, creative scheduling is important—as important as appropriate content. Managers may need to provide additional staffing for patients to maximize resources. A longer program is likely to be more complex. An example might be discharge planning for the psychiatric population. Skills to be acquired include persuasion, advocacy, documentation, and principles of outpatient psychiatric care. The number of expert faculty required to teach the content may equal the number of participants. Therefore, it is important that the program is offered as few times as possible to as many persons as possible. Providing variety throughout the day will help learners remain engaged in the program. Often a small group loses its motivation quickly if there is not a lot of energy moving within the audience.

Consortiums

A consortium can satisfy the problem of offering an expensive course to only a few persons from one employment setting. Specialized programs, such as collaborations between several counties to provide a school health nurse certification review course, are suited to consortium participation. By sharing planning, teaching, and enrollment expectations with other institutions, the resources of a larger program can be enjoyed, with the expenses of only a smaller one. SDSs benefit from the shared responsibility and a less-demanding teaching assignment (Sammut, 1994).

Longer Programs for Many

Larger space and a more complex agenda are necessary to handle many learners over several days. Planning can begin more than a year in advance to publicize the program. Learners require ample time to budget for more expensive events. Coordination should be done by someone experienced in conference planning, supported by a flexible team of content and education experts. Many types of learners will attend the conference; therefore, offerings should be geared toward their varied levels and disciplines. Various templates can be used for organizing the days, mixing general content and concurrent sessions. Added learning opportunities can be realized by audiotaping the conference and organizing a proceedings book. Hosting a conference requires creativity, flexibility, and organization (Brady, 1996).

Courses for Continued Development

Collaboration with schools of nursing can provide the opportunity to teach new skills to experienced nurses as needed to retool them for changing delivery systems. A course designed by the SDS and faculty from the school of nursing can encourage further enrollment in a baccalaureate completion program or entry into graduate studies while teaching new skills to current practitioners. Operating room, critical care, and home health nursing continue to be areas in which managers prefer to recruit experienced practitioners.

Using Resources

Gone are the days when drug companies' dollars were freely distributed to educators for use in designing learning activities. The policy for commercial support of educational activities (ANA, 1995) provides guidelines for circumstances under which money can be donated and how it can be used (Display 10-3). However, contracts negotiated with equipment and supply companies can include a requirement for training. Teaching samples can be provided by the vendor as part of the purchase agreement. The SDS should retain responsibility for coordinating the learning activities provided by vendors to ensure that they are in line with agency policies and meet learning objectives.

DISPLAY 10-3

ANA Policy on Commercial Support for Continuing Nursing Education (CNE)

Excerpt from Guiding Principles

- CNE is conducted for the education of the audience and for the benefit of the health care consumer. It builds upon the knowledge and competence levels of nurses. It should not be primarily for the benefit of commercial supporters, providers, or presenters involved in the activity.
- CNE programs should be objective and, where legitimate differences or contrasting views exist, balanced. The assurance of objectivity and balance is the responsibility of the provider.
- Factors that can result in the introduction of bias must be avoided. These may include monetary inducements beyond necessary expenses, gifts of more than nominal value, or personal amenities.
- Presenters, topics, course materials, and "enduring materials" must be subject to the approval of and be the responsibility of the provider and not be at the discretion of commercial sponsor(s).
- Disclosure of affiliations, sponsorships, financial support, and other potentially biasing factors must routinely be made to the audience by the provider and participating presenters.
- The educational activity records document evidence of compliance.

ANA. (1995). *Position statement. Guidelines for commercial support for continuing nursing education.* Washington, DC: ANA.

DESIGNING THE ACTIVITY

Following the educational process (Holmes, 1989), once needs have been assessed and learning objectives established, the design can begin. Three questions useful to validate these objectives and guide the design are:

1. How many people will drive to your institution or leave their work area to hear this particular program?
2. How many people will pay money or invest their time and energy to hear this particular program?
3. From whom will learners value hearing the message?

Applying these questions to each objective and content area will help planners differentiate what content is designed for all learners and what is designed for only some, how long learners may choose to address a specific aspect of the content, and how much to invest in faculty.

Concern should be directed to the learners' attention span. Most health care workers are accustomed to long hours and constant stimulation and movement. Placing them in a classroom can be counterproductive, resulting in restlessness and inattention. Breaks should be planned frequently to allow movement and increase energy. Teaching strategies should involve activity and increase participation. It is not unreasonable to require novice faculty and some others to rehearse to ensure that their delivery is enthusiastic and engaging.

Length of time is as important as timing. Whenever possible, programs should be planned to coincide with the introduction of new knowledge, policies, or products. A lag time between the training and the initiation date can decrease the usefulness of the training. Too many new programs begun at the same time can cause staff to have concern that there is no strategic plan guiding the organization's activities, and chaos may ensue.

MARKETING

When marketing a staff development activity, the SDS is doing more than just promoting a program to ensure good attendance. Ideas and organizational changes are being sold to learners before they set foot in the door. Exciting (but not cute) titles are used to grab the attention of potential learners. Scheduling nontraditional start times for presentations, like 10:06 a.m., are sure to cause people to take a second look. Promoting the primary benefit of attendance as increased, improved, or enhanced clinical competence is one approach that will engage potential participants. Writing an intriguing, relevant question and placing it in a prominent place in large type on a flyer or electronic message will catch some potential learners' attention. Promoting the other perks of attendance, like food, prizes, and credit for attendance, will attract others. Marketing is a key component to the planning process and must be given special consideration early in the process.

Whether marketing within the organization or externally to other communities, programs must be seen as originating from within the sponsoring department and organization. One of the principles of promotion is name recognition, implying quality and credibility. Many staff development departments have been renamed to represent their total organizational focus or a clinical versus professional focus. This is an opportunity to develop a departmental logo and adopt a certain "look" for printed materials. Even a one-person department deserves the attention that comes with name recognition. The logo should be used on all printed materials because it may be the distinguishing factor that draws attention to promotional efforts.

Internal Marketing

Marketing within the agency, internal marketing, involves subtle and direct approaches to get the attention of learners and their managers. Managers must find the promotion appealing and sensible, because they are the ones who may or may not release the learners to attend. Initial internal marketing begins with involving the right people in the planning process, from needs assessment through faculty selection. Key informants in the organization as well as possible opponents to the event should be involved in planning. Conflicts with other major organizational programs that compete for learner time should be avoided. Key informants also become the early marketers of the event. It is reasonable to expect persons on the planning committee to play a fundamental role in "selling" the program to their constituencies. They will serve as salespeople within the organization, providing credibility and support for the program.

The timing of internal marketing depends on the distribution of staffing schedules. If the staff's schedule changes every 6 weeks and is posted 2 weeks in advance, and requests must be in 4 weeks before posting, then programs requiring a requested day off should be promoted at least 12 weeks in advance. This includes workshops, teleconferences, and special presentations. A 15-minute introduction to a new feeding pump can be promoted with only a week's notice, and many may be available for the short offering. Organizational norms will prescribe promotional schedules and may need to be adjusted as new administrators are introduced to changing health care systems.

Fliers can be developed for each program. However, each brightly colored sheet with multiple fonts is competing with every other announcement that is taped, stapled, or tacked to walls and bulletin boards. The key is to offer a timely announcement that provides enough information without contributing to information overload and chaos.

In a large facility, there may be enough programming generated that an annual or semiannual calendar of events in the form of a catalog may best suit staffing and programming needs. Fliers become supplemental then, once staff become used to looking for learning opportunities in the catalog. In a smaller facility, a monthly or bimonthly calendar may be sufficient. Program promotions can be placed on a home page on the Internet or a computerized administrative bulletin board, or scrolled across the patient information system screen as the screen saver.

Announcements over the paging system can serve as reminders and alert patients to the fact the staff members are continually learning. Presentations at staff or administrative meetings provide opportunities for key persons to ask questions about the event. Notes included with paychecks or "table tents" in the dining room may offer reminders for annual mandatory training sessions.

Constant salesmanship is the key to success in increasing participation in programs. It will allow learners, managers, and other customers to view SDSs as responsive providers.

External Marketing

If the mission of the organization supports participation in programs by external communities, then clear goals about external marketing must be set. External marketing will require a budget and the commitment of staff for the tasks required. Brochures can cost 30 cents to $1.50 each and should not be wasted on an outdated mailing list or an inexperienced mailing service. Brochure design can be accomplished using desktop publishing software or through a graphic artist employed at a local printer. Some large health care organizations and systems have internal design capacity and the ability to handle all their external marketing tasks. These organizations usually have guidelines for SDSs about the parameters and limitations of those internal services.

A successful brochure includes all the essential information but must compete with all other mailed information. Color, font, and white space are as important as accuracy, completeness, and quality of content.

There is considerable disagreement regarding the number of brochures that should be mailed to market a planned event. Marketing sources indicate that only a 1% to 2% response rate can be expected—for every 100 brochures mailed, only one or two potential participants may respond (assuming the brochure is well designed, appeals to the learner, and fits the participant's perceived needs). Mailing labels with names always yield the best results; however, maintaining or buying an accurate list can be costly. Mailing lists can be purchased from the American Hospital Association, the ANA, a specialty organization, publishers, and others. These lists reflect persons who are members or buyers of books and journal subscriptions. Not all persons on those lists will be interested in the promoted event or service. List purchases are for one-time use only and carry associated royalty fees as well as printing fees. Lists should be checked for accuracy and usefulness before accepting the order for use. Cover letters to key leaders in an organization may encourage brochure distribution to appropriate persons.

Choosing to use a service or volunteers to label and sort brochures for mailing may be a time management or a financial decision. Many novice SDSs have spent hours "saving money" by completing this task. After a few times, most people yield to the information age and go with a computerized service. At a penny per label and sort, the SDS can spend time on tasks requiring his or her educational expertise.

Advertisements in the appropriate journals can be purchased or placed at no cost in continuing education calendars. Organization newsletters offer space for workshop information as a member benefit. Internet discussions and postings offer a wide-reaching advertising strategy. Cosponsorship with another organization enhances marketing potential, as does an educational grant by a vendor. The more persons involved in planning, the more potential participants will be contacted by the planners.

PROJECTING COSTS, EFFECTIVENESS, AND BENEFITS

Projections are only as good as the planning. Variables such as other agencies' programs or acts of God are uncontrollable. Projecting costs can be accomplished using formulas and estimates as described in Chapter 14. Projecting effectiveness is based on following the educational process. Projecting benefits will depend on the audience and their needs. Swanson and Gradous (1990) offer formulas for calculating the benefits of training and translating them into dollars for the organization. This is a very useful strategy to employ when training dollars are being cut. Demonstrating the financial effects and benefits of training can show that training makes money for the organization rather than serving as an expense center.

Costs for the program can be real or assumed within the departmental budget. It depends on the type of reporting and accountability of the department as to how detailed a cost analysis should be completed. Leaning toward more detail would require that planning time, secretarial time, faculty time, each sheet of paper, and equipment depreciation be listed. Using less detail would require that actual expenditures requiring a check request, a purchase order, or interdepartmental fund transfer be noted, as these are not costs that are necessarily part of departmental operations, and may need to be offset by income (Kelly, 1985). Knowing the current costs of items, from soft drinks to binders, helps in planning a program within budget and handling the unexpected during the program.

Program effectiveness refers to the anticipated effects or outcomes of the program being measured after the event. Analysis of impact provides one approach to viewing effectiveness (de la Cruz and Bickerton, 1996). Three themes emerged from their comparative analysis of participant evaluations:

- "Earthquake effect": implies that learning is triggered by a variety of forces during spontaneous moments
- "Effective debunking": uncovering or unmasking assumptions or patterns—in other words, unlearning
- "Bushfire effect": information that is learned can move like fire if it is exciting to the learner.

This is only one method for describing program effectiveness. The method used within each agency should align with its mission and goals.

GENERATING REVENUE

The decision to generate revenue must be in line with the institution's mission and policies. A nonprofit organization can generate revenues; however, the funds must be directed as the organization desires.

When making the choice to generate revenue, a decision must be made about how much income in excess of expense is desired. Care must be taken not to overprice the program in an effort to turn a profit. However, a program that appears to be underpriced may not be valued as highly and therefore may not generate the interest it deserves. Some think that if something is free, it must have no value (these people probably don't clip coupons either).

If a fee is assessed, then there must be provisions for a refund policy. Under what circumstances would a prepaid registration fee be returned to the participant? Perhaps refunds can be given before a certain date, in case of a personal emergency, and if staffing is required. Will cash, checks, and credit cards be accepted? Cash requires that receipts be given; checks may be returned for insufficient funds; and credit cards require special arrangements and fees through the bank.

Consideration should be given to setting up fee schedules, providing discounts to employees or members of participating organizations. An early-bird rate can be offered to encourage early registration; a late fee may be assessed for registration the day of the event. Keep the fee schedule simple while offering incentives as appropriate.

Some departments assess a fee to hold a participant's place in class, only to return it when the participant actually attends. A policy such as this must be in accordance with the administration's philosophy of staffing and education. What if the employee cannot attend because of a staffing change?

If funds are generated, a clear path for their deposit should be established. Does the department have a provision for collecting funds and keeping them within the department? What are the parameters for using these funds? Or does all income go into a general operating account (and therefore would not be available to offset expenses)?

DOCUMENTING THE EVENT

Records should be kept based on the type and amount of information that may require retrieval later. Clinical staff development providers, specialists, and other groups should have a recordkeeping system. For example, the Joint Commission on Accreditation of Healthcare Organizations (JCAHO) seeks information about problems within the organization and how they have been resolved through education. Records of programs offered in the past and planned for the future will satisfy this JCAHO request. Records are also required to document competence of new and continuing employees related to required job skills. An account of the educational process including all critical criteria must be recorded. Information about the percentage of the intended audience that participated and achievement of the desired effects should be noted.

Risk management departments need documentation that a problem has been resolved or information that a person has been deemed competent to perform a specific task. Attendance records, course outlines, and competency validation plans can all be called for to defend an employee or the agency in malpractice litigation. Most nurses are quite good at creating forms and tools to answer these requests for information—sometimes so many forms exist that they serve as a detriment rather than a benefit.

Software for recordkeeping is readily available for customizing and reporting. Professional journals regularly carry ads for new documentation packages. The SDS should evaluate them and select one that will meet the organization's needs.

Specific records (e.g., contact hours) are required to be on file for educational accreditation bodies such as the American Nurses Credentialing Center, the primary accrediting agency for nursing continuing education credits. These records must be kept in an area that can be secured (double-locked in some situations) and are accessible only to authorized persons. The same principle of confidentiality used with patients' medical records applies to staff development records.

Recordkeeping Systems

Records can be kept manually or with an automated system and relevant software. They may also be kept by learners or by selected departments. It is not uncommon for an organization to set a policy and guidelines for storage and retention of all records. The recordkeeping system should reflect the ease and frequency with which information must be retrieved. The system should reflect where the responsibility for education lies, with the learner or with management. An employee may have primary responsibility for documenting when learning has occurred, making note of attendance at programs, dates of clinical check-offs, and annual repetition of mandatory programs.

In our future is a recordkeeping system installed on chips and inserted onto a new employee's body part that records movement and activity as he or she comes in contact with a learning activity (approved for contact hours, of course); it may even record the evaluation of that activity for eventual downloading. Reports would then be designed and generated to produce data for all those who need to know. SDSs would be responsible for creating those meaningful reports. Imagine the paperlessness of that day!

Today, bar-code and scanning technology can be used to record employees' participation in scheduled learning activities. Data in the form of reports can be retrieved in a variety of formats, some more sophisticated than others.

A computer-based system can be a mere extension of a paper-and-pencil system, with all of its problems. Or an automated system can be integrated so that registration at a program and subsequent attendance allows an employee's record to be updated automatically. Tying the computer system to the time and attendance system allows for even more sophisticated data links. Using magnetic strips on identification badges permits quick data entry for some events.

Need-to-Know Principle

Access to records should be clearly identified in agency policy and may depend on the recordkeeping system in addition to the accountable bodies. Persons making staffing assignments are required by JCAHO to have access to clinical competence assessment records. However, because education records reflect competence as well as "incompetence," the principle of confidentiality must again be applied to develop a policy and guideline describing who may have access to which employees' records under specified circumstances. The Student Privacy Act has also been applied to the education of employees.

Judgment must be exercised when giving out information about participation. The American Nurses Credentialing Center requires that a copy of a contact hour certificate be requested in person or in writing, not over the telephone. It also suggests handing certificates to course participants only at the end of the learning experience. This is to prevent fraudulent acquisition of certificates, because they are valuable for relicensure in 30 states (Yoder-Wise, 1997).

According to JCAHO, when the surveyor is reviewing the education records of selected employees, other information must be excluded from this record, such as disciplinary actions, salary information, and vacation requests. A specially organized and labeled folder should be available for JCAHO review.

Reports

Most staff development departments are overloaded with information. It is important to identify what reports should be generated to represent the work of the department. A candid conversation with the leadership of the organization can guide identification of data sets and reports required to satisfy the needs of department personnel as well as management and administration. Questions to consider include:

- Are numbers (*e.g.*, of participants, of programs, of cancellations, of no-shows) most important?
- Is program effectiveness and benefits information that is reported to accrediting bodies and boards more important?
- Can the computer-based system generate the reports that are needed when, for example, Medicare surveyors make unannounced visits? Or will clerical staff need to hand-tally data to answer their safety training participation question at the time of the visit?

Designing the reports to meet the stated needs will permit clear communication with decision-makers.

PLANNING THE COMPETENCE EVALUATION METHOD

When planning a program that addresses a particular skill or process, it is necessary to identify the strategy by which competence will be evaluated and documented at the end of the program. If a new feeding pump is introduced to the organization, should training address the operation of this new pump only, or is this a good time to assess the competence of staff regarding tube feeding management? This is not to imply that every in-service requires a great amount of effort, but because evaluation of competence is required in most quality management programs and accreditation guidelines, the savvy SDS should consider how to tie the two projects together while the employee is focused on tube feedings.

Competence evaluation can be combined with skills training or considered part of managerial or educational rounds. A team comprising the manager, the educator, and staff can physically move from patient to patient with the intent of evaluating care and assessing competence in a particular area—growth and development, documentation, or physical assessment. This provides opportunities for the manager to participate in competence evaluation and for the educator to provide teaching during a receptive moment. Organizations that accept and promote learning and improvement will also recognize the teaching role of every professional.

Another strategy used for competence evaluation is participation in an annual skills fair. When multiple skills must be checked off, it can be cost- and time-effective to set up stations where demonstrations and return demonstrations of certain skills can be performed. This works well for the manipulation of equipment, such as blood glucose monitoring, sequential compression devices, infusion pumps, and drainage systems. Instruction can occur when necessary, but staff members who are competent can move on quickly to the next station. Annual mandatory training can take place during this event as well.

IMPLEMENTING EDUCATIONAL PROGRAMS

Good planning is the key to implementing a sound educational program. The actual implementation takes creativity and flexibility, as events occur that may change the original plan. Patient care always takes priority over education; staffing is beyond the educator's control. Planning for a program can be analogous to preparing a holiday meal. It takes hours, even days, to prepare all the foods, which will be eaten in the space of only an hour. Careful planning allows guests to savor and remember a delicious and delightful holiday; lack of planning can mean a disaster.

Step-by-Step Process

Following the educational process is important to the program's success. The Holmes model provides a classic, well-recognized approach. The approach *assess, plan, implement, and evaluate* is the classic scientific method for problem solving and is sometimes recognized by nurses as the nursing process. Like all processes, activities are dynamic rather than stable or linear. Once needs are documented, then learning objectives are written. These are shared with potential learners to validate their appropriateness. The length of the program can then be determined based on how long it will take for learners to accomplish the objectives and how long the agency will allow for the program. A date is selected to provide the learning at an opportune moment. The room or facility is reserved. Identified faculty are contacted. The design and content are negotiated with the faculty. An appropriate method for evaluation is chosen. Time is allowed for development of promotional and learning materials to support the program.

Once the program is delivered, evaluation occurs to ensure that goals were met, transfer of learning to work-related performance expectations occurred, and learners were satisfied. Recordkeeping is completed and accessible for future reference.

Gaining Administrative Support

The premise to planning any educational program is to maintain alignment with the philosophy, mission, and expressed values of the organization. Thus, gaining administrative support is easier if the program meets the needs of the institution, the patient population served, and the learners. Administrators are most interested in how the organization will benefit from the time and investment spent on the training. Administrative support is easier to gain if the concept is presented verbally or in writing within an outcome framework—that is, the outcome of the learning activity will:

- Decrease errors, infections, or exposure to risks
- Improve processes or systems
- Change customer impressions of the organization.

In presenting the concept to the administration, the educator should be able to demonstrate that this is the right program, providing the right outcome, using the right design, at the right time in this organizational environment. The educator should recognize which programs require administrative support and which can be planned as a matter of routine.

Right Program

Delivering the right program can be ensured by including a learner, an expert, and an accountable person on the program-planning committee to help the educator identify appropriate objectives, content, and faculty. For example, a staff nurse, a clinical nurse specialist, and a nurse manager are often the right team to plan a program addressing the nursing care of most conditions. Of course, adding persons from other disciplines or someone who disagrees with the concept may be helpful as well. Content must be current and appropriate for the setting.

Right Design

The right design can make or break a program. Creativity and fun are necessary components of a program in today's world. Television has led society to seek entertainment while learning. However, more traditional learners may resist strategies such as games, group work, and active participation. The design will depend on the resources, time, and characteristics of the learners. Mimicking popular game shows has been quite successful for many topics, especially during annual mandatory training. Many educators have gotten the facility's maintenance department to build a "Jeopardy" board for multiple uses throughout the year. Additional teaching techniques designed for a variety of health care workers use games ranging from crossword puzzles to variations on popular board games (Deck, 1993).

Design, in terms of length and sequence of the day, is important: a balance needs to be achieved between active or sedentary learning sessions and other activities. Providing breaks long enough to allow movement, refreshment, and networking is important, but breaks that are too long make learners feel that the day is less productive than it could have been. Multiple-day workshops may be spread across several weeks or completed as a continuous series. This depends on the nature of the scheduling of the particular audience and the costs to travel to the site of the education.

Right Timing

When introducing a new procedure or equipment to a facility, the training should occur as close to the actual implementation date as possible. When several new processes are scheduled for implementation around the same time, the educator can suggest that they be staggered so that staff are not overwhelmed with changes and unable to learn one concept before dealing with another.

If a documentation problem has been known for some time, the educational intervention to improve it might best be done after a citation or before an accreditation visit to "rally the troops" around a common cause. Staff may have little incentive to learn after a commendation, although the need may still exist. Specialty courses should be offered when the specialists are generally available.

Right Outcome

The right outcome can be achieved by asking initially, Can this problem be solved by teaching, or is it a supervision or system problem that needs to be addressed? Indeed, it is rare that education alone will solve a situation. This is difficult to convince others: it is often easier to direct that an educational program be planned than to identify that a manager has work to do. It is also often cheaper to provide initial teaching than to redesign a work system.

The key to achieving the right outcome is to address the right learning need. This supports the premise that the learning needs assessment must be thoroughly and accurately accomplished, then validated, before any other planning. If the situation changes between the planning and the delivery of the program, the desired outcome may no longer be the right outcome. Being flexible and aware of changes as they occur is important to providing the right outcome. The measurement of achievement of the right outcome must be planned before the educational intervention is delivered, so that success or failure can be defined.

DEVELOPING PLATFORM SKILLS

Many health care educators get their start as Basic Life Support instructors, as defined by the American Heart Association's standards, guidelines, and manual. Others may have had opportunities to teach for their professional or personal communities. Others may come to clinical staff development with formal academic preparation and credentials. A few come to staff development practice as recognized expert clinicians. All should bring characteristics that they acknowledge and others that can be developed and improved.

Practice

Practice can be achieved in a variety of ways. When a novice faculty member has been invited to present a course, it can be with the understanding that a rehearsal will be scheduled before the presentation. The rationale is to validate that the content that is expected will actually be delivered. Practice can occur in front of the planning committee or experienced educators. Videotaping the presenter is a successful way of delivering feedback while highlighting examples that support the need for improvement. Second videotaped practice sessions often demonstrate significant improvement.

Many ideas are available in the popular literature regarding techniques useful in relieving anxiety before making a presentation. Doing deep-breathing exercises and imagining the audience naked are two of the most popular. However, a little anxiety is actually helpful before a presentation: it heightens the senses and keeps the presenter on edge enough to be quick-witted.

Teaching an already scripted presentation several times will give developing speakers the opportunity to hone their presentation skills without the need to focus on content development. In the same way, writing a script to use for a presenter's first few presentations will allow the presenter to focus on the style of presentation rather than the content.

Practice is important to help the presenter identify how long sentences can be without pausing for breath. If the presenter gets a dry mouth or scratchy throat, he or she should feel comfortable sipping water during the presentation. If props will be used, then practice using the prop is necessary. Just as important is practice using audiovisual equipment. Placing a transparency correctly on an overhead projector can be viewed as a sign of credibility, just as much as good content.

Trying New Approaches

Once they learn about new educational approaches, excited educators are often eager to try them out. For new approaches to be successful, staff within the agency must be willing to try something new, too. Asking a group of managers to engage in small-group discussion may be unsuccessful if they are under an autocratic leadership and never asked for their opinions. This strategy must be used with a topic that is not threatening or closely linked to their current job responsibilities for the first few experiences. This approach assumes that the agency will be shifting to a more participative style of management. Thus, the efforts spent on the learning activity will translate into new behaviors in other ways.

The first time that a game situation is used, the educator may have to choose the game players beforehand so that volunteering to be silly does not become an issue. Game rules can be complicated, so playing the game a couple of times outside the classroom will be helpful before getting in front of the audience.

Creativity

The classroom is a stage, so anything that is appropriate for the stage may be appropriate for the classroom. Use of music, movement, acting, props, light, or darkness can enhance the learning environment. Celebrating the completion of agency orientation may call for a welcoming ceremony, complete with a reception with cake and punch and a ceremonial pinning of name tags by the chief executive officer. Creating a skit to demonstrate the perceptions of a patient when faced with myriad health care workers in a typical day can capture learners' attention, because the learners may not know much more than the patient does about their full contributions to the team.

Creativity can mean preparing colorful transparencies using a variety of clip art, using props to demonstrate a point, or letting learners lead the session by contributing their own experiences. However, in an effort to be creative, some presenters go beyond the norm and create elaborate visuals and use many props and background music. Some learners will find this distracting and will have a difficult time engaging in the learning activity. Knowing the audience members and their preferred learning styles and activities will help the creative presenter prepare an appropriate array of innovative strategies.

EVALUATING THE PROGRAM

The educational process closes with evaluation of the program. Evaluation is a word used in many ways by various people with different agendas. It is important to differentiate evaluation of the individual educational activity provided from the total departmental educational program. It is also important to identify what is being evaluated. Many persons equate the participant feedback or learner satisfaction tool with evaluation of the program. Evaluation in clinical staff development can be significantly enhanced if supported by a model, several of which are discussed below. These models are generally applicable to both the overall educational program and individual programs.

To choose an appropriate model for the evaluation process, it is important to determine the focus of the evaluation. Asking the following questions will guide the process:

- For whom is the evaluation being conducted? Learners? Administrators? A specific community? A combination of the preceding groups?
- Why is the evaluation being conducted? To determine transfer of learning? Benefits to the organization? Impact on the budget? A combination?
- What questions will be asked in the evaluation? Are the questions specific? Measurable? Related to the purpose of the evaluation process?
- What is the scope of the evaluation? Will each objective be measured? Every faculty member or instructor? Every skill or step in a procedure?
- What resources are available to conduct the evaluation? How much time? What are the specific resources needed to collect, analyze, and report data?

A model that has been in use for more than 20 years emerged from the work of Kirkpatrick (1975), who analyzed the evaluation methods used in the 1950s. This classic model (1975) takes a comprehensive four-level approach to evaluation of total programs or individual activities within a total program:

1. Reaction: the participant's reaction to the program. This can be measured with learner satisfaction instruments or participant feedback questionnaires.
2. Learning: the facts, principles, or techniques that were understood by the participants. This can be measured with skills performance checklists, written tests, or a review discussion.
3. Behavior: transfer of learning and desirable behaviors actually demonstrated on the job as a result of the learning experience.
4. Results: outcomes, both individual behaviors and the effect of the aggregated change in behaviors on the patients served. Results can be measured by reduction of costs, improved clinical outcomes, decreased turnover, and other measures of productivity (Kirkpatrick, 1975).

Chapters 6 and 8 also discuss the Kirkpatrick approach to evaluation.

In 1991, the International Association for Continuing Education and Training published *Assessment of Learning Outcomes in Continuing Education and Training: A Practical Guide to Assessment Plans*. This model focuses on the evaluation of learning outcomes, the behaviors that were established as the end product of the learning experience. The measures include:

● Changes in the learner's knowledge, attitude, and skill
● Subsequent behavioral change
● Impact of behavioral change on the learner's environment.

Participant feedback questionnaires, pre- and post-assessments, plan of action, follow-up assessment of application of learning, ongoing support, ongoing interventions with the learner's environment, and assessing the impact of the application of learning are key evaluative methods in the IACET model. These methods are chosen based on the complexity of the program and the intended change in the learner and environment.

The model allows for one of 10 plans to be selected after use of the "assessment plan decision survey." Program planners answer eight questions (Display 10-4) regarding the intended learning outcomes, rating each on a scale of 1 to 10. The responses are then averaged, yielding information to help the SDS select a plan from among those provided. To allow for flexibility, the designers suggest that if plan 6 is selected, then plans 5 and 7 be given consideration as well. The guide is not prescriptive; planners may alter, add, or delete components from any plan to match program needs and objectives. The assessment plan has applicability for clinical staff development within any specialty as well as patient and community education.

A major component of any of the plans is the participant feedback questionnaire. This tool is intended to determine how satisfied the learner is with the learning experience. These questionnaires are sometimes known as "smile sheets" or "happiness indices." The participant feedback questionnaire can be used to determine how pleased the learner was with the content, faculty, setting, and time frame. A key point to determine is if the learner met the original objective for attendance. Because learners have different reasons and goals for learning, the learner must have a clear goal in mind when assessing if the goal has been met. Motivation for participation in learning can range from completing an activity to social support to fulfilling a relicensure or recertification requirement. The learner's satisfaction depends on his or her motivation.

The models described above can be used to evaluate an individual program, too. The

---

DISPLAY 10-4

Questions from Assessment Plan Decision Survey

1. What level of responsibility does the instructional design require to help ensure the transfer of learning back to the job, community, or family?
2. Where does the assessment of learning outcomes fall in our list of priorities for this particular program?
3. How much money can we devote to assessing learning outcomes in this particular program?
4. How much time/human resources can we devote to assessing learning outcomes in this particular program?
5. How crucial will it be that we know that learners have applied what was taught in this particular program?
6. How crucial is it that we know the impact of learning at the workplace, in the community, and/or the home?
7. What degree of structured feedback must we provide participants regarding their learning during and subsequent to the program?
8. How much evidence do we need to show that it was this particular program that really made a difference in the learner's life, work, community, or family?

From International Association for Continuing Education and Training. (1991). *Assessment of learning outcomes in continuing education and training: A practical guide to assessment plans.* Washington, DC: IACET.

---

following is a discussion of the components of the "Assessment of Learning Outcomes" model and how they are developed.

General Test Construction Guidelines

Although many adults do not like to take tests, they do provide a measure of learning that can be used for evaluation purposes. The SDS must be sensitive to adults' discomfort with taking tests and choose this option only when it will be useful. Changing the name from "test" to "assessment of learning" or "evaluative method" may or may not relieve test anxiety. Understanding what the data derived from the test will be used for will help the learner frame this evaluation experience.

All testing, evaluations, and assessments should occur in a nonthreatening environment, using support and reinforcement. An example of how the SDS can integrate these concepts into learning can be found in the American Heart Association's instructor manuals. Recognizing the anxiety caused by performance tests, the association suggested guidelines to adapt testing situations for Basic Life Support and Advanced Cardiac Life Support courses to include group testing and the use of real-life scenarios. Participants report better feelings about the testing, and faculty report good results in performance.

WRITTEN TESTS

When using a written test as an evaluation technique, the test should be planned using a test blueprint. A test blueprint identifies how many questions are planned per topic and can help ensure that content and objectives are reflected. Only critical topics should be addressed, and the number of questions per topic should reflect the relative weight of that topic in relation to all others. Test questions should be written for areas that can be addressed cognitively, rather than those best addressed by performance. Chapter 11 describes these concepts in detail.

PERFORMANCE TESTS

Performance tests are primarily used to measure the psychomotor domain. They can also be used in combination with written or verbal questions to provide richer data about the learner's capacity. Design of the performance checklist should follow the procedures already developed and approved within the organization. In some cases, the performance test or checklist has become the organization's approved policy and is incorporated into other manuals as documentation and a resource for staff.

Participant Action Plan Approach

A classic option suggested by Salinger is the "Participant Action Plan Approach" (OPM, 1980). Participants are asked to describe what they will do with the content learned from the program. This description is written in the form of an action plan. This plan is taken home or back to the workplace for later reference and self-evaluation at specified intervals. Copies of the original may be mailed to the participant in 3 to 6 months as a reminder of the goals set during the education activity. Some organizations use pressure-sensitive paper to provide copies for the SDS and the learner's manager or supervisor as part of a comprehensive employee evaluation program that uses competence development data as part of the performance appraisal system. The primary intent of PAPA is to stimulate the learner to take responsibility and use the knowledge in the best way possible for self-growth. PAPA can also remind the SDS and manager about a learner's stated intentions.

TRANSFER OF LEARNING

The effect of learning one skill on the later performance of other related skills is known as transfer of learning. For example, once aseptic technique is mastered, then it should be readily applied to all types of dressing change techniques. For transfer of learning to be successful, the practice situation should be designed to include a situation similar to real-life conditions. Patterns should be identified for the learner. Personality conflicts and other barriers to learning should be eliminated. The more positive the learner is about success, the more likely it is that transfer of learning will occur. Virtual reality technology has great promise to provide realistic simulations for learner assessment and development.

As in the Assessment of Learning Outcomes model discussed above, the intent is for one learning activity to have long-term effects for the learner and the community served by the learner. Using today's competence models, it is expected that learners will apply their experiences to current learning activities or employment requirements. Whenever possible, learners can be reminded where content or skills may have been introduced before, to help them organize the meaning of the new content or skill.

SUMMARY

Program planning is an important component of success in developing learning experiences. Using the scientific method of problem solving, this chapter has addressed needs assessment, domains of learning, various types of activities, marketing, recordkeeping, and evaluation. The key to success is to design the right program, with the right outcome, offered at the right time, and using the right design. Variety in planning is vital to keeping learners interested. SDSs engaged in the multitude of activities required to keep staff current on health care developments will benefit from the suggestions offered in this chapter.

Applying the Method in Daily Practice

BARBARA J. DALEY

When I started working in continuing nursing education and staff development, program planning was one of those areas of practice that I thought made perfect sense. I was schooled in the classic scientific problem-solving method of program planning. This meant the planner assessed the learning needs of the participants, used those identified learning needs in planning the program, implemented the program using a step-by-step process, and then evaluated the results. This type of program planning meant specifying objectives, outlining teaching methods, and articulating time frames needed to cover content. It all seemed logical, linear, and very organized. I think I could relate to this model of program planning because to me it seemed so similar to using the nursing process in clinical practice. The nursing process steps of assess, plan, implement, and evaluate were the same steps that I learned to use in program planning.

However, over the course of my career I learned that program planning is not such a neat, clean package. Program planning involves an integrated understanding of nursing as a profession, the context in which the program is being planned, and the persons whose needs are being served by the program. The complexities in program planning arise because of the variety, scope, and individuality of the people involved.

I think the first time that I became aware of the complexities involved in program planning was when I was asked to prepare and present a program on medication administration. The director of nursing told me that medication errors had once again been on the increase, and she wanted the staff development department to review the correct procedure for giving medication with all clinical nurses in the hospital. It seemed like a simple request and one that would not involve a large amount of detailed planning. So my first step was a short needs assessment of staff nurses. My intent was to find out which parts of the medication procedure they needed to have reviewed or did not understand.

Much to my amazement, staff nurses thought the entire idea was ridiculous. They said they were fully aware of the procedure for medication administration and said the problem was not the procedure, but the recently changed medication administration forms. The nurses said the forms were unclear and difficult to read, used nonstandard abbreviations for dosages, and required duplicative documentation. One head nurse reported that the change in the medication administration form was made to satisfy the pharmacy department and meet its documentation requirements. This change did help pharmacy, but at the same time it had increased and complicated the nurses' work. This ultimately led to more errors.

At this point, I recognized that my nice, clean, neat program was going to be more difficult than I had imagined. I could see three different perspectives or ways of defining the issues around medication administration. The director of nursing thought the need was to prepare a review program; staff nurses thought there was no need for a program but wanted the medication system changed; and pharmacy said that their job was complete once the medications were sent to the floor. How could I possibly plan a program in the midst of this turmoil?

I felt I had two choices. One, I could continue on and plan a medication administration program as requested. The intended consequences of this action would be that my boss was happy and the task that I had been asked to do would be complete. The unintended consequences of this action could be that nothing in the system would change. Second, I could try to come up with a way to meet the needs of the various constituencies involved. Because I believe that the role of continuing nursing education and staff development is to promote learning and foster changes that positively affect client care, I chose the second option.

My next step was to interview staff nurses, head nurses, and pharmacists to find out the specific details of the medication administration system that were problematic from each perspective. I then presented all these issues to the director of nursing and suggested that we needed to pull together a group of professionals to recommend how to improve the entire medication administration system. After numerous meetings, discussions, and negotiations, recommendations for a new system that would meet the needs of nursing and pharmacy were forwarded to both departments. With further review and modification, a new system was implemented. The staff development program that I ultimately planned was geared to help nurses and pharmacists understand the changed, upgraded system.

I think I remember this case because it was the first time I recognized that program planning could not exist in isolation from the context or environment in and for which the program is being planned. I found it necessary to balance the interests of three distinct groups, generate discussion on a system-wide issue, and then plan the program to promote system change. Since that time, whenever I am planning a program, whether it is a single offering or an entire sequence of offerings over a period of time, I ask myself these questions:

1. Is this a single learning issue or a more complex system issue?
2. Whose needs and interests are being served with the program I am planning?
3. How do I include and balance all those needs and interests in the program planning?
4. Will the program as planned foster improvement in the delivery of patient or client care?
5. How will the program planning fit within the context or environment for which it is planned?

I have found that these questions help me focus on the content of the program I am planning, the planning process, and the relation of that process to everyone involved.

REFERENCES

Alspach, J. G. (1995). *The educational process in nursing staff development.* St. Louis: Mosby.

American Nurses Association. (1995). *Position statement: Guideline for commercial support for continuing nursing education.* Washington DC: Author.

Bastable, S. B. (1997). *Nurse as educator.* Boston: Jones & Bartlett.

Brady, M. (1996). So you want to host a nursing conference? *Journal of Continuing Education in Nursing, 27*(2), 89–94.

Care, W. D. (1996). Identifying the learning needs of nurse managers. *Journal of Nursing Staff Development, 12*(1), 27–30.

Dave, R.H. (1970). Psychomotor levels. In Armstrong, R. J. (Ed.). *Developing and writing behavioral objectives.* Tucson, AZ: Educational Innovators Press.

de la Cruz, L. A. D., & Bickerton, M. (1996). The 12-1/2 minute learning session: Some examples and analysis of impact. *Journal of Continuing Education in Nursing, 27*(2), 85–88.

Deck, M. L. (1993). *Instant teaching tools for healthcare educators.* St. Louis: Mosby.

Dyche, J. (1982). *Educational program development for employees in healthcare agencies.* Calabasas, CA: Tri-Oak Education.

Francke, A. L., Garssen, B., Abu-Saad, H. H., & Grypdonck, M. (1996). Qualitative needs assessment prior to a continuing education program. *Journal of Continuing Education in Nursing, 27*(1), 34–41.

Holmes, S. A. (1989). Getting started: Educational offering design model. *Journal of Nursing Staff Development, 5*(2), 94.

House, G. (1972). *The psychomotor domain: A guide for developing behavioral objectives.* Washington DC: National Special Media Institute.

International Association for Continuing Education and Training. (1991). *Assessment of learning outcomes in continuing education and training: A practical guide to assessment plans*. Washington DC: IACET.

Kelly, K. J. (1985). Cost-benefit and cost-effectiveness analysis: Tools for the staff development manager. *Journal of Nursing Staff Development, 1*(1), 9–15.

Kelly, K. J. (1992). *Nursing staff development*, 1st ed. Philadelphia: Lippincott, p. 128.

Kirkpatrick, D. L. (1975). *Evaluating training programs: A collection of articles from the Journal of the American Society of Training and Development*. Madison, WI: ASTD.

Krathwol, D. R., Bloom, B. S., & Masia, B. (1964). *Taxonomy of educational objectives, Handbook II*. New York: David McKay.

Office of Personnel Management (OPM). (1980). *Assessing changes in job behavior due to training: A guide to the Participant Action Plan Approach (PAPA)*. Washington, DC: US Government Printing Office.

Puetz, B. (1992). Needs assessment: The essence of the staff development program. In Kelly, K. J. (Ed.). *Nursing Staff Development*. Philadelphia: Lippincott.

Rittman, M. R., & Sella, S. (1995). Storytelling: An innovative approach to staff development. *Journal of Nursing Staff Development, 11*(1), 15–19.

Sammut, N. A. (1994). Critical care education: A consortium approach. *Journal of Nursing Staff Development, 10*(4), 219–222.

Simpson, E. J. (1966). *The classification of educational objectives: Psychomotor domain*. Chicago: University of Illinois.

Swanson, R., & Gradous, D. (1990). *Forecasting financial benefits of human resource development*. San Francisco: Jossey-Bass.

Yoder-Wise, P. S. (1997). State and association/certifying boards CE requirements. *Journal of Continuing Education in Nursing, 28*(1), 5-9.

11

Competence Development: Critical Thinking, Clinical Judgment, and Technical Ability

BETTE CASE

When staff development specialists (SDSs) talk about "developing competencies," they may be talking about crafting competency statements and criteria (Gurvis & Grey, 1995) or they may be talking about educating and training staff to improve personal job performance and quality care outcomes (Kelly, 1992). This chapter explores the latter meaning with respect to cultivating, enhancing, and producing clinical judgment and technical abilities among clinical care providers.

Critical thinking, clinical judgment, and technical capabilities predominate among the essential competencies that experts (Shugars et al., 1991, Swansburg, 1995) predict for the health care workers and professionals of the future. Staff will need to learn to participate more fully in the "big picture" of patient care and the health care organization. This chapter defines critical thinking as:

> Purposeful thinking that takes into consideration focus, language, frame of reference, attitudes, assumptions, evidence, reasoning, conclusions, implications, and context when they matter in deciding what to believe or do. . . . The relevance of these components of critical thinking varies according to the situation. (Miller & Babcock, 1995, p. 8)

Therefore, critical thinking includes the judging and deciding that clinical care providers do when they engage in aspects of their roles outside of direct patient care. Activities such as delegating, collaborating with other disciplines, and improving performance require critical thinking skills. Caregivers apply critical thinking skills when gathering and analyzing patient data and planning and evaluating direct patient care. For the purposes of this chapter, clinical judgment is making patient care decisions in all phases of the nursing process. In this discussion, clinical judgment is used to apply critical thinking skills in the context of patient care.

The distinction between critical thinking and clinical judgment is not always clear or meaningful. Aspects of the caregiver role outside of direct care still affect patient outcomes. Most of the strategies presented in this chapter that support critical thinking also support clinical judgment, and vice versa. Separating the two for the purposes of discussion is not meant to imply an exclusive placement of certain strategies with one or the other.

To perform their roles as developers of critical thinking, clinical judgment, and technical competence, SDSs exercise skills outside the traditional educator role. For most SDSs, this presents no problem, because in many ways the SDS exemplifies a prototypical multicompetent practitioner. The staff development needs in today's health care environment highlight the consulting skills of the SDS.

The competence development program must go beyond ensuring each year that all staff still have their competencies, and correcting any deficiencies discovered. In the first place, new technologies, treatments, policies, practices, and accreditors' mandates are continuously creating new competency requirements. Second, changes in care delivery and populations served require new competencies. Finally, and significantly for the staff development role, the retooling of caregiver roles offers SDSs a magnificent consulting opportunity. Health care organizations need staff development expertise to design and describe new jobs (National Nursing Staff Development Organization, 1996). SDSs play a leading role in planning restructured care delivery.

After planning, organizing, coordinating, delivering, and evaluating training to prepare staff for their new roles, staff educators again activate their consulting skills. In organizations that have restructured and retooled effectively, educators and others have acted as performance coaches or performance consultants. These consultants function on the units to troubleshoot restructured delivery of care and facilitate continuing staff compliance with the new model.

Every health care organization needs a sensible system for assessing, validating, and documenting staff competencies. Departments in the health care organization need education about competency and the organization's system for managing competency requirements. They also need assistance in crafting competency statements, criteria, and training programs to develop and maintain staff competency. For some SDSs, the scope of competency management services extends throughout a multihospital network.

Since the Joint Commission on Accreditation of Health Care Organizations (JCAHO) first mandated competency assessment and documentation, competency statements and checklists have burgeoned. More recently, SDSs have recognized the need to streamline and refine them to improve the credibility and manageability of competency assessment and development systems. Evidence of this need was Grey's (1996) tongue-in-cheek suggestion that the critical care nurse job description needed to include the ability to carry a 50-pound competency checklist. Jutsum (1996) referred to the need to define the essentials as "truth-telling in competency." SDSs apply their own critical thinking skills in facilitating the shift from long lists to essential competencies.

This chapter suggests strategies for developing essential critical thinking, clinical judgment, and technical competencies, identifies the effects of retooled clinical care provider roles, and examines measurement issues in relation to critical thinking, clinical judgment, and technical competencies.

DEVELOPING THE CLINICAL CARE PROVIDER

"Gurus" of competency (Benner, 1982, Del Bueno, 1990) emphasize the importance of defining competency in the context of the real world of practice. The real world of practice today includes new definitions of established caregiver roles and newly created caregiver roles.

Managers and educators identify needs to develop staff competency in preparation for introducing new organizational initiatives such as patient-focused care, new policies and practices, and new technologies. JCAHO standards also stimulate competency development in particular aspects, such as skills and attitudes related to patient satisfaction, patient and family education, and specific variations in practice related to the age of the patient. Analysis of risk management and quality management data also define needs for competency development. Competencies selected for training usually include those that are high-risk, problem-prone, or of low frequency.

The Caregiver Team

The real world of practice today revolves around teamwork. Teamwork does not happen automatically when a group of persons assemble and receive an assignment. Teamwork competencies belong in the staff development curriculum as well as in performance appraisals. Some teamwork competencies and methods used to develop them are closely related to critical thinking, clinical judgment, and technical competence.

Teams function in interdisciplinary performance improvement and quality management committees, task forces, and standing committees and at the unit level, as caregiver teams. Teams apply critical thinking skills in an interpersonal mode. When team members collaborate, each shares his or her own perspective. When solving a problem, each presents the factors he or she considers most important for a successful solution. The team uses these to create the specifications for a solution to the problem. To collaborate effectively, team members must be willing to express their perspectives in a manner that other members can understand. For members who are new to participation on a team, particularly those in ancillary roles, the notion of speaking up and challenging and thinking beyond the viewpoint of specific tasks may be threatening. For the team to work effectively, the leader needs to enforce the expectation that all members will participate. The leader must also elicit perspectives and ask members to clarify their statements if needed.

For the caregiver team, collaboration is goal-directed. To improve communication and work toward common goals, members need a common language and knowledge base. Each member brings unique information, but all must share core values and a common language to collaborate effectively.

Teamwork also has a technical component. Each member must know the roles of all other members. Members need to know who performs specific duties, who has responsibility for various aspects, and who helps with specific duties.

Teams can function more effectively if they receive this information as intact teams. This presents some difficulties for the educator, because members may represent very different educational backgrounds and language skills, as well as different roles. However, it is important that members have the opportunity to operationalize statements of philosophy, values, and description of care models into meaningful actions that they will take in the course of their daily work. Many hospitals have made their values highly evident in training at all levels. For example, Nyack (NY) Hospital emphasizes the values of competence, courtesy, efficiency, and safety in training. Saint James Hospital and Health Centers (Chicago) defines and integrates Franciscan values in job-specific performance standards (American Health Consultants [AHC], 1996). Training with intact teams permits team members to share their perspectives and expectations of themselves and one another in relation to the organization's philosophy and values.

To generate alternatives and approaches to organizational performance improvement, team members need a common concept of the big picture. This must go beyond the limitation of the specific role and duties of each member.

When new roles are introduced to the patient care scene, as is the case in patient-focused care, all caregivers need orientation to these roles and how to interact with them (NNSDO, 1996). Members need to know not only what each role does with the patient, but what one role can expect from another (e.g., support, assistance, coaching). In a survey by the American Association of Critical Care Nurses (AACN), 56.6% of the RNs responding said they had received no training concerning the scope and standards of practice for unlicensed assistive personnel (UAPs) (AHC, 1996).

The sharing of perspectives is vital to interpersonal critical thinking. Sharing, respecting, and integrating perspectives is important to working effectively with a diverse group of persons and developing cultural competence. In teamwork and in patient-focused care, the roles and experiences of team members add another dimension of culture to ethnicity, national origin, education, and so forth.

Cultural competence builds first on an awareness of one's own cultural perspective and then adds knowledge about the perspective of another culture on the same issue. Next, the person acquires the skills to be effective when working and communicating with a member of the other culture. Finally, the person seeks encounters that will provide occasions for culturally sensitive practices (Campinha-Bacote, 1994). Team members need awareness of each others' cultures as well as the predominant cultures represented in the patient populations they serve.

The diversity of backgrounds and disciplines represented on teams underscores the importance of the educator's role as a translator of concepts such as time management, managed care, and business aspects of care delivery into terms that all team members will find meaningful.

Organizations take various approaches to team building, but many have recognized the importance of conducting interactive training and group exercises with intact work teams. However, in AACN's 1996 survey, only 19% of the RNs responded that UAPs receive training in collaboration (AHC, 1996).

St. Luke's Episcopal Hospital in Houston used an eight-step team-building process (AHC, 1995):

1. Team identity, embracing the patient as a team member
2. Team building (strength in diversity)
3. Dealing with change
4. Action planning
5. Analyzing work processes
6. Solving quality problems
7. Participating in quality problem-solving sessions
8. Ongoing facilitation.

Community Hospital of Central California uses a six-level corporate orientation for caregiver teams. Clinical partners (RNs) receive all six levels, technical partners three levels, and service partners two levels (AHC, 1995). An important emphasis in team training as well as training in separate roles is goals and outcomes for the patient, rather than tasks. Common patient-focused goals become rallying points for integrating individual roles.

Although the team concept and team training are central in today's practice environment, there are certain competency concerns specific to nurses, to therapists, to technicians, to UAPs, and to nonclinical support staff.

Nurses

Managed care has brought changes in patient acuity and length of stay that have greatly affected the competencies required of RNs. Economic drivers, as well as concerns for quality and compliance with standards for patient satisfaction, patient and family education, and interdisciplinary approaches have propelled many health care organizations to restructure their models of care delivery. These restructured models feature patient-focused care. The models also involve the use of UAPs and expanded skills sets for many other job descriptions, including RNs. Nurses must develop new competencies in clinical judgment and technical skill to function effectively in restructured care delivery.

When giving direct care, the RN employs critical thinking skills to make clinical judgments. This is nothing new. The nurse approaches the patient with knowledge gained through education and experience and selectively collects knowledge about the patient.

The nurse critically reflects on this knowledge and identifies, gathers, and organizes additional information needed to assess the patient. After analyzing the information, the nurse plans and acts. Then, the nurse critically reflects on the results of the action taken and adds this knowledge of patient response to a working knowledge base for continuing care (Ford & Profetto-McGrath, 1994). The process has not changed, but the context has.

The current context of higher patient acuity and shorter length of stay implies greater complexity, higher risk, quicker responses, and more emphasis on discharge planning. Educators must factor in these elements when constructing learning activities to develop critical thinking and clinical judgment. The current context also emphasizes outcomes: patient outcomes as well as those obtained from initiating various practices in the organization. Nursing practice has always placed the RN in a position of interacting with many departments and coordinating many services and aspects of care. RNs naturally encounter many sources of organizational performance data while practicing nursing. However, RNs do not automatically think in these terms. The nurse who displays exceptional critical thinking skills in direct patient care does not automatically transfer these skills to the organizational performance improvement arena. To contribute to their full potential, nurses need training not only in data collection but also in suggesting meaningful indicators of quality outcomes.

Learning experiences must provide opportunities for RNs to practice the skills that patient-focused care requires. Patient-focused care frees the RN from direct care and clerical duties that others can perform so that the RN can concentrate on higher-level skills of assessing and planning for a greater number of patients. Planning involves:

- Planning for continuity over time (discharge planning)
- Planning for coordinating care (case management)
- Planning for delivering direct care through UAPs (delegation).

Developing the competency to delegate effectively has proven to be a great challenge for RNs and educators. According to a patient-focused care coordinator at Saint James Hospital and Health Center, Chicago Heights, IL, "Eighty percent of our problems are due to RNs unable to lead [the UAPs]. RNs need to understand their role as leaders and problem-solvers" (AHC, 1996, p. 72). Developing RNs' competencies in delegation usually includes examining the parameters of the state's Nurse Practice Act and standards of care and practice established by professional organizations and by the health care organization. Developing the delegation competency also includes skill in competency assessment, supervision, direct communication, and feedback. The most effective training sessions include exercises requiring RNs to make appropriate assignments for UAPs, using a simulated patient census and condition report. Part of the ongoing role of the RN is to help the UAP develop competence not only in performing a skill, but also in recognizing:

- When a skill is, or is not, indicated
- When assistance from another caregiver is needed
- Whom to call for various kinds of assistance and services
- How to obtain the assistance of others.

Because RNs lead the patient care team, they must develop leadership competencies in addition to delegation. Many training programs include coaching skills and situational leadership.

Competency in clinical judgment and critical thinking grows with practice. Developing competency statements to reflect differences in novice, competent, and expert practice helps define a competency development continuum that attends to the learning needs of experienced nurses (McGregor, 1990, Jeska et al., 1995, Herbert-Ashton, 1996).

Therapists

For the purposes of this discussion, therapists include professional staff who specialize in disciplines other than nursing (*e.g.*, pharmacy, respiratory therapy, physical and occupational therapy). This discussion focuses on the needs of therapists in developing clinical judgment and technical competencies and on ways in which therapists can contribute to the competency development process in the organization. In other words, therapists both receive educational services to develop competencies and serve as resources for competency development.

The disciplines of pharmacy, respiratory therapy and physical and occupational therapy are experiencing many of the same changes that are affecting nursing. Leaders in these disciplines note that new graduates come "without knowledge packaged the way you want it" (Witte, 1996) and all lack some of the same skills (*e.g.*, "they want to tell the patient what to do" [Wcislo, 1996]), and that "when first hired, nobody knows what to do" (Beaver, 1996). Strategies are needed to help new graduates develop clinical judgment and technical skills and to help develop preceptors who can assist in the development process. These disciplines also have sound approaches in use and can provide a rich collaborative resource.

Therapists can also serve as both resources and recipients in developing competencies in clinical judgment. For example, pharmacy departments often have excellent learning materials related to patient education and age-specific care.

Interdisciplinary quality monitoring leads to interdisciplinary educational opportunities (*e.g.*, medication errors, neonatal protocols, use of physical therapy appliances such as the quad cane). Therapists need to develop critical thinking competencies in relation to data collection and analysis and in creating new practices and techniques to address opportunities for improvement. They also have effective strategies to share.

For the individual therapist, cross-training consists largely of applying skills with less-specialized patient populations than in the past. However, in some cases a particular unit's need for the therapist's services is sufficient to justify assigning a therapist to the unit. For example, in some patient-focused models, a physical therapist "resides" on a orthopedic unit and provides services there to eliminate the need for scheduling and transporting patients to a central department. This physical therapist may perform selected patient care skills in addition to physical therapy services needed by the patients on the unit. In some neonatal intensive care units, respiratory therapists feed infants and take vital signs. In some emergency departments, respiratory therapists draw blood. However, state professional regulations may prohibit cross-training in even closely related disciplines; for example, cross-training physical therapists to provide occupational therapy services may be prohibited in some states.

Therapists can teach the skills of their discipline in organization-wide educational programs. For instance, physical therapists can teach body mechanics, back safety, and prevention of cumulative trauma disorder. Therapists also provide technical competency training for UAPs, usually in training programs designed and coordinated by SDSs.

In general, these disciplines are quite self-reliant in developing the competency of their staff in clinical judgment and technical skill. They often blend those sets of competencies; as described by one expert, "education [in physical therapy] is technique-based. We review what was done and what could be done differently or better" (Wcislo, 1996).

To be a responsible and effective collaborator, the SDS must learn about the therapists of other disciplines, including their educational preparation, state and professional organization regulations, and continuing education requirements.

Technicians

Planners of patient-focused care models sometimes target technicians in disciplines other than nursing for cross-training as UAPs. In response, SDSs must apply their own critical thinking skills and encourage a thorough assessment before proceeding. Some EKG or lab technicians may be eager to learn nursing skills and take responsibility for broader aspects of care than their technical roles have permitted. However, others may have chosen their technical field because they prefer technical aspects and do not want to perform hygienic and comfort care or take on broader responsibilities for patients. When designing critical thinking and clinical judgment competency development for UAPs who have technical backgrounds, SDSs must address the difference between performing narrow technical skills with patients and taking on responsibility for the broader context of patient needs.

Unlicensed Assistive Personnel

UAPs actively perform patient care duties under RN supervision. A survey of AACN members found that the top five tasks performed by UAPs were bed baths, feeding patients orally, taking temperatures, assisting patients with bedpans and urinals, and transporting patients (Varro, 1996). Many institutions have added skills such as phlebotomy, administration of nasal oxygen, and selected physical therapy techniques. The controversy surrounding the use of UAPs is fueled by the conviction of opponents that UAPs lack sufficient training to perform their duties. Despite strong differences of opinion about the role, all agree that training is essential to the safe use of UAPs.

In most hospitals, SDSs have planned and controlled UAP training. Most have used the services of other departments to develop the technical competencies of the UAPs. For example, phlebotomists and respiratory therapists have taught UAPs specific technical competencies using the procedures and criteria their departments have used for training their own personnel.

Because of the diversity of UAP backgrounds, many training programs have used a competency-based approach. Many have also used the entering skills of UAPs to assist in training their peers—for instance, allowing those who have worked as EKG techs to demonstrate the skills and coach their peers.

Most hospitals recommend prehire screening for literacy and basic computation skills. Many hospitals have collaborated with public schools or other community resources to provide remedial education for prospective UAPs. Although some members of a UAP training class may have marginal basic language and math skills, others may be medical students, nursing students, paramedics, and EMTs. This diversity presents a great challenge for the SDS, but he or she can face the challenge and make diversity part of the training process by eliciting the various perspectives that the UAPs represent, rather than making assumptions about their backgrounds and viewpoints. Every UAP has a skill set and some previous experience that fellow UAPs can value and appreciate. Building a good working relationships during training can help UAPs prepare for building relationships on the job.

Some recommend that training begin with a broad approach and role definition before getting into details and procedures (AHC, 1996). This allows UAPs to place skills and specifics within a context of overall responsibility for patient care. The training contains many details that may appear unrelated without knowing the context of patient care.

Some report that UAPs at first felt "petrified of the patients" (Biemolt, 1996). Beginning with the patient and refocusing on the patient during training may reduce this fear.

Although this chapter concentrates on clinical judgment and technical skills, the interpersonal skill component is very important in UAP training. Because UAPs spend a great deal of time with patients, they encounter many opportunities to respond to the questions and concerns of patients and families. They must learn the skill of reflecting concerns to gain a clear understanding, and then referring the concern to the appropriate caregiver. (See Chap. 14 for a communication model.)

One deficiency that often emerges as UAPs begin to practice in their roles is failing to know the names of things. Various games, treasure hunts, and similar approaches using real items during training helps them learn proper terminology.

One source of controversy about the UAP role is a lack of standardized UAP training. NNSDO (1996) advocates a standard curriculum. AACN designed an educational program for UAP orientation, training, and assessment called *The Competency-Based Skill Building Curriculum for Unlicensed Personnel* (Turner, 1996).

Most UAP training lasts 6 to 8 weeks, plus 2 weeks of on-the-job precepted practice. Some recommend excluding any skills that will require more than 6 weeks of training (AHC, 1995). Of course, licensing, credentialing, and union rules also influence the selection of skills for cross-training. Specialty areas such as the operating room, emergency department, or critical care require additional training.

Nonclinical Support Staff

Although this chapter focuses on caregivers, service associates and business associates complement the direct care team. Business associates' duties include unit secretary responsibilities, business office functions dealing with the admission, transfer, and discharge process, and responsibilities related to medical records. Business associates in some settings transport patients and orient patients to the unit. Although service associates and business associates have less patient contact than the UAP who is giving direct care, they also need to develop judgment and technical skills relative to their roles. The caregiver team members need to understand the roles of these associates and their own roles in relation to these associates.

Shorter training programs suffice for service associates. The usual skill set for service associates includes environmental duties, selected dietary duties, and transportation duties.

STRATEGIES
....

SDSs exercise their own critical thinking skills when they create strategies for developing others' clinical judgment and technical skills. They discriminate when they select relevant competencies. Long lists of technical skills have proliferated and must be weeded out to be useful. Because critical thinking and clinical judgment competencies are more elusive than technical competencies (Del Bueno, 1990), they are frequently not stated or stated in terms too general to be useful. SDSs must consult with clinical experts and managers to operationalize critical thinking in terms of practice competencies. SDSs apply the skills of organizing information and identifying appropriate resources when they construct competency-based models in which they identify skills, objectives, resources, and target dates for developing particular competencies.

Del Bueno et al.'s (1987) well-known competency model divides competencies in three categories: critical thinking, technical skill, and interpersonal skill. She sees these sets of competencies as interlocking circles because many practice activities tap more than one set of competencies. For example, critical thinking comes into play when a patient's condition requires the nurse to modify the usual technical procedure.

This section first addresses development strategies that apply to all sets of competencies and then identifies strategies specific to critical thinking, clinical judgment, and technical competencies.

Assessing Needs for Competency Development

After staff complete the orientation process, their direct supervisors validate their competencies through the ongoing process of performance appraisal. Summarized performance appraisal results then should indicate the particular competencies staff need to develop further. Many hospitals are working toward integrating their performance appraisal and competency management systems (Jeska et al., 1995, Herbert-Ashton, 1996).

Most hospitals have integrated quality management and organizational performance improvement into the competency development program. Often SDSs include the competencies involved in problem-prone aspects of care in the annual mandatory education program. Competencies that often make the list include falls, medication errors, documentation, chest tubes, pain management, restraints, and blood administration. Usually, different competencies are selected for each year's program, based on quality management findings.

Many hospitals use self-assessment findings to identify the competencies that staff feel they need to strengthen. Some use performance appraisal statements and criteria to design a self-assessment format. In some restructured delivery systems, staff who perform newly created multiskilled jobs respond to open-ended questions about their level of comfort and feeling of safety in performing their duties (AHC, 1996). When obtaining self-assessment findings, it is critical to ensure that staff members are reporting directly and specifically about their own appraisal of their job performance and what training can improve their performance (Puetz, 1992).

As noted earlier, many competencies that emerge as needs for development contain both clinical judgment and technical skill components. Therefore, training approaches must address the judgment difficulties as well as the technical deficiencies.

Ensuring Validity

As Del Bueno et al. (1987) noted, competency assessment measures what staff can do, not necessarily what they will do when the occasion arises. To ensure the validity of competency development, the SDS creates training situations that approximate actual practice to the fullest extent possible. This requires creating a context for learning activities, integrating the clinical judgment and technical components of competencies, and collecting and replicating clinical situations that have actually occurred. The process of gathering practice situations brings the SDS into close collaboration with nursing managers, clinical experts, preceptors, and staff. The process also helps to incorporate the real tools of practice into training. For example, training situations can present excerpts of real findings of chart audits, challenge participants to judge excerpts as acceptable or unacceptable, and require participants to correct any deficiencies. Chart audits can focus on documentation or on critique of the assessments made and the care given. Other tools, in addition to medical records, might include standards, performance appraisal criteria, risk management reports, financial reports, and any other sources of information that the organization compiles.

Incorporating a Variety of Approaches

In the context of patient care, critical thinking, clinical judgment, and technical skills are all active processes; all result in actions. Therefore, developing competency requires active practice. However, most competencies also operate on knowledge bases. Because most hospitals find it necessary to limit class time, most rely more on self-directed methods for building this knowledge base. Fortunately, instructional technologies offer many useful products for computer-assisted learning, closed-circuit television, and self-instruction packets. SDSs can then reserve the majority of class time for placing knowledge in clinical contexts and putting knowledge into action.

The term "just-in-time learning" captures today's emphasis on efficiency. One annual education extravaganza cannot possibly meet the staff's ongoing needs for competency development. Just-in-time learning implies not only offering training close to the time of introducing or improving the competency in practice (not too far in advance), but also providing staff with on-the-spot corrective feedback. Feedback becomes more effective if it is part of a targeted competency development program rather than if it comes from managers, educators, clinical nurse specialists, and preceptors about whatever they have happened to observe in the course of delivering care. Paying attention to selected competencies during selected time periods and giving on-the-spot corrective feedback can improve performance dramatically. SDSs can train staff as participant observers and deliverers of feedback, much as they train staff as quality improvement data collectors. Empowering staff in this manner leads to some of the same benefits of peer review without requiring staff to judge one another and document their judgments. Monitoring quality indicators already in place will document the improvement that occurs as a result of this approach.

Using Interdisciplinary Resources

When using the services of other disciplines, SDSs must plan carefully. Although other disciplines have their own competency statements and training methods, these resources may or may not be appropriate for interdisciplinary education and cross-training. SDSs must apply their own critical thinking skills to determine how to use these resources to meet the objectives of interdisciplinary education and cross-training. Most SDSs can recall using at least one physician as a guest speaker who failed to address the objectives of the program. Part of the coordinating role of the SDS is to fit resources to the objectives and to communicate expectations to all experts and preceptors who participate in the competency development program. These personnel may need assistance with instructional technique.

When incorporating other disciplines into the process of developing competencies, SDSs must be sensitive to concerns that these disciplines may have about training others to perform their job skills. Therapists and technicians may perceive "multiskilling" as a threat to their jobs and to the viability of their own departments. These perceptions have some validity and may cause these therapists and technicians to feel less than enthusiastic about participating in training.

Empowering Preceptors

Effective preceptors are important to ongoing competency development. Preparing preceptors presents challenges for the SDS. Patient-focused models, interdisciplinary education, and the training needs of other departments require effective preceptors. SDSs have conducted highly successful programs for training nurse preceptors. Today's mandates require critical thinking to compress the time frame for training programs and at the same time create training that will prepare preceptors who practice disciplines other than nursing. In addition to training, the effectiveness of preceptor programs rests on compensation, recognition, and preceptor-friendly assignments and unit practices. SDSs can consult with managers and others to create an environment that supports effective precepting. The adventurous SDS might consider how competent preceptors might be cross-trained to float among several units, departments, or disciplines.

Addressing the Literacy Deficit

When developing competencies with UAPs, the SDS may discover literacy deficits. Some organizations have introduced prehire screening or use the resources of the local public schools for remedial assistance. Even when screening and remedial training are in place, the SDS must explore effective strategies for developing competencies with staff who have lesser mastery of reading comprehension and arithmetic concepts than the nursing staff who have typically been their primary audience. Dillon (1995) suggested partnering readers with nonreaders, using videotapes and audiocassettes rather than written materials, and using pictures, graphics, and games such as poker and bingo. She also recommended protecting the confidentiality and self-esteem of nonreaders by offering them anonymity—in other words, by using strategies to meet their needs without requiring them to disclose their status as nonreaders to fellow classmates.

Following Up on Training

Experience has taught most SDSs that education and training have little impact unless managers value the outcomes of training and expect the staff to practice newly acquired behaviors (Rath et al., 1996). Follow-up has proven particularly important in implementing competency-based systems (Staab et al., 1996) and in introducing patient-focused care. Patient-focused care profoundly changes care delivery, and these care delivery changes and the accompanying role changes do not remain in place without ongoing reinforcement. One of these changes is the expectation that UAPs will practice critical thinking and clinical judgment—in other words, that they will notice cues that suggest exceptions to the rules, that they will be alert to the total context of patient care rather than just to "lockstep" thinking and task-oriented performance, and that they will make decisions within the parameters of their job descriptions. The change that allows these competencies to develop is the reciprocal change on the part of RNs—that they will expect and permit UAPs to exercise critical thinking and clinical judgment.

Managers have an active role to play in follow-up. They need training to develop coaching skills and support in making the transition from traditional manager to "coach" (Whitman, 1996). Managers also must reframe more traditional views of supervision to incorporate concepts of competency and competency development.

Many hospitals have formalized a coaching component to reinforce their continuing commitment to patient-focused care. At St. Joseph's Hospital and Health Care Center in Chicago, staff educators maintained a continuous presence on transformed units and served as models for the RNs on the use and expectations of UAPs. They raised questions that led to revising approaches, such as, "Why isn't delegation happening?" Exploring this question led to the consistent pairing of particular RNs with particular UAPs. Biemolt (1996) recommended tapering off the coaching involvement rather than abruptly discontinuing it.

St. Charles Medical Center in Bend, OR, included healing health care coaches in their patient-focused redesign. After a 2.5-day seminar entitled "People-Centered Teams: Healing the Workplace," selected caregivers functioned as healing health care coaches (AHC, 1995). St. Luke's Hospital in Houston followed up a team-building series by revisiting functioning teams and facilitating teams for up to 1 year (AHC, 1995). Community Hospital of California designated a coach on each patient-focused care unit (AHC, 1995). University of Chicago Hospitals used "position champions" in its redesigned system (Nick, 1996). Coaches on the unit also perform observational audits to identify competencies for retraining or re-emphasis.

Critical Thinking

This section explores ways to operationalize characteristics of critical thinking in staff development and to develop critical thinking competencies. For the purpose of this discussion, a set of characteristics is considered to make up critical thinking. Caregivers reflect on, reframe, and analyze situations, generate solutions, and make decisions in the course of their practice. The situations and decisions involve direct patient care, indirect care, and interdisciplinary collaboration. The next section, Clinical Judgment, explores strategies for developing the judgment process involved in direct patient care.

Experts agree on certain characteristics of critical thinking. Most would agree that the critical thinker:

- Reframes problems; explores situations
- Generates alternatives and ideas
- Assembles evidence to support conclusions
- Reflects critically
  - On knowledge base (organizes, infers, selects relevant data, thinks in terms of concepts, makes connections)
  - On actions taken
  - On his or her own thought process
- Examines assumptions
- Critiques
  - Develops and uses criteria
  - Evaluates credibility of sources
- Inquires (clarifies, challenges)
- Shows openness to challenge and other perspectives
- Collaborates; examines assumptions and perspectives and generates integrated solutions in an interpersonal process.

The first step toward developing staff competency in critical thinking is to specify the desired practice behaviors. To do this, the SDS places the characteristics in the context of caregiver roles and makes the behaviors more specific. For example, "reflects critically" can be placed in the context of the nursing process with an orthopedic patient. Desired behaviors might include selecting relevant assessment data to support a particular nursing diagnosis. The act of selecting relevant data itself requires reflecting on one's own knowledge base. Desired behaviors might also include reflecting on actions taken with the patient:

- Were the actions effective?
- How does the nurse judge effectiveness or ineffectiveness?
- What are the criteria for effectiveness in this situation?
- What could have been done differently to yield a more effective outcome?

Another series of questions stimulates reflecting on one's own thought process:

- Where did I look for evidence to support that particular diagnosis?
- What did I look at first?
- What did I decide was irrelevant?
- What did I fail to notice that might have helped me choose a more effective action?
- How will I change my approach to a similar situation next time?

The SDS can begin the process of developing critical thinking competencies with staff only after operationalizing the characteristics. In collaboration with managers and other unit-based clinical experts, the SDS must find answers to questions such as:

- What exactly does a nurse on this unit do when he or she "develops and uses criteria"?
- What specifically does a UAP do when he or she "shows openness to challenge and other perspectives"?

To design learning experiences in which participants can develop critical thinking skills, the SDS must have a clear picture of what critical thinking "looks like" for particular caregiver roles and on particular units. As a further step in developing these competencies with staff, the SDS, in consultation with clinical experts, specifies differences in critical thinking among levels of expertise, such as novice, competent, and expert practitioners.

The context for critical thinking characteristics may be examining assumptions in relation to policies, procedures, and practices (*e.g.*, visiting hours), considering all perspectives, generating alternatives, and creating new policies. For RNs, other contexts might be specifying indicators of quality and making assignments to UAPs. For UAPs, contexts might include troubleshooting equipment, balancing priorities, and deciding what information to report and when and to whom to report it. For all levels of staff, an important context is workplace advocacy—in other words, exercising vigilance to workplace safety hazards, finding potential hazards, and proactively addressing safety issues (Young et al., 1995).

Critical thinking is not appropriate in every situation. In certain situations, usually emergency or high-risk situations, only one answer is acceptable; exploring alternatives and arriving at a collaborative solution could prove dangerous. The instructor's responsibility is to communicate clearly which situations are of the "one right answer" type and reassure learners that they will receive support for following through with the prescribed action in those situations, but that in all others they are expected to reflect on the situation and consider alternatives.

Having specified the critical thinking behaviors that staff must develop, the SDS designs learning situations in which staff will practice the specified behaviors. To develop their critical thinking skills, staff must actively practice critical thinking behaviors. The heart of all strategies for developing staff critical thinking competencies is to engage staff actively in posing and responding to open-ended questions.

Well-designed questions can elevate lower-level cognitive learning into opportunities to develop higher-level critical thinking skills. Educators can show videotapes on topics such as age-specific patient needs, customer service, or organizational core values and then follow up with questions designed to elicit specific actions and behaviors that apply the material to on-the-job situations. Such learning is enhanced with an interdisciplinary group. Sharing perspectives helps all involved to gain broader and multiple perspectives.

One reason for asking open-ended questions is to obtain feedback about the learner's thought process. In psychomotor skill training, the instructor can observe step-by-step performance and offer corrective feedback. However, when the skill is thinking, often only the results can be observed. The instructor must prompt the learner to "think out loud" to identify weaknesses or misinterpretations and offer corrective feedback. To assess the thought process, the instructor can ask questions such as, "What did you notice first?" or "What other information did you collect?" Questions such as these make the thought process explicit. The instructor might also ask the caregiver to draw a flow chart or decision tree to display the thought process. This is analogous to "showing your work" when answering a math problem.

Multiple-choice tests provide a useful classroom tool for group work on critical thinking skills. The instructor can ask participants to select the answer, at first individually and then as groups. Each member then describes how he or she chose. The participant describes not only the content-related rationale, but also the test-taking process and strategy (*e.g.*, "I eliminated certain choices" or "I tried to answer without looking at the options, then matched my answer to the options"). When each option describes a nursing action in response to a situation, the group can be asked, "What would happen if you did #1? #2?" The group can then identify the thinking that led to its selection. This helps clarify faulty conclusions and may proactively prevent mistakes in practice.

The questions can also be given minus the answers. The group can then come up with all the answers it can and figure out how to choose the best one. After the group members believe they have identified every possibility, the leader can ask, "What else?" and then wait until a new idea emerges.

Corners of the room can be designated for each answer. Participants go to the corner they choose and construct a rationale with other participants who gather there. Each group then presents its choice and rationale. This works best with ambiguous or controversial questions in which there is not clearly one best choice, such as situations of ethical conflict.

Scenarios and cases can be used to help develop critical thinking skills. The SDS presents direct or indirect patient care situations to caregivers. Mahlmeister (1996) suggested categories of such situations:

- A critical incident requiring immediate action
- One problem with multiple dimensions
- A situation for delegating care—a multidisciplinary team
- A situation for evaluating care.

She recommended that the instructor provide only selected information and ask probing, open-ended questions to help the learners analyze the situation. For example, in a critical incident, the instructor might provide a brief description, including major cues or classic signs of a problem that requires priority action. Some questions might include:

- What is the immediate threat?
- What will happen if it is unresolved?
- What led you to identify that as the problem?
- How can you help this patient?
- How can you reverse the problem?
- How quickly do you have to act?
- How long can the patient tolerate this?
- What will you need?
- What will happen if you (perform a certain act)? (Mahlmeister, 1996)

Critiquing is an important facet of critical thinking. Situations reported to risk management present excellent material for critiquing situations, identifying problems, and suggesting approaches.

Another important part of critical thinking is determining the criteria for assessment and evaluation. Staff can practice this skill in a number of situations simply by stating the criteria they would use to assess the patient or evaluate the patient's response to treatment. Presenting a series of limited situations and asking the same question with respect to each situation provides practice with a particular critical thinking component. For example, the question might be whether or not a situation as described was problematic from the standpoint of the patient's rights, or infection control, or another aspect of care.

Jigsaw cases offer an approach to analyzing more complex cases and situations. In jigsaw cases, the group receives a case study and each group member investigates one aspect of care. For example, one member might gather information about medications and another about discharge needs. The cases must be constructed to yield equitable assignments for the group size. The SDS assembles appropriate reference materials, including those resources available on the unit. After completing their individual assignments, group members discuss the case. Questions should include some that require integration of the separate assignments.

Problem-based learning (Gordon, 1996), a method that some medical schools have adopted, can be adapted for use in staff development. The method, as used in the medical schools, completely substitutes for the traditional curriculum of courses in biochemistry, pathophysiology, and others. Instead, students meet all the objectives of the curriculum by analyzing patient problems, searching for and validating the information needed to solve the problem, hypothesizing, and testing their solutions. In problem-based learning, the faculty member provides patient information in segments. After receiving the first set of limited information, students identify what they know, what they must know, and where to find it. They hypothesize about the patient's problem and the relation of the pieces of information to one another and to a diagnosis and plan. At the next class session, the faculty member discloses more information about the patient. The students then validate their hypotheses in light of the new information and the information they have gathered in the interim. The cycle continues until the students have solved the problem.

The technique of providing a patient situation in segments may provide a useful simulation of the course of a hospitalization. The method need not be limited to a direct patient care situation. Problems in teamwork, quality improvement, staffing, delegating, or other areas of concern could also be presented segmentally.

Group interaction is a useful strategy for developing critical thinking skills because of the opportunity to learn the perspectives of others. When using group activities, the educator should provide time for the learners to formulate their viewpoints alone before sharing. This increases the likelihood that all will participate and that minority viewpoints will be expressed.

Another useful group assignment is to create a policy or procedure for some technique performed in patient care or some indirect aspect of care. The current policy or procedure should not be available during the learning exercise.

Pike's *three-group review* technique (1989) creates an opportunity for learners to write and reflect on questions. The instructor asks each group to write a question that addresses the objectives of the workshop or concerns a particular topic. Each group passes its question to another group, which must critique, revise, and clarify the question. In the third step, the revised questions are passed to a different group, who must answer the questions.

A useful variation of the three-group review technique gives the learners practice in describing and solving problems. In round one, the instructor asks each group to set out a problem (*e.g.*, your biggest problem in delegating, or precepting, or teaching patients and families). In round two, the problems are passed to another group, "giving away" the problem. The receiving group discusses the problem and may consult the group who composed the problem to ensure that they understand it. In the third round, the problem is passed to another group, who comes up with as many solutions as possible. The problem, with solutions, is then returned to the group who originated it, and that group chooses a solution.

Mind-mapping (Buzan, 1991) and *concept-mapping* (Daley, 1996, Baugh & Mellott, 1996) also provide opportunities for group work and collaboration in identifying and correlating multiple aspects of a concept or problem. Both of these formats are nonlinear outlines or graphic representations of concepts, problems, or plans of patient care. Learners begin by creating a colored image that represents the topic in the center of the paper. The next step is to do a "mind dump," or write down all ideas related to the topic on a large piece of paper. Self-sticking notes make a convenient vehicle for jotting down ideas and affixing them to the paper. At this stage, no attempt should be made to organize the items. Using self-sticking notes allows the participant to rearrange and cluster ideas in various configurations before settling on the most useful arrangement. Buzan (1991, p. 85) listed the following additional steps in creating a mind map:

- Place images throughout your mind map.
- Print words.
- Place each word on a line.
- Connect each line to another line.
- Use one word per line.
- Use color.
- Don't obsess over organizing the information or deciding "where things go."
- Let size and nearness to the center indicate importance.

Mind maps can serve a variety of purposes in addition to exposing learners to a new method of organizing and relating ideas. When groups share their mind maps, they can identify and attempt to account for differences in perspectives among groups.

Before one preceptor training program, groups of managers and educators created mind maps of the characteristics of effective preceptors, and during the introduction to the course, groups of participants did the same thing. During the course, participants compared the maps and discussed their different perspectives.

Other group techniques can be used to develop critical thinking in indirect aspects of care. De Bono (1985) suggested using *colored hats* to represent different perspectives that one might take on an issue. Each color represents a viewpoint:

- White: information
- Red: feelings
- Yellow: optimism
- Black: pessimism
- Green: creativity
- Blue: clarification, facilitation.

Colors may be assigned to group members or to groups. In response to a controversial issue, each person or group develops the assigned perspective, and a group discussion follows. For example, to consider the issue of assisted suicide, the white hat would decide what information was needed and gather that information; the red hat would decide whose feelings needed to be considered and identify the feelings of those persons. When discussing an issue, the feelings may be determined through readings or speculation on the part of the red hat. However, when discussing a real patient's situation, such as a discharge planning situation, the red hat must validate feelings with the real people involved. The yellow hat would develop the perspective that assisted suicide is a great kindness. The black hat would develop the opposing viewpoint, including legal and moral objections and emotional issues. The green hat develops creative ideas, in this case alternatives and perhaps ways of regulating the practice. The green hat is intended to raise wildly creative ideas, not restrained by practical considerations. The ideas may be modified to become more practical through later discussion. Being rather practically oriented, clinicians often present green-hat thinking already adapted for feasibility. However, impractical ideas should be considered so that the group can determine whether there may be ways to reframe and adjust a seemingly impractical idea into a practical one. The blue hat functions in the discussion as a clarifier and facilitator. In preparation for the discussion, he or she identifies as many aspects of the issue as possible to ensure that all are considered during the discussion. This technique can help groups to deliberate about quality management issues, staffing proposals, and other courses of action. It provides a means of discovering perspectives and ensuring that no perspective is neglected.

Brookfield (1994) recommended a technique for *examining assumptions* that applies well to patient care situations and other problem-solving situations. One member of a group describes a problem-solving process that he or she has recently done. Members, while listening without interruption, identify assumptions or factors that the storyteller seems to have taken for granted in pursuing the solution. When the storyteller has finished, listeners discuss the assumptions they heard. With the storyteller, they identify ways in which these assumptions were or could have been validated. Validating assumptions is usually a matter of asking questions or gathering additional information. Based on the assumptions examined, the group proposes at least one alternative interpretation of the problem and a new solution.

Another method suggested by Brookfield (1994) calls for reflection on experience to develop an *action plan*. This method also can be applied to patient care situations and other planning needs, such as the introduction of a new service, policy, or program. This method involves identifying the best and worst practices one has ever experienced in relation to the subject of the plan. The subject may be caring for a particular type of patient, introducing a new staffing plan, or, in Table 11-1, fostering critical thinking. Learners think about the best and worst practices they have ever seen by the persons listed at the left. It is important to keep the list very specific and related only to the subject at hand! This technique may be used as an individual activity, but the planning process is greatly enriched when a group develops a plan together. One method to promote group activity is to label flip charts with each of the levels (*e.g.*, supervisor, peer, me) and display them on the walls of the room. The number of charts used should allow three or four participants to use each chart. The participants go to each chart and list the best and worst practices they can recall for the level indicated on the chart. After a few minutes, they move to the next chart, and so on until they have discussed all the levels. Then the group members read all the charts as a sort of "gallery tour" and check or star the points they believe to be most important and those that recur frequently. The group discusses ways to obtain as many best practices as possible and to eliminate or prevent the worst practices.

Ulsenheimer (1996) described a method for developing critical thinking integrated with the quality improvement process. The method involves training about a model of critical thinking for all staff. Preceptors follow up the training with staff at the bedside on a one-to-one basis. Nurses use the critical thinking process to make a decision, to reflect on a decision that has been made to see if a better decision or outcome can be achieved, or to reflect on situations in which a poor decision has been made to obtain a better decision or outcome. Laminated cards and posters reinforce the visibility of the critical thinking process. The model involves the following questions to prompt reflection:

TABLE 11-1

THE CRITICAL THINKING ACTION PLAN: PUTTING INTELLIGENCE INTO ACTION

	The BEST Practices I've Ever Seen for Fostering Critical Thinking	The WORST Practices I've Ever Seen for Fostering Critical Thinking

By a(n):
   instructor
   supervisor
   boss
   authority figure
   past or present		

By a colleague or peer:
   past or present
   classmate
   coworker
   my department or another		

By me:
   past or present
   with nursing students
   with practicing nurses
   with children
   with students in other settings
     (religious education, club
     leadership, etc.)		

Action plan: Strategies to obtain the most best practices and eliminate or prevent worst practices

Used with permission.
Adapted from Brookfield, S. D. (1994). *Understanding learning organizations*. Creating learning organizations: Moving beyond the competencies, sponsored by Marquette University Continuing Nursing Education, Milwaukee, May 1994.

- What circumstances are involved in this event?
- What else must I know?
- Why did I think that, or do that?
- What did I do? Did it work?
- What is happening?
- How can I apply this to clinical practice?
- What did I learn from this experience?
- How could I have acted differently?

One of the most effective techniques for developing critical thinking competency is *modeling*. Modeling requires that the SDS display the characteristics of critical thinking when relating to learners. Some of the modeling may occur in interactions with patients, but much occurs in the process of teaching:

- Encouraging the expression of multiple perspectives
- Maintaining an open attitude
- Thinking out loud to demonstrate priority setting or examining assumptions
- Assembling evidence to support conclusions about the teaching process
- Encouraging learners to challenge the instructor.

At times the critical thinking environment creates feelings of discomfort and unpopularity for the critical thinker: most people prefer a steady state and accepted routines rather than continually challenging and examining assumptions. Brookfield (1993) describes ways to cope with the discomfort.

Regardless of the particular approach used in the classroom, the instructor must make an ongoing effort to ask questions rather than give information. At intervals, the instructor might ask learners to teach each other. The instructor designates one participant (using a numbering system or some other means, such as the person who got up earliest that morning) to teach a small group or a partner a particular piece of information or to give an example of a particular concept. Even when the instructor asks a question and only a few participants volunteer to share their answers, usually many others have formulated answers to the question.

During the orientation process, educators and preceptors can use questions to facilitate developing critical thinking skills. Orientees can be instructed to complete sentences such as, "I didn't understand what was going on when . . ." or "When my patient said . . . , I assumed . . ." Various sentence completions about the unit, patients, or the preceptor relationship ("I wish my preceptor would stop . . .") stimulate alertness to the environment and reflection.

Orientees might also be assigned to compare and contrast the responses of patients on the unit to medication or treatment. The orientee identifies a few patients who are receiving the same medication, treatment, or self-care education and compares the responses of these patients, using either criteria provided or criteria that he or she develops.

Educators and preceptors can use the performance appraisal tool to help clarify expectations for the orientee. The educator or preceptor refers to specific items contained in the performance appraisal and asks the orientee, "What will I see you doing when you are accomplishing this criterion?"

Many of these strategies lend themselves to interdisciplinary sessions on topics such as mandatory safety education (which Blickensderfer calls "bugs, plugs, and other ughs" [1996]). The SDS can present scenarios in words, pictures, or simulations as the stimulus for group deliberation and problem solving. Some of these scenarios may re-enact situations reported to risk management or in the press. Other suitable interdisciplinary topics include customer service, patient rights, and patient and family education. Among the goals of interdisciplinary education are to present and clarify the perspectives of each discipline (and ideally the patient and family as well) and to arrive at solutions that are "antidisciplinary" (Blickensderfer, 1996): the solutions are integrated and represent neither the approach of only one discipline nor a disjointed composite of each discipline's approaches.

Clinical Judgment

By using patient care situations, some of the strategies suggested in the previous section may be useful in developing clinical judgment skills. This section recommends additional strategies for applying critical thinking skills in direct patient care to make clinical judgments.

Jeska et al. (1995) described the use of exemplars to assess and develop clinical judgment skills. An exemplar is an example that displays judgment in the practice of the particular caregiver. Caregivers may present exemplars in written or oral format. The SDS prepares questions that will require the caregiver to reflect on the exemplar.

Questions should be limited in number so that they lead the caregiver to thorough reflection. The questions should focus on whatever aspects of judgment are the objectives of development. The focus may be gathering information, relating historical information, or priority setting. The example here is an RN exemplar, but the method can be adapted easily to examples of clinical judgment by UAPs and other caregivers.

The SDS can construct simulations at stations for caregivers to view and analyze. The caregiver might receive questions about the simulation in written form, and the station might include a receptacle to collect the written responses from caregivers. Questions must be limited and focus specifically on the objectives. For example, "Is there a problem here? If yes, what is the problem? If no, what follow-up or ongoing monitoring is indicated?" or "What must you find out before proceeding?" or "What will you do first?" Sometimes the SDS should present situations in which there is no problem—for instance, the patient is responding to treatment as desired. This gives caregivers practice in discriminating situations needing intervention from situations that do not.

For UAPs, simulations might include a series of tube set-ups, such as the "In and Out" assignment (Biemolt, 1996). This assignment requires the UAP to identify the name and purpose of particular tubes, and whether or not and when the UAP should clamp or discontinue the tube. The "how" or technical component need not be included with the same simulation.

Ongoing development of clinical judgment with UAPs should be directed toward aspects that have proved problematic. Hospitals that have implemented the role have found they must re-emphasize the UAPs' interpersonal responses to patients and family— for instance, how the UAP should respond to questions such as, "Why are you wearing gloves?" or "What happened to the patient in the other bed?" (Biemolt, 1996, Weber, 1996). The response that demonstrates good judgment and accountability must offer more assistance than, "Ask your doctor," "Everything will be all right," or "I have no idea."

UAPs also must practice determining how urgent particular situations are and how to readjust their priorities when various situations occur. Sometimes the correct response in readjusting priorities should be to report the situation to the RN and ask for direction.

Several books provide good resources for patient care situations and cases. These include Alfaro-LeFevre, 1995, Collier et al., 1995, Miller and Babcock, 1995, and Rubenfeld and Scheffer, 1995. All include exercises and case study materials and questions. The book by Collier et al. is oriented toward developing skill in making nursing diagnosis, but the cases might also be useful for developing other aspects of critical thinking and clinical judgment. The book presents cases for caregivers at three levels of proficiency in writing nursing diagnoses and provides model answers written by experts. The model answers might serve as material for developing the critiquing skills of experienced nurses.

Vendors of educational materials are constantly developing new computer-assisted learning products to develop critical thinking and clinical judgment. The critical care nursing series available from Mosby is one example. Other educational products companies, such as Williams & Wilkins, also produce clinical simulations in various specialties.

Technical Skill

SDSs have a great deal of experience developing technical skills for effective, safe, and accurate performance. The process is quite straightforward. Procedures, protocols, and texts define skills in a step-by-step fashion. Expert staff abound in the environment, and SDSs can consult them. Evaluators can observe directly to assess and evaluate performance. Caregivers learn skills through practice, practice, and more practice, shaped with constructive corrective feedback. In today's environment, emphasis on cross-training and ensuring competency highlight certain aspects of skill development.

Efficiency and competency-based learning are both important in today's environment. Both are served when SDSs assess and validate entry skills and then provide training only for the skills the caregiver lacks. Packaging skill training in self-directed practice modules permits this kind of flexibility. In the group learning situation, a caregiver who has previous experience and whose performance has been validated can assist his or her classmates with practice.

Some roles that formerly did not include performing skills with patients have been retooled to include skills such as vital signs, specimen collection, phlebotomy, EKG, and screening for cholesterol and glucose. Outpatient scheduling clerks cross-trained in these skills perform the new outpatient care technician role at Riverside Medical Center in Kankakee, IL (AHC, 1995). The new role combines customer service and the clerical duties of preregistration, registration, and order entry with selected caregiver skills.

In cross-training and developing skills with experienced caregivers, SDSs work most effectively when they incorporate previous skill learning in the process. Following up a demonstration with the question, "How does this differ from your previous experience?" helps the learner integrate new learning and shows respect for his or her previous experience. If the caregiver has previous experience with the skill, identifying differences increases the chances that he or she will continue to practice the skill as newly learned rather than reverting to previous practices.

SDSs have valuable input to offer in the process of selecting skills for "multiskilling" and cross-training. One widely accepted redesign rule is to include only skills that can be learned in 6 weeks or less. Many redesigned organizations have refined their retooled roles, deleting skills that caregivers were not performing with sufficient frequency to maintain competence.

For efficient and flexible skill training, many organizations compile menus of technical competencies, complete with performance criteria and training materials (Biemolt, 1996). Some technical skill training modules are also available for purchase; for example, the ADD-A-COMP program (Makely, 1994) sells packets for EKG, rehabilitation technician, telemetry testing, and other skills.

Learners can also assist one another with skill development. Instructors create triads in which learners alternately take the roles of caregiver, patient, and coach. For this method to work effectively, the instructor must prepare and expect learners to function as coaches—in other words, emphasize what they are to look for in the skill performance.

Videotaping may be a luxury few can afford, but when feasible the opportunity to critique the performance of oneself and one's classmates enhances learning. Providing succinct self-assessment checklists for learners to use when practicing may help. These checklists take the form of, "Did you remember to . . .?" and contain the same features that instructors look for when observing practice.

Part of the SDS's role in skill development is to identify and use practice opportunities. Traditionally, nursing education has emphasized skill learning in the context of total patient care. The total patient orientation is important in UAP training also because these caregivers spend most of their time in direct, consistent contact with patients. However, while bearing the total patient orientation in mind, the SDS must often seek skill practice opportunities in addition to the lab and the usual unit opportunities. Otherwise, UAPs may not get enough practice to become proficient.

Greater proficiency may result from concentrated practice in one skill at a time. Most organizations that have implemented a UAP role that includes venipuncture skill have found they must provide additional training and practice. Seeking areas of the health care facility where the skill is performed in high volume and at a high frequency and arranging for precepted practice there will pay off in greater competence.

Often caregivers are anxious about performing new skills and when giving care may tend to focus on tasks rather than the overall context of the patient's needs. The SDS may address this problem by building confidence in skill performance through intensive practice and then revisiting the overall context of the patient.

To feel comfortable in the role of supervising and delegating to UAPs, RNs must learn the skills that their UAPs perform. All those who assess and validate competencies and evaluate performance need training to ensure that they implement standards and criteria consistently. The SDS must develop approaches to orienting and training managers and all who will function as preceptors, including representatives of other disciplines. Representatives of other disciplines who teach skills may need assistance with techniques of demonstrating and thinking out loud.

SDSs must apply their own critical thinking skills to the process of skill training. By reviewing past cross-training efforts for failures, deficiencies, and mistakes, problems can be avoided. Brookfield (1994) refers to this process as "making our mistakes into our instructional friends." Educators also must reflect on the process of skill learning as they observe it and continually refine the strategies they use.

RETOOLING ROLES

Staff development forms the foundation for successful retooling. Yale-New Haven Medical Center began patient-focused care in May 1994. There,

> The commitment has been and continues to be, while adhering to the principles of adult learning, to provide a training framework which promotes employee effectiveness and supports desired performance outcomes across all organizational roles . . . [Patient care associate training was designed] to minimize concern about patient safety and to maintain the reputation for quality care that the organization enjoys. (American Hospital Association, 1995)

The consulting firm Booz-Allen Hamilton Healthcare, Inc., identified functional role training as one of the eight key elements for effective redesign (AHC, 1994). "People think re-engineering is equipment and facility redesign, but it's primarily people and training," said a care center vice president at St. Mary's Medical Center in Long Beach, CA (AHC, 1995). Wilson (1992) advocated including the education department in restructuring from the preplanning phase forward. She noted that educators are in key positions to sabotage or impede implementation of new models and might do so if not incorporated into the process.

Augusta Medical Center in Fisherville, VA (AHC, 1996), suggested five steps to set the stage for successful training:

1. Gain total administrative support to get people in class.
2. Involve all in-house educators from the beginning.
3. Conduct frequent and ongoing evaluation of the effectiveness of training from a wide range of sources.
4. Organize a means of tracking employee attendance during training.
5. Encourage communication among groups and departments involved in training.

More research is needed to identify the effects of retooling roles. Some evidence suggests that it has positive effects on staff. Physicians appreciate the timely services available from UAPs and particularly "love phlebotomy" (Nick, 1996). Physician dissatisfaction decreased from 47% to 13% at Orlando Regional Medical Center in Orlando, FL (AHC, 1995). One physician there said that staff knew what was going on with his patients, when to call him, and where things were located. He added that those factors made his practice much easier.

According to a 1996 survey by *Revolution: The Journal of Nurse Empowerment*, job satisfaction for many RNs is decreased by concerns about delegation, job security, and the competency of UAPs (Elsasser, 1996). RN satisfaction is higher where RN partnerships with UAPs have matured, RNs feel comfortable with UAP training and competency, and RNs feel they can attend to patient needs that require RN skills.

Further research is needed to describe RN satisfaction with patient-focused models. Some hospitals, such as Lehigh Hospital and Health Network in Allentown, PA (AHC, 1996), and Dixie Regional Medical Center in St. George, UT (AHC, 1995), have reported overall gains in staff satisfaction since implementing patient-focused care. Other systems have developed incentive programs based on productivity of service centers, such as the Heart Institute at St. Joseph's Medical Center in Towson, MD (AHC, 1996).

Further research is also needed to describe the effect of retooled roles on patient care outcomes. The ANA, other professional organizations, and individual hospitals are pursuing this effort. A great deal of controversy surrounds the impact of retooled caregiver roles on the quality and safety of patient care. ANA opposes extensive retooling, expressing concern about patient safety, quality of care, and elimination of RN positions. The American Organization of Nurse Executives believes that these concerns can be managed. Its executive director cited the results of a National Hospital Panel Survey showing a greater increase in the number of RN positions than in nursing assistant positions between 1994 and 1995 and a decrease in LPN positions during that period (Varro, 1996). One point of agreement between the professional factions appears to be that training, continuing education, and ongoing competency assessment for UAPs are crucial.

According to Press-Gainey, one of the largest surveyors of patient satisfaction, the four leading contributors to patient satisfaction are the patient's perception of comfort, patient education and information, friendliness, and cleanliness (AHC, 1996). UAPs are positioned to address these needs or at least to acknowledge the need and readily obtain the appropriate assistance.

Many hospitals also report gains in patient satisfaction with the implementation of patient-focused care. One hospital experienced a 12% gain in patient satisfaction in 6 months (AHC, 1995). Some report decreased patient falls, decreased medication errors, and decreased nosocomial infections, along with reduced lengths of stay and increased nursing care hours (AHC, 1995, 1996). Some report maintaining quality levels despite downsizing. Others identified an increase in quality indicators while maintaining morbidity and mortality at the levels that existed before patient-focused care was instituted (AHC, 1995). In most hospitals, financial considerations drove the introduction of patient-focused care. However, some hospitals took the patient-focused direction as a means of enhancing quality (Whitman, 1996).

In addition to initial and continuing training, other supports in which staff development plays a role include communication, quality improvement, and evaluation. "The new model doesn't automatically work and keep working," said the project director of Patient Care 2000 at the University of Alabama—Birmingham (AHC, 1995).

Most working programs consider communication vital to implementing and evolving retooled roles and patient-focused models (AHC, 1994). Miniace and Falter (1996) described the "ready, aim, communicate, evaluate" model that they successfully implemented at New York University Medical Center. As in all change processes, those involved must hear and hear again about the change, the reasons for it, and what it means to them. This sort of reinforcement is the only way to keep a new model in place. Fears and anxieties usually accompany change. The profound change and job threats (both real and perceived) that accompany retooling heighten fears and anxieties. Leaders at one hospital believed that an advantage of a quick roll-out was that people in the organization had less time to worry, observe, and wonder (AHC, 1996).

Roles of the SDS in Retooling

As experienced communicators who traverse the organization, SDSs play a major role in clarifying information, translating information for various stakeholders, and feeding back information to organizational leaders. Reports of working programs, including all the programs referenced in this chapter, reveal ongoing improvements. Continuous quality improvement (CQI) is integral to working programs; the approach is one of revising and revisiting a work in progress. Most salient for SDSs are revisions in skill sets (*e.g.*, due to the needs of some units, combining environmental and transportation duties has proven problematic) and training emphasis (*e.g.*, more venipuncture, less class and more hands-on, more intact team training, more follow-up).

Retooling roles is but one component of a constellation of changes taking place when patient-focused care is instituted. The concomitant changes and complexity of the data generated make evaluation difficult. SDSs can draw on their expertise in evaluation to suggest strategies. One important first step is to review the evaluation processes others are using. One ambitious evaluation process examining retooled roles, training, and patient care outcomes is currently underway at the Ohio State University Medical Center in Columbus (Whitman, 1996).

Because of the CQI ongoing in retooled systems, the organization continually retools the retooled roles. Some skills may be dropped from the package of one role because they are not working. Different skills may be selected for cross-training. Some skills may be redistributed to other roles or back to centralized services. Staff development must have input into this process because of the training implications. The observations and experience that SDSs obtain in the initial training process are valuable pieces of information.

Another important implication for SDSs is the need for continuing education for UAPs (Varro, 1996). To participate more fully in patient care, UAPs need a broader knowledge base. They also need the opportunity to update their new skills and stay abreast of new developments in patient care.

Managers also need new skills in retooled environments. They must create the expectation that retooled caregivers will perform their new skills regularly. They must develop coaching skills—in other words, "how to listen to people and get them to think about a problem without directly telling them what to do about it" (University of Chicago Hospitals, 1996, p. 3). Because some management positions are usually eliminated in restructuring, managers who remain must develop skills in reframing their responsibilities to accommodate accountability for broader services and groups of personnel.

SDSs also must think about their own role, new applications of the expertise they have, and what new skills they must acquire to remain viable and vital to their organizations.

One new attitude that hallmarks retooled roles and organizations redesigned for patient-focused care is the elimination of the "It's not my job/problem" attitude. The new attitude is, "If a problem comes to my attention, that makes it my problem." This does not mean that it is the person's problem to solve, but that he or she must bring it to the attention of someone whose scope of practice or duties includes solving this problem. This attitude can be put into play only when all team members know the roles and resources of the organization and how to gain access to them.

Another important attitude for the RN involves delegation. Many RNs who have learned how do delegate do not consistently do so in practice. One educator reported that in the course of following up work transformation on the units, she and her colleagues asked nurses why they could not do it on the unit after having demonstrated their ability to do it in training. The RNs' simple, elegant response was, "We don't want to" (Biemolt, 1996). The staff development responsibility is to assist RNs to eliminate whatever barriers they have toward delegation.

The attitude that makes retooling work and also supports effective staff development is the attitude of inquiry. The attitude of inquiry, one of three major components of critical thinking that Watson and Glaser (1985) identified in their critical thinking work, continues to stimulate and guide effective critical thinking (Miller & Babcock, 1995). The attitude of inquiry raises questions about assumptions and challenges caregivers and SDSs to search for new ways to frame and approach situations.

MEASUREMENT

Measuring competence is a complex issue. Inaccurate or insufficient measurement and documentation of staff competence creates risks to quality and safety in patient care, legal risks, and incomplete compliance with accreditation standards. The most valid means of evaluation is to use a variety of measures, including performance appraisal, peer review, and formal observation and testing. Some hospitals also include demonstration, testing within self-learning modules, observation, audits of documentation, and exemplars to measure competency (Keane & Pistone, 1996). The soundest approach, and the preference of accreditors, is to ensure that all essential competencies are clearly stated and identified in the performance appraisal. Other documentation provides supportive evidence for performance appraisal ratings but should not function as a separate or parallel system. Many organizations use summary formats that present competencies in a table format with expectations, resources and strategies, and methods and demonstration dates for each competency.

Some institutions incorporate not only peer review but also 360° evaluation. The 360° evaluation incorporates feedback from as many persons who interact with a role as is feasible. In the case of the RN, these persons might include peers, UAPs, and representatives of other disciplines, in addition to peers and managers. The use of different sources of information and different measures to evaluate competence increases validity. In research, this integration of different measures is referred to as triangulation. Some trainers (Pike, 1989) refer to the concept as nonredundant, repetitive measures.

Many organizations are working on closer integration of competency assessment and performance appraisal systems. Some are working toward incorporating a structural scheme that separates competencies into critical thinking, interpersonal, and technical domains (Jeska et al., 1995). Others are developing tools to rate the knowledge, interpersonal, technical, and problem-solving dimensions of competencies (Weber, 1996).

This section focuses on written tests and performance ratings, popular measures of competency. The discussion matches measures with the appropriate domain of learning (cognitive, affective, psychomotor) and the appropriate level within the cognitive domain (primarily differentiating knowledge, comprehension, and application from critical thinking skills). One caveat to the discussion: these measurement techniques are not appropriate for all competencies, nor do they substitute for performance appraisal. "Measurement techniques, no matter how refined, cannot overcome mistaken identification of competencies" (Benner, 1982, p. 303). This section also addresses the use of published and standardized tests and various concerns related to using and refining tests.

Constructing, using, and improving tests is a complex and well-studied field. For more detailed treatment of the subject, readers are referred to Alspach (1995) and Gronlund and Linn (1990).

Testing in the Cognitive Domain: Knowledge and Thinking

The levels of the cognitive domain described by Bloom (in Gronlund & Linn, 1990) have become the classic and widely accepted standard for progressive development of cognitive skills. These levels, and the key words to capture the behavior that demonstrates achievement in each domain, are:

- Knowledge: recall
- Comprehension: explain
- Application: transfer
- Analysis: separate
- Synthesis: combine
- Evaluation: make a judgment.

Gronlund and Linn (1990) provided an extensive description of these levels and suggested general instructional objectives and specific learning outcomes associated with each level. (Chap. 10 also discusses program design and objective development.) Critical thinking and clinical judgment belong in the three highest levels of the cognitive domain.

Behavioral statements of learning objectives or competencies drive the measurement process. Testing and measuring is simply creating a means for learners to do or perform the behaviors specified by the objectives and specifying the criteria and standards that will indicate successful performance. Although technically criteria and standards come into play when evaluating or making a judgment about the results obtained in measurement, the test-maker also must consider the criteria and standards when designing a test.

For example, if the learning objective or competency states that the nurse will identify contraindications for administering tissue-type plasminogen activator, the testing situation could ask the nurse to choose the correct option in a multiple-choice item, to select contraindications contained in the description of a patient who presents in the emergency department, or to locate contraindications in the medical record of a real or simulated patient. The critical point is that the test must require the nurse to "identify." When the objective or competency states that the nurse will "describe" something, the testing situation must require the nurse to describe it orally or in writing and not simply select a description from a set of multiple-choice options.

A written test gives evidence of what a test-taker knows but not necessarily what he or she will do when a situation arises that requires the use of that knowledge. This is the question of validity in testing for the purpose of competency validation. Is the response on this test a true and meaningful indicator of the desired competency? The question implies that test situations must represent practice situations as accurately as possible and that competency must be evaluated and documented in ongoing performance appraisal in addition to whatever supportive evidence testing supplies.

KNOWLEDGE, COMPREHENSION, AND APPLICATION

Lower-level cognitive objectives are amenable to objective testing with the use of matching or true/false test items. SDSs prefer to use objective testing when appropriate because objective responses can be scored more quickly and easily than open-ended responses and because scoring is more reliable. Reliability means consistency: the instructor who scores the test will evaluate responses consistently from one test-taker to the next or, if more than one instructor were to evaluate a given test, the instructors' evaluations would be consistent. Obviously, objective responses lend themselves to greater consistency than do open-ended responses.

Objective testing has a reliability advantage, but there may be problems with validity. Complex decision making is not as easily measured as are knowledge, comprehension, and application of facts and principles. As Del Bueno (1990) noted, "Unfortunately, few patients present nurses with four possible options to solve their health problems" (p. 5). In practice, caregivers must collect information, make decisions, and act, not simply choose from a limited range of four choices.

CRITICAL THINKING AND CLINICAL JUDGMENT

Although testing of higher-level cognitive skills is less objective, it is no less driven by learning objectives. The SDS must have a clear vision of exactly what the caregiver will be doing when giving evidence of critical thinking or clinical judgment. Once the behavior is defined, the challenge is to set up a situation that will call for the caregiver to display the behavior. The situations presented must replicate practice as closely as possible. Educators must collaborate closely with clinical experts and managers to ensure that the problem-solving situations that occur most commonly in practice are well represented in testing.

The test can present the situation in a variety of formats: a written description, a videotape or audiotape, a live simulation or equipment set-up, or printed or projected still pictures. Computer formats allow for CD-ROM and laser disc presentations.

The test must present specific questions to which the test-taker can respond. The questions presented previously with strategies for developing critical thinking offer some examples. Although the same questions can be used for testing as were used for practice in learning sessions, the test must present new situations. To test critical thinking and clinical judgment, the situation must be new to the test-taker; otherwise, he or she may simply recall previous discussions and solutions rather than actively solving the problem.

Although objective testing does not fully test critical thinking and clinical judgment, it can measure some aspects of critical thinking. For example, the true/false type of item can ask for dichotomous responses such as safe or unsafe, urgent or not, legal risk or not, appropriate or inappropriate delegation, competent or not competent (in a test item for RNs in which the situation describes examples of UAP performance). This style of item can be used efficiently by presenting a number of brief situations (a sentence or two) and asking the test-taker to choose between the same responses for each situation. The items can test critical thinking more fully by asking the test-taker to state the evidence to support one choice or the other—how the unsafe situation can be made safe, what else a caregiver must know, and so forth.

Multiple-choice items can ask the test-taker to identify the assessment data in a situation that supports a particular nursing diagnosis, or to select the most appropriate first action. The limitation as a full test of critical thinking is that the test-taker is not generating an answer based on all the possible thought processes and solutions he or she might generate. Instead, he or she considers only the relative merits of the four choices presented. The action he or she might actually do may be one that the test-writer did not include.

Before using test items that ask for an open-ended response (e.g., fill-in-the-blank, a few sentences, a written plan of care, a decision tree), the test-writer must establish the criteria for evaluating the responses. To do so, the test-writer creates a model response or correct answer and decides what elements of that response must be included in the test-taker's response for the response to be considered correct. A test-writer can assign points to certain key elements of a model answer so that the test-taker can earn partial credit. However, in the practice setting (as compared with the academic setting), a pass/fail scoring system is more useful than points, scores, and grades. Therefore, it is important that the test-writer establish what a test-taker's response must contain to be considered correct. Clear and simple criteria ensure reliable evaluation across a number of test-takers or evaluators. The test-writer can protect validity in the process of determining the criteria by consulting with clinical experts and managers to establish essential elements. The test-writer also ensures validity by asking the question in such a way that the criteria are clear to the test-taker. This includes communicating the essential elements of the response to the test-taker (*e.g.*, "You must state which action takes priority.").

TABLE OF SPECIFICATIONS

The table of specifications (Table 11-2) may also be called the test blueprint or the test plan. its purpose is to ensure content validity—in other words, to make sure a test accurately represents the behaviors and content areas desired. The most important feature of any test is that it tests the objectives or the competencies that the teacher intends it to test, or that the test is valid for its intended purpose. Whether the SDS is writing the test, using standardized questions, or combining the two, he or she must make sure that the test measures the objectives of the course or the competencies of interest.

A table of specifications identifies the behaviors and content for the test and the number of points or test items allocated to various objectives. Each column is designated for a cognitive level. It may not be necessary or practical to distinguish among "Analyzes," "Synthesizes," and "Evaluates" in every test; a suitable alternative is to label the columns "Knowledge," "Comprehension," "Application," and "Critical Thinking." For each objective, the number of points or number of items that will measure each level is entered in the appropriate column. For example, if one objective is, "Plans patient teaching for the

TABLE 11-2

TABLE OF SPECIFICATIONS

Objectives	Cognitive Levels (The behavior that the test-taker will exhibit when answering the question)						
	Knows	Comprehends	Applies	Analyzes	Synthesizes	Evaluates	TOTAL
TOTAL							

hip replacement patient," there may be some items that ask for facts about anatomy or the surgical procedure. Questions about facts measure what the test-taker knows, and the number of fact questions is entered in the "Knows" column. There may also be some questions that require the test-taker to apply principles of adult learning. The number of questions that measure the test-taker's application of principles is entered in the "Applies" column. Some questions may require the learner to analyze a patient teaching situation or develop criteria for evaluating the patient's learning. The number of these questions is entered in the "Analyzes" and "Evaluates" columns respectively; if "Critical Thinking" is used as an alternative to the "analyzes, synthesizes, evaluates" model, both types of questions would be entered in the "Critical Thinking" column.

It is important to measure only one objective with each item. If answering an item correctly depends on knowing terminology and solving a problem, the test-taker may answer incorrectly due to a deficiency in either terminology or problem solving. From that one answer, it will not be possible to ascertain which deficit was present. If knowledge of terms is important, that knowledge should be tested separately, perhaps using a matching item to test knowledge of a number of terms. Those terms can then be used in problem-solving situations in another portion of the test. The table of specifications would reflect different items measuring each objective.

The numbers used in the table may be the number of items on the test or the number of points. If the convention of giving one point per multiple-choice item is being followed, or if all items have the same point value, it is convenient to use the number of items. However, if not all items on the test have the same value, it is more meaningful to use point values.

The process of figuring out numbers of items or points begins with determining how many will be designated for each objective and then dividing the number for each objective into the appropriate cognitive levels. It is not necessary to have items at each level for each objective. In advanced courses for experienced RNs, most of the items should be at the higher levels. The determining factor is the objectives. The objectives, in turn, are formulated to reflect the performance expectations of the caregiver, or the caregiver's competencies.

The instructional emphasis determines the allocation of items. The greatest emphasis is given to the most important aspects of the content and objectives. Instructional emphasis is usually reflected in the amount of instructional time devoted to a topic. However, caregivers may be expected to read information, view videotapes, or acquire information in ways other than direct instruction from the teacher in the classroom.

The SDS uses the table of specifications in several ways. First, it is used to specify the number of items or points devoted to each objective and each cognitive level. Then it serves as a guide, whether the test-maker is constructing items or selecting items from sources of test questions. If certain test items must be replaced because they are outdated or were found to be faulty through item analysis, the item chosen to replace the discarded item should fit the same specifications. Finally, the SDS should share the table of specifications with test-takers to help them allocate their study time, identify priorities, and prepare for the test.

TEACHER-MADE TESTS

In addition to using a table of specifications, following certain guidelines in constructing test items and assembling and administering tests improves validity. These guidelines are intended to ensure that the test as a whole and the particular items measure the intended objective in a straightforward manner. Although multiple-choice items are most commonly used, other types of questions are useful as well and may be more efficient or more consistent with the cognitive level to be measured. For all types of items, certain rules apply:

- Keep items brief, succinct, and free of extraneous information.
- Avoid using absolute determiners such as always, all, only, or never.
- Underline, italicize, capitalize, or otherwise emphasize the focus or determining factor in choosing an answer.
- Limit the use of negatively stated questions. When used, underline, italicize, capitalize, or otherwise emphasize negatives (*e.g.*, ALL EXCEPT; which of the following is NOT). Negatively stated questions are more difficult for the test-taker to process. Try to find a way to state the question positively. For example, if asking an RN which of the following duties a UAP should not perform, phrase the question to ask which of the following is beyond the scope of practice of the UAP, or which of the following is reserved for the RN, or which of the following will require assigning a licensed person.
- When the choices for answers are letters or numbers, require the test-taker to circle the letter or number, or fill in a space on a scanning sheet. Clever but uncertain test-takers may make letters indistinguishable.
- Be sure that directions are clear and complete. Include the point value. For open-ended responses, specify the criteria for awarding points. Include instructions for how and where to record answers.
- When presenting lab values, box them and use the format of the agency rather than writing them in a narrative, sentence format.
- Use language consistent with the reading level required in practice. Use the simplest word that communicates the meaning (*e.g.*, use, not utilize).
- Make choices (true/false statements, multiple-choice options) of equal length.
- If terminology is part of the knowledge to be tested, test it separately and not in the context of a situation in which another level, such as analysis, is also tested.
- Use random order for correct responses.
- Proofread carefully.
- Ask a colleague to review the items. Because the test-taker knows what he or she had in mind, another person will be better at detecting ambiguous or confusing statements.
- Be sure each item is complete on one page and does not continue onto the next page.

Observing these guidelines for each item type improves test validity by ensuring that the test-taker focuses on the objective being tested and not on extraneous or confusing artifacts. For true/false items:

- Be sure that statements are absolutely true or false and not dependent on circumstances. This is especially important if the test-taker will not be correcting a false statement.
- Make the number of true and false answers approximately equal.
- If the statement is a matter of opinion, be sure to identify the source.

For matching tests:

- Within each column, make the list homogeneous (*e.g.*, all are drugs, all are lab values, all are side effects) and label each list ("Generic Names of Drugs," "Lab Values," "Side Effects").

- Make directions clear as to the basis for matching and the number of times each choice may be used.
- Place the responses in the right column, the premises on the left.
- Make one list longer than the other (either more responses than needed, or only five or fewer responses that must be used to label or categorize the premises).
- Place responses in a logical order—time sequence, ascending order if numbers, alphabetical order if there is no other logical order.
- Keep responses brief and of same length, one word if possible.

For multiple-choice items:

- Present a clear, concise stem that poses a meaningful problem—in other words, if the options are removed, the stem presents a meaningful question or an incomplete statement.
- Make sure that only one option is clearly the best answer.
- Write options that are grammatically consistent with the stem, of similar length and form, free of any verbal clues to the answer (*e.g.*, words from the stem repeated only in the correct answer), and free of unnecessary words (rather than repeating words, place more words in the stem). The options should begin with active verbs if they are actions.
- Make incorrect options plausible to test-takers who have not mastered the objective. Use common misunderstandings as distracters rather than ridiculous alternatives. When computations are involved, write distracters that would be obtained by carelessness or by missing a step in the computation procedure.
- Preserve any logical order in listing the options (*e.g.*, time sequence or ascending order if numbers).
- Make questions independent of one another. The answer to one question should not depend on the answer chosen for another question.
- Limit the number of questions posed about each patient situation. If using situations, be sure that the information in the situation is required to answer the question. For instance, do not write a long story about a diabetic patient and then ask the test-taker to choose the normal value for blood glucose.
- Avoid using "all of the above," "none of the above," and "multiple-multiples." Multiple-multiples present a list of choices and then create options that are combinations of the choices (*e.g.*, "1, 3, and 5"). If the objective requires a combination answer, make the options all short series.

An interpretive exercise presents a picture or a graphic such as a rhythm strip or set of lab values. The questions that follow may be of any type (true/false, matching, multiple-choice item, fill-in-the-blank, or short answer):

- Make sure that the material is new and not the same set of information used in class or in a reference. If the material is not new, the test-taker can answer correctly by rote without interpreting the information.
- Ensure that the test-taker must interpret the information to answer. In other words, the test-taker must do something with the material, not simply recall facts.

For fill-in or completion items:

- Be specific about the nature of the answer. For instance, the answer to "The agency that accredits hospitals and health care agencies is . . ." could be answered in a number of ways, such as "in Oakbrook, IL" or "a bureaucracy." If the name

or acronym is the intended answer, then the question should ask for the name of the agency.
- Use blanks for the most significant words only.
- Word the question so that only one answer is correct.
- Place the blank at the end of the statement.
- Make sure items are free of clues, such as "a" or "an."
- Make scoring easier by placing blanks to the left of the item so that written answers will appear as a list (Alspach, 1995) and by preparing a list of acceptable answers as a key.

For short answer, essay, and other freeform responses, such as decision trees or diagrams:

- Decide in advance what the criteria will be for scoring, and communicate them to the test-takers.
- Develop a model answer and decide which elements are essential.
- Decide on and communicate the criteria related to writing skills. Will grammar and spelling be evaluated? Must the answer be expressed in complete sentences, or is a list acceptable? Is any particular agency-specific format to be used?

ASSEMBLING AND ADMINISTERING TESTS

Following certain procedures when assembling and administering tests helps focus the test-taker on the material being tested and therefore improves validity.

- Make the test long enough to sample the content adequately.
- Leave plenty of white space for the answer.
- Arrange items from easy to difficult.
- Consider using a matching item at the beginning to summarize a number of fact questions rather than presenting multiple-choice items for a number of different facts (*e.g.*, lab values, definitions, drugs).
- Allow sufficient time—1 minute for multiple-choice items, more for high-level complex items and responses that require organizing and writing. Give the test a trial run with staff who are as similar to the test-takers as possible. The time that the test-writer needs to take the test will not indicate how much time a person unfamiliar with the test will require.
- Eliminate cheating.
- Make and abide by rules about giving assistance. It is better to give none during the test. Announce in advance that no questions will be answered during the test. Let test-takers know that they may write questions for the educator on the question paper or on other paper provided. Responding to test-takers' questions is distracting and gives an advantage to those assertive enough to ask.
- Minimize distractions, including physical and psychological ones.
- Make scoring of open-ended responses objective, as much as possible. Conceal names. Skim all the papers first for a typical response. Score one item at a time across all papers, reshuffling papers to avoid a "halo" effect. Either apply the same criteria to all and score each one, or rank the papers on each question.

STANDARDIZED TESTS

A standardized achievement test has certain distinctive features, including a fixed set of items designed to measure a clearly defined achievement domain, specific directions for administering and scoring the test, and norms based on representative groups of individuals like those for whom the test was designed. (Gronlund & Linn, 1990, p. 266)

SDSs have a variety of published tests at their disposal. Some of these tests are standardized and some are not. For tests that have been standardized and evaluated for validity and reliability, the publisher makes this information available, usually in a test administrator's manual.

The information about the evaluation of the test includes statements about validity and reliability. Both validity and reliability are expressed as correlation coefficients, ranging in value from -1.00 to $+1.00$. A negative value indicates a negative relation (as one value increases, the other decreases); a value of zero indicates no relation; and a positive value indicates a positive relation (as one value increases, the other value also increases). The closer the value is to 1.00, the stronger the relation.

Validity studies establish a relation between results on the test and some other measures. Two types of validity are not statistically determined: face validity and content-related validity. Face validity is determined by experts who judge a test to represent the content and behaviors that it purports to represent. Content-related validity is the extent to which the test represents the instructional outcomes and cognitive levels intended. Content-related validity is ensured by adhering to a table of specifications. The SDS consults with clinical experts and managers to judge face validity and to establish the appropriate relative emphasis of instructional outcomes and cognitive levels. To evaluate a published test or standardized test for use in measuring caregiver competency, the SDS must determine, usually in consultation with others, to what extent the test measures the competencies that are important in the caregiver roles.

Criterion-related validity and construct-related validity are statistically determined. Criterion-related validity establishes a relation between the results on the test in question and the results on some other test. Criterion-related validity may be predictive in nature, in which case the relation is one between the results on the test in question and the results on a test to be taken in the future. The relation is established with groups of test-takers who have taken the test (*e.g.*, the National League for Nursing [NLN] Achievement Tests taken during nursing school) and then later taken another test (the NCLEX-RN after graduation from nursing school). Based on this reference, a student taking the NLN Achievement Test can project how he or she will do on the NCLEX-RN.

Concurrent validity refers to the extent of the relation between the results on two tests taken at approximately the same time. For example, the results on the NLN Long-Term Care Nursing Assistant Test might be positively related to the results on the NLN Nursing Assistants in Acute Care Settings Test for a group of certified nursing assistants taking the examinations at nearly the same time.

Construct-related validity is the extent to which a test represents a global construct such as intelligence or self-esteem. This type of evidence for validity is more of a research interest than a concern of the SDS in competency testing.

The most important type of validity in the staff development setting is content-related validity, ensuring that the test measures the desired outcomes and competencies in a representative fashion.

Reliability refers to consistency of results obtained with a test. Types of reliability include stability or test/retest reliability, parallel or equivalent forms reliability, and internal consistency reliability. SDSs sometimes become concerned with the type of internal consistency reliability known as interrater reliability when they determine the similarity between ratings by two different raters using the same tool. For example, if two different preceptors use the same performance checklist to evaluate the performance of a UAP performing venipuncture, how closely will their ratings agree?

Gronlund and Linn (1990) recommended assessing the following features when deciding whether to use a particular standardized test:

- General features
  - Author credentials
  - Stated purpose of the test
  - Intended test-takers
  - Publication date
  - Type of scoring
  - Administration time
  - Cost
- Technical features
  - Validity
  - Reliability
  - Norms (particularly the similarity of the norming group to the group with whom the test would be used)
  - Criterion-referenced interpretation
- Practical features
  - Ease of administration (procedure and timing)
  - Ease of scoring and interpretation
  - Adequacy of test manual and accessory materials
- General evaluation
  - Comments of reviewers (*e.g.*, experts or colleagues who have used the test)
  - Summary of strengths and weaknesses
  - Recommendations concerning local use.

The most important criterion for selecting a published or standardized test is that the test actually tests the desired competency. The group to be tested should be similar to the norming group if any claims will be made related to norming information.

Human resources professionals often stress the importance of using standardized tests, particularly for prehire screening. Standardization does offer some protection against claims of discrimination, but it is also important that the test be related to job competencies and expectations.

Tests are supplied by vendors in sets containing a number of test booklets, a scoring guide, and an administrator's manual. The manual explains the analysis conducted in developing the test.

Before using published or standardized tests, it is wise to pilot the test with a small sample of nurses to make sure that the test measures competencies pertinent to the organization's practices. These tests, particularly the medication administration tests, are widely used. Therefore, the SDS can consult with colleagues in other organizations and learn about their experience with the tests.

The Basic Knowledge Assessment Tool, a popular standardized test, measures basic knowledge in critical care nursing. Jean Toth, the principal author, has evaluated the test extensively and published her results in the nursing literature. Versions are also available for progressive critical care and pediatric intensive care. The test is supplied with an answer sheet, a score sheet, information concerning the validity, reliability, uses, and scoring of the test, and selected references. Inquiries should be directed to Dr. Toth at The Catholic University of America School of Nursing in Washington, DC.

Some hospitals use published tests purchased from vendors of educational products, such as the cancer chemotherapy certification preparation course and the pain management series available from Williams & Wilkins. Many other publishers and vendors of educational resources offer educational programs that contain tests. Professional nursing specialty organizations may also be sources of relevant testing materials. Again, the important factor in choosing to use such tests is how closely the information tested corresponds to the competencies required to practice in a given setting.

The Performance-Based Development System offers a battery of assessment materials and a system for their use in assessing and developing competencies for RNs in selected clinical specialties, management, and precepting and for UAPs. The system requires the nursing staff within the user organization to develop model answers appropriate to practice in their organization. Performance Management Systems, Tustin, CA, can supply further information about this system. Dorothy del Bueno, who developed it, has written and coauthored several articles about the use of the system (Del Bueno, 1990, Del Bueno et al., 1990, Del Bueno, 1987).

Standardized measures of critical thinking are also available. Some of these are The Critical Thinking Disposition Inventory and The California Critical Thinking Skills Test (California Academic Press, San Francisco, CA), The Cornell Critical Thinking Skills Test Level Z (Critical Thinking Press & Software, Pacific Grove, CA), and the Watson-Glaser Critical Thinking Appraisal (Psychological Corporation, Dallas, TX). Standard tests of critical thinking have not shown a consistent relation to clinical nursing judgment (Beck et al., 1992, Bechtel et al., 1993). Continuing research with nursing samples (Facione et al., 1994) may yield useful relations. Although these tools have interesting research potential, they do not offer a valid, practical approach to assessing practice competency.

TEST EVALUATION

SDSs must continually ensure the validity of competency tests. This means ongoing comparison of test results with other indicators of competence, such as reports of medication errors, other reports of accidents, injury, or risk situations, performance appraisals, patient outcomes, patient satisfaction, and results of quality monitoring. Competency tests have no value if they do not produce results that are consistent with other indicators of quality.

Competency testing does not produce the range of scores that result from achievement tests. However, testing used in the learning process to develop competency produces a range of scores. For example, pretesting will usually produce a range of scores because there will be differences in knowledge about the subject within the group.

For tests that produce a range of scores, test results are often described by a frequency distribution, measures of central tendency, and variability (Appendix C). These may be produced by a computer or constructed and calculated by hand. For further information about these characteristics of a set of scores, see Gronlund and Linn (1990) and Alspach (1995).

For tests that produce a range of scores, item analysis procedures can be applied to evaluate test items. Three characteristics are useful in evaluating test items: difficulty, discrimination, and distracter effectiveness (Display 11-1). Of course, these characteristics describe how a test item performed with only a particular group of test-takers.

Difficulty is the percentage of test-takers who answered the item correctly. Difficulty ranges from 0% to 100%; the higher the percentage, the more test-takers answered correctly. Therefore, an item that all answered correctly has 100% difficulty. If all answer an item incorrectly, the difficulty is 0%. In achievement tests, most sources suggest a difficulty level of 25% to 75%; others recommend a range of 30% to 70%. Some suggest that ideal difficulty is 65.5%. However, competency testing measures essential competencies. Although pretest and formative tests may yield many incorrect answers, on final tests of competency most items will be answered correctly.

Discrimination compares the number of test-takers who scored high on the test overall and answered a particular item correctly with the number of test-takers who scored low

DISPLAY 11-1

Sample Test Item Results for Computing Difficulty and Discrimination

High 10	Low 10	1. Your patient required intubation and was placed on a ventilator. Which of the following is the most valid indicator that your patient no longer requires mechanical ventilation?
1	4	A. Your patient is assisting ventilation at regular intervals.
9	4	B. Your patient's arterial pH value is WNL at a reduced FIO_2.
0	1	C. Your patient's respiratory rate averages 32 breaths per minute during weaning.
0	1	D. Your patient frequently attempts to extubate himself.

Difficulty

$$\frac{\text{Correct Responses, high} + \text{low}}{\text{Total responses, high} + \text{low}} = 13/20 = 0.65, \text{ expressed as } 65\%$$

If 10 per group:

$$\frac{\text{Correct responses, high} + \text{low} \times 10, \text{ add } \% \text{ sign}}{2}$$

$$= 13/2 \times 10 = 6.5 \times 10 = 65, \text{ add } \% \text{ sign} = 65\%$$

Discrimination

$$\frac{\text{Correct Responses, high} - \text{low}}{1/2 \text{ Total Responses, high} + \text{low}} = \frac{9 - 4}{10} = 5/10 = 0.50$$

If 10 per group:

$$\frac{\text{Correct responses, high} - \text{low} \text{ add a "0"}}{10}$$

$$= \frac{9 - 4}{10} = 5/10 = 0.5, \text{ add a "0"} = 0.50$$

on the test overall and answered the item correctly. The high group includes the highest 30% of scores, the low group the lowest 30%. In groups ranging in size from 20 to 40, the highest 10 scores and the lowest 10 scores are used to form the two groups. Possible values for discrimination range from -1.00 to $+1.00$. A negative value indicates that more test-takers in the low group answered correctly than did test-takers in the high group. Negative discrimination indicates a need to examine the item and probably revise or discard it. Zero discrimination indicates no difference between the number answering correctly in the high group as compared with the low group. Discrimination greater than 0.30 is considered desirable.

Item analysis identifies items the SDS should examine. Zero, near-zero, and negative discrimination indicate a need to revise or discard items. The way in which test items function is influenced by the instructional process. Sometimes item analysis identifies aspects in which instruction and instructional materials created confusion or lacked clarity.

The effectiveness of distracters is determined by comparing the number of test-takers in the high-scoring group and the low-scoring group who selected each option in the item. Distracters that more high scorers than low scorers selected are ineffective and indicate a problem with the distracter or with the stem. Distracters that are not chosen by either group are not functioning and should be replaced. Nonfunctioning distracters reduce the number of choices in a four-choice item to three and therefore make the item easier—in other words, test-takers have a 33% chance of guessing the correct answer as opposed to only a 25% chance of guessing correctly if all four choices function.

TEST IMPROVEMENT

Test improvement should be an ongoing process. The SDS should continually update test items and situations presented in testing to ensure that the test reflects current practice and patient care situations that are currently high-volume, high-risk, and problem-prone.

When results of item analysis suggest a need to replace an item, the SDS should refer to the table of specifications and replace the discarded item with another item that measures the same objective. When replacing distracters, construct choices that reflect common misunderstandings or common mistakes of caregivers in the situation the question presents.

Feedback from test-takers can also identify unclear statements. The test-writer should always submit items to a colleague or caregiver for review before presenting them on a test. Because the test-writer knows what he or she intended the item to communicate, ambiguity may not be evident to him or her.

Testing in the Psychomotor Domain: Technical Skills

To test psychomotor skills, the SDS observes and rates performance. Usually skills are evaluated first in a lab or simulated setting, then with a fellow caregiver assuming the role of patient (if feasible), and finally with an actual patient. Often different evaluators will observe and rate the performance—the instructor in the lab simulation and the preceptor or manager in actual practice.

Criteria for safe, effective performance must be clearly defined, and all who will participate in the evaluation process must have a common understanding of the criteria and the basis for assigning ratings. The SDS must provide training for evaluators to ensure this common understanding. Training should include opportunities for evaluators to observe and rate performances, either videotaped or simulated, compare ratings with the instructor, and clarify any discrepancies.

For the purposes of competency testing at the conclusion of training, performance must ultimately be judged as acceptable or unacceptable (competent or not competent). This judgment is usually based on safety and accuracy in performance. A performance checklist that indicates whether each step in a procedures is done or not done may be used to document competence. During training, ratings such as "needs improvement," "not yet competent," or "needs more practice" are useful to identify areas to improve.

For ongoing measurement of competency in practice, preceptors, managers, and performance coaches might rate a caregiver's performance considering other factors in addition to accuracy, such as consistency and amount of assistance needed.

Essential criteria and characteristics of performance may be generated in collaboration with clinical experts and experienced nurses. Published rating scales and checklists may be applicable but should be validated for local use. The validation process requires using the tool with practicing nurses. To be useful, lists of criteria must be limited to only the essential items.

Rating scales may take a number of forms. Three- or four-point scales are most common. These points should be labeled with some descriptive information that identifies the basis for rating, such as, "Rarely distinguishes between normal and abnormal findings," "Usually distinguishes between normal and abnormal findings," "Sometimes identifies subtle deviations," and "Consistently distinguishes between obvious and subtle deviations from normal." For some aspects of technical performance, it may be desirable to identify outstanding performance, but usually this category is reserved for evaluating only a few selected competencies in the performance appraisal process.

Testing in the Affective Domain: Feelings, Beliefs, Values, and Attitudes

Although this chapter has focused on critical thinking, clinical judgment, and technical competence, the affective domain deserves mention. Feelings, values, beliefs, and attitudes are often reflected in making decisions and taking actions. SDSs work with staff to develop feelings, values, attitudes, and beliefs consistent with the values and philosophy of the organization and professional standards. This affective component often is reflected by incorporating respectful consideration of the values, beliefs, and rights of others (both patients and coworkers) into care delivery and other aspects of practice. These affective behaviors may be incorporated into tools used to measure critical thinking, clinical judgment, and psychomotor competence. For example, performing treatments with patients might include protecting patient privacy and explaining in terms the patient understands. Chapter 12 provides additional information about teaching and testing in the affective domain.

Reporting

SDSs must preserve the confidentiality of the measurement information they collect while assessing and validating competencies. Caregivers are entitled to receive the scores, ratings, and interpretation of competency tests they have completed. SDSs should inform caregivers about what information concerning their performance will be shared and with whom and how it will be shared. Policy and procedure governs this process to protect all concerned.

SDSs should share competency testing results only with those who will make legitimate use of the information. Whatever recordkeeping system is used, including computerized storage, must be able to protect confidentiality. Usually the SDS shares such information only with colleagues directly involved in the assessment process, the caregiver, and the direct supervisor of the caregiver. The competency management system should provide for an objective, written means of reporting the results of competency testing to the caregiver and the caregiver's manager.

SDSs who are experienced in orienting caregivers often form intuitive impressions about their potential for success. Often these impressions elude description in specific documentation formats. When this occurs, SDSs should reflect on their impressions and attempt to identify the objective data that led to the impression. The impression and observations that support it can then be documented and shared with the caregiver and manager. To maintain credibility and professional ethics and to protect against potential charges of discrimination, SDSs must resist the temptation to share unsupported impressions that could bias a manager against a newly hired caregiver.

SUMMARY

This chapter explored the role of the SDS in developing caregivers' competencies in critical thinking, clinical judgment, and technical skill. It identified the roles of various members of the caregiver team, new models of care delivery, and the implications of these roles and models for competency development. Finally, it presented general concerns in measuring competency in critical thinking, clinical judgment, and technical skill.

Expertise in Everyday Practice

KAREN KELLY-THOMAS

SDSs assess and develop the competence of nurses who work in complex health care environments. We often speak of specific staff development strategies to help others develop skilled practice. As we consider strategies to develop others, we often talk of "knowing of the possibilities." Our conversations also include an understanding of individual and group potential for improvement, and we identify our choice of actions based on this knowledge.

SDSs take action in specific situations but continue to dwell in other situations, listening for new information, looking for new possibilities, and using their knowledge to transform everyday staff development practice. In my dissertation about the nature of intuition in staff development, expert SDSs said they trusted their intuition but were frustrated in trying to finding the right words to articulate this form of knowledge. Knowledge was made whole by the experts' understanding of the entire staff development situation. Subtle cues and nuances informed their whole-knowing. In the following narrative, Carole, an expert SDS, reflects on the use of intuition, or trusting one's inner voice, in staff development practice (Kelly, 1994).

> It's hard to explain intuition about staff development when you have to go up before logical people who want to know the rationale for why you are making a particular decision. It's not that I can't look at other alternatives. I have looked at other alternatives; it's just that it makes so much more sense. I do the analysis, I do all the logical pieces, but it's my feeling that says, "In this institution, this one won't work, and this one will work." I go with my gut instinct.
>
> Intuition means knowing your people well enough to handle them. For example, you know intuitively that with some people, you cannot bring up a certain topic in a group; you must talk to them ahead of time. In the case I'm thinking of, I brought something up in the group, and then it clicked on me that I had missed a cue. The woman in question didn't say anything, but her body told me that she wasn't happy with what was going on. I said, "Mary, is there something you'd like to

> say?" and she withdrew. I went to her afterwards and said, "I think I made you uncomfortable," and she told me that's what I did.
>
> I know how the directors think and I know what they are willing to buy. In my own mind, I put all the pieces of the puzzle together, and that's what my intuition is built on. Intuition comes first, and the logic is used to back it up.

Carole's expertise is evident as she continues:

> I think you learn as much from something that doesn't work as something that does work. When you see those things again, the same type of person or the same type of situation, you have a reference bank. You go back and find out what you've sorted out and what has worked, and that's how you move forward. As you're working through it, the person gives you enough clues so that you know you're right. It's almost like if you watch enough, and you're close enough, you can read it. The critical issue is, how do you read it right? You have to go closer to find out if you're reading it right. You continue that relationship back and forth.

Carole describes the "reference bank" formed by her experiences. This reference bank became a source of knowledge that was difficult to describe in linear, step-by-step procedures. She trusts her intuition as she goes with her gut instinct, her inner voice. She relies on her inner voice and counsel to figure out how to handle different situations, and she continues to monitor the situation to validate her intuition. She does not simply make a snap decision and act; rather, she retains a reflective stance to make sure she is "reading it right." She knows she must connect with others in the institution to accomplish mutual staff development goals, which she refers to as "handling" those whose support she needs to implement programs. Carole seeks clues and messages to inform her inner voice. Her trust in her intuition is developed over time as she gains perspective through myriad staff development situations with persons and groups. Her decisions are fluid and dynamic in each situation.

Staff development practice requires a constant vigilance to every opportunity to develop competence. In some cases this occurs purely in the classroom setting, but often everyday interactions in meetings and groups provide important opportunities for staff development to take place. Experts use everyday situations to promote staff development and are sensitive to the whole organization and its members continuously.

This SDS represents a level of expertise that will serve patients, care providers, and the organization well. Magnificent outcomes can be realized with this kind of "big picture" thinking.

REFERENCES

Alfaro-LeFevre, R. (1995). *Critical thinking in nursing: A practical approach.* Philadelphia: W.B. Saunders.

Alspach, G. (1995) *The educational process in nursing staff development.* St. Louis: Mosby-Year Book.

American Health Consultants. (1994). *Patient-focused care.* Atlanta, GA: Author.

American Health Consultants. (1995). *Patient-focused care.* Atlanta, GA: Author.

American Health Consultants. (1996). *Patient-focused care.* Atlanta, GA: Author.

American Health Consultants. (1996). *Patient satisfaction management.* Atlanta, GA: Author.

American Hospital Association. (1995). Creating the future workforce. Teleconference, Feb. 2, 1995. Chicago, IL: Author.

American Society of Healthcare Educators and Trainers. (1992). *Competency assessment: Challenges and opportunities for healthcare educators.* Chicago, IL: American Hospital Association.

Baugh, N., & Mellott, K. (1996). *Clinical concept mapping.* Nursing Education '96, sponsored by The Medical College of Pennsylvania and Hahnemann University (now Allegheny University), Washington DC, June 1996.

Beaver, C. (1996). Interview with author.

Bechtel, G., Smith, J., Printz, V., & Groneth, D. (1993). Critical thinking and clinical judgement of professional nurses in a career mobility program, *Journal of Nursing Staff Development,* 9(5), 218–222.

Beck, S., Bennett, A., McLeod, R., & Molyneaux, D. (1992). Review of research on critical thinking in nursing education. In Allen, L. R. (Ed.). *Review of research in nursing education,* volume 5. New York: National League for Nursing.

Benner, P. (1982). Issues in competency-based testing. *Nursing Outlook, 30*(5), 303–309.

Biemolt, M. (1996). Interview with author.

Blickensderfer, L. (1996). Interview with author.

Brookfield, S. D. (1993). On impostorship, cultural suicide, and other dangers: How nurses learn critical thinking. *The Journal of Continuing Education in Nursing, 24,* 5.

Brookfield, S. D. (1994). *Understanding learning organizations.* Creating learning organizations: Moving beyond the competencies, sponsored by Marquette University Continuing Nursing Education, Milwaukee, May 1994.

Buzan, T. (1991). *Use both sides of your brain.* New York: Plume, a division of Penguin Books.

Campinha-Bacote, J. (1994). Cultural competence in psychiatric mental health nursing: A conceptual model. *Nursing Clinics of North America, 29*(1), 1–8.

Collier, I. C., McCash, K. E., & Bartram, J. M. (1995). *Writing nursing diagnoses: A critical thinking approach.* St. Louis: Mosby-Year Book.

Daley, B. (1996). Concept maps: Linking nursing theory to clinical nursing practice. *The Journal of Continuing Education in Nursing, 27*(1), 17–27.

de Bono, E. (1985). *Six thinking hats.* Larchmont, NY: The International Center for Creative Thinking.

Del Bueno, D. J. (1990). Evaluation: Myths, mystiques and obsessions. *Journal of Nursing Administration, 20*(11), 4–7.

Del Bueno, D. J., Griffin, L. R., Burke, S. M., & Foley, M. A. (1990). The clinical teacher: A critical link in competence development. *Journal of Nursing Staff Development, 6*(3), 135–138.

Del Bueno, D. J., Weeks, L., & Brown-Stewart, P. (1987). Clinical assessment centers: A cost-effective alternative for competency development. *Nursing Economic$, 5*(1), 21–26.

Dillon, S. (1995). Posttesting the nonreaders. *Nursing Staff Development Insider, 4*(4), 1.

Elsasser, G. (1996). Nurses rally in D.C.: Protest RN replacement, "unsafe conditions." *NursingNews,* May 29.

Facione, N., Facione, P., & Sanchez, C. (1994). Critical thinking disposition as a measure of competent clinical judgment: The development of the California Critical Thinking Disposition Inventory. *Journal of Nursing Education, 33*(8), 345–350.

Ford, J., & Profetto-McGrath, J. (1994). A model for critical thinking within the context of curriculum as praxis. *Journal of Nursing Education, 33*(8), 341–344.

Gordon, P. (1996). *Problem-based learning: Introduction to an innovation in education.* Nursing Education '96, sponsored by The Medical College of Pennsylvania and Hahnemann University (now Allegheny University), Orlando, FL, January 1996.

Grey, M. T. (1996). *Evaluating the effectiveness of education: The performance improvement approach.* Challenges, changes, choices: The evolving role of staff development, sponsored by the National Nursing Staff Development Organization. Boston, July 1996.

Gronlund, N., & Linn, R. (1990). *Measurement and evaluation in teaching,* 6th ed. New York: Macmillan.

Gurvis, J.P., & Grey, M. T. (1995). The anatomy of a competency. *Journal of Nursing Staff Development, 11*(5), 247–252.

Herbert-Ashton, M. (1996). Interview with author.

Jeska, S. B., Anderson, L., & Bach, M. (1995). *Blueprint for competence: The University of Minnesota Model.* Pensacola, FL: National Nursing Staff Development Organization.

Jutsum, V. (1996). *Education planning for competency: A neurological nursing competency program* (poster session) Challenges, changes, choices: The evolving role of staff development, sponsored by the National Nursing Staff Development Organization, Boston.

Keane, A., & Pistone, C. (1996). *Multidisciplinary competency assessment.* Nursing staff development/ New horizons in case management '96, sponsored by The Medical College of Pennsylvania and Hahnemann University (now Allegheny University), Baltimore, May 1996.

Kelly, K. (1992). *Nursing staff development: Current competence, future focus.* Philadelphia: J. B. Lippincott.

Kelly, K. J. (1994). *The nature of intuition among nursing staff development experts: A Heideggerian hermeneutical analysis.* Unpublished doctoral dissertation. George Mason University, Fairfax, VA.

McGregor, R. J. (1990). Advancing staff nurse competencies: From novice to expert. *Journal of Nursing Staff Development, 6*(6), 287–290.

Mahlmeister, L. (1996). *Case studies: A method to stimulate critical thinking.* Nursing Education '96, sponsored by The Medical College of Pennsylvania and Hahnemann University (now Allegheny University), Orlando, FL, January 1996.

Makely, S. (1994). ADD-A-COMP program. Indianapolis: Methodist Hospital of Indiana.

Miller, M. A., & Babcock, D. E. (1995). *Critical thinking applied to nursing.* St. Louis: Mosby-Year Book.

Miniace, J. N., & Falter, E. (1996). Communication: A key factor in strategy implementation. *Planning Review, 24*(1), 6–30.

National Nursing Staff Development Organization. (1996). *Position statement on the role of staff development in the education of unlicensed assistive personnel.* Pensacola, FL: Author.

Nick, S. (1996). Interview with author.

Pike, R. (1989). *Creative training techniques handbook.* Minneapolis: Lakewood Books.

Puetz, B. (1992). Needs assessment: The essence of the staff development program. In Kelly, K. (Ed.). *Nursing staff development: Current competence, future focus.* Philadelphia: J. B. Lippincott.

Rath, D., Boblin-Cummings, S., Baumann, A., Parrott, E., & Parsons, M. (1996). Individualized enhancement programs for nurses that promote competency. *The Journal of Continuing Education in Nursing, 27*(1), 12–16.

Rubenfeld, M. G., & Scheffer, B. K. (1995). *Critical thinking in nursing: An interactive approach.* Philadelphia: J. B. Lippincott.

Shugars, D., O'Neil, E., & Bader, J. (Eds.). (1991). *Healthy America: Practitioners for 2005: An agenda for action for U.S. health professional schools: A report of the Pew Health Professions Commission.* Durham, NC: Pew Health Professions Commission.

Staab, S., Granneman, S., & Page-Reahr, T. (1996). Examining competency-based orientation implementation. *Journal of Nursing Staff Development, 12*(3), 139–143.

Swansburg, R. C. (1995). *Nursing staff development: A component of human resource development.* Boston: Jones and Bartlett.

Toth, J. D. (1996). Personal communication, September.

Turner, S. O. (1996). *Competency-based skill building curriculum for unlicensed assistive personnel.* Aliso Viejo, CA: American Association of Critical Care Nurses.

Ulsenheimer, J. (1996). Thinking about thinking. *The Journal of Continuing Education in Nursing, 28*(4), 150–156.

University of Chicago Hospitals. (1996). Management development: Turning insights in the classroom into actions in the workplace. *UCH Academy Quarterly.* Chicago: Author.

Varro, B. (1996). UAPs. *NursingNews,* Sept. 18.

Watson, G., & Glaser, E. M. (Eds.) (1985). *Critical thinking appraisal.* Cleveland, OH: Psychological Corp.

Wcislo, K. (1996). Interview with author.

Weber, M. (1996). Interview with author.

Whitman, N. (1996). Interview with author.

Wilson, C. K. (1992). *Building new nursing organizations: Visions and realities.* Gaithersburg, MD: Aspen Publishers, Inc.

Witte, K. (1996). Interview with author.

Young, S. W., Hayes, E., & Morin, K. (1995). Developing workplace advocacy behaviors. *Journal of Nursing Staff Development, 11*(5), 265–269.

Creating an Environment of Learning: An Opportunity

LORRY SCHOENLY

This chapter discusses the opportunity that clinical staff development specialists (SDSs) have to create an environment of learning at an organizational, classroom, and unit level in a health care organization. Educational and interactional models provide frameworks for viewing the learning environment in the physical, psychological, mental, and social spheres. Domains of learning guide the application of learning environment strategies.

AN OPPORTUNITY

No matter what his or her location on the organizational chart, the SDS is an integral part of the organization, with far-reaching impact in all patient care and support service areas. SDSs shape and maintain an environment of learning for health care providers. They play a pivotal role in creating an organizational environment that can adapt to external and internal forces.

Through the use of self and the application of learning theory and principles, SDSs encourage an environment that promotes continuous learning, critical thinking, and caring. Health care organizations provide a particularly challenging, high-stake, and risky arena for learning; opportunities and challenges abound.

Two major themes specific to a health care organization—the context of health care and issues of gender—should be considered when endeavoring to create an environment of learning. SDSs are encouraged to consider these issues as they move forward.

Unlike organizations in industry, government, or agriculture, health care organizations are geared to serve people in need. Staff members are involved in activities that affect people's lives and health. The common saying, "We don't make widgets, you know" identifies the need to look carefully at the impact of learning and change on patient outcomes in the environment where care is given. An environment of learning where mistakes can cost life and limb is a highly charged environment with little tolerance for error, and the impact of a learning mistake can be far-reaching.

Learning, however, requires some measure of trial and error. Care providers need to move from novice to expert practice and develop skill. The challenge for the SDS is to understand the health care environment and provide a protected learning experience for the novice. This will enhance learning while maintaining a safe environment for the patient.

The health care field is predominantly populated by female workers. Excluding the medical profession, fully 86% of health care professionals and 81% of health service workers are female (U.S. Government, 1996). This gender imbalance affects the ordering of the learning environment. Women think and learn in unique ways (Belenky et al., 1986), and their learning needs should be considered when creating an environment of learning in a health care organization.

Women learn best in a supportive environment based on community (Gallos, 1995). They place importance on relationships and an ethic of caring (Gilligan, 1977). Women learn best in an environment that fosters a pattern of "confirmation, evocation, and more confirmation" (Belenky et al., 1986).

Experiential learning methods are especially appropriate for female-dominated groups. Small-group work fosters interaction and reflection, both of which help to produce community and relationship.

Teaching methods that foster confirmation while challenging the participants to further growth help create an effective environment of learning for women. SDSs should take time to acknowledge good or thought-provoking answers to questions. They should reinforce participation by referring to specific participant comments later in the presentation (Gallos, 1995). Quality feedback that is not evaluative but that supports and encourages the learner should be chosen over criticism. Participants should be encouraged to learn with and from their peers as well as from the SDS. This in turn fosters a community of learners in the organization.

Taking into consideration the gender-based needs of the learners will enable SDSs to create an effective environment of learning in a health care organization. Attention to gender issues should occur at the organizational, classroom, and unit levels.

CREATING AN ENVIRONMENT THAT PROMOTES LEARNING: ORGANIZATIONAL LEVEL

The Organization as Ecosystem

An ecosystem is a complex, interdependent life-supporting web. In this integral network, each element interacts directly and indirectly with all other elements; each element affects the function of the whole. The two major elements of an ecosystem are the living community and the physical environment, composed of the climate, soil, water, air, nutrients, and energy (Tudge, 1991).

A health care organization can be viewed as an ecosystem. The living community of patients, family members, professional care providers, support staff, and administrative personnel are interrelated and interact in a complex, interdependent web. The activities of one group within the web, even the activities of one person, have an impact on the whole. The physical environment of an organization may not include soil, but there is certainly an organizational culture or climate, air or atmosphere, and energy flow pattern. There is also dirt, in different forms, in organizational ecosystems. An organization has methods of nourishment (nutrients) and refreshment (water).

Continuing this analogy, SDSs can affect an organization's ecosystem at several points. As a member of the community, the communication patterns of the SDS can have a direct impact on the whole. Through the educational process and by serving as a role model, SDSs can alter other community members, thereby creating a greater environmental impact. SDSs are often involved in the nurturing and refreshment activities of an organization. Strategic retreats, organizational celebrations, and public events frequently require educational services. Finally, SDSs can affect the climate and atmosphere of the ecosystem by creating a learning environment. An atmosphere of continuous learning can direct the flow of energy to respond to the challenges of the future.

Creating a Learning Organization

A learning organization is a place "where people continually expand their capacity to create results they truly desire, where new and expansive patterns of thinking are nurtured, where collective aspiration is set free, and where people are continually learning how to learn together" (Senge, 1990, p. 3). A learning organization is the ideal work environment for an SDS, but most health care organizations do not start out that way. SDSs have a great opportunity, by virtue of their position and influence, to foster the development of a learning organization.

A learning organization engages in organizational learning. This refers to the process of collective learning that goes on in an organization as it grapples with daily, cyclic, and emergent challenges. Although all organizations learn during these times, a learning organization finds ways to make learning intentional and systematic. The learning organization continuously transforms itself through adaptation and innovation.

SDSs can encourage organizational learning through their educational efforts. Calvert et al. (1994) identified key strategies that encourage organizational learning. A major strategy involves the use of a tangible organizational need to muster a cohesive group effort. Continuous learning opportunities abound in the health care organization. An upcoming survey by the Joint Commission on Accreditation of Healthcare Organizations or a state inspection can provide an impetus for collaborative efforts. Another excellent opportunity to enact organizational learning would be the implementation of a system-wide change such as a new computerized documentation system or a major product change. In each instance, the SDS has an opportunity to take a leadership role in molding an environment of learning.

Another strategy involves the creation of structures and processes that support the learning environment. The creation of regular "town meeting" sessions for education and information sharing provides such a structure. Other structures could involve written communication—say, an educational newsletter or electronic mailing lists for sharing information with a wide range of employees.

Organizational learning is encouraged when ongoing and orderly dialogues are created across organizational barriers. SDSs have an opportunity to encourage dialogue through the educational programs they offer, the participant mix they determine in an offering, and the participant interaction they foster.

Inquiry and dialogue should be encouraged at every opportunity (Marsick & Watkins, 1996). Dialogue should go beyond advocating a certain position: SDSs must encourage participants to discuss and explain the reasoning behind the position while inquiring about others' reasoning. Active listening skills should also be fostered. Learning can be achieved through personal interaction, and SDSs have the opportunity to enhance this personal interaction during group sessions and educational programs.

This moves staff development into the area of communicative learning. Unlike instrumental learning, which focuses on a specific area of content with predictable learner outcomes, communicative learning engages the participant in a dialogue involving understanding, intentions, feelings, and reasoning (Marsick & Watkins, 1996). In this situation, outcomes are fluid, based on the subject under discussion, the participant mix, and the skills of the teacher.

As active participants in facilitating organizational change, SDSs can encourage the use of debriefing sessions to capture lessons learned during the experience. Participants from various departments and levels in the organization share information, which can prove helpful for future learning opportunities. In this way an organization can avoid making the same mistakes again and again. The health care organization may deal with an emergent situation that reveals weaknesses in its systems and processes. A debriefing session can create an organizational plan of action that leads to changes that improve the organization's readiness for the next emergency.

External Environment

A health care organization's external environment affects organizational learning by creating perceived needs. Economic trends, including governmental interventions, drive organizational changes. Organizations are restructuring organizational charts, moving to product lines and services, and initiating patient-focused care and self-directed work teams to meet external demands for quality and cost-effective health care. SDSs are called on to create programs and initiate processes to meet these organizational changes.

In his landmark work *Technotrends* (1993), Daniel Burrus paints a picture of organizational change marked by fundamental technological discoveries. He identified a major need: organizations must move from a state of status quo, "sameness," and incremental innovation to one of redirection and rapid, fundamental change. SDSs, by virtue of background and skills, are positioned to play a major part in moving an organization into the future. Creating an organizational learning environment is key to meeting the demands of the technological future.

Internal Environment

In addition to educating staff members and initiating change, SDSs are also part of the internal environment of the organization and interact within it. SDSs find themselves interacting at all levels within an organization through committee participation, project management, consultation with persons and groups, and facilitation of organizational change. SDSs function in a staff role, providing advisory and support services to line managers with accountability to meet organizational goals. In this role, an SDS can affect the decisions made in the organization. Being neither a line manager nor a direct care provider, SDSs can often be the glue that binds the organization together. They can interpret management positions to staff members while providing much-needed feedback to management regarding the impact of organizational decisions on staff members. In this process, SDSs can model collaborative behaviors to management and staff alike.

Virtual Environment

The environment of learning has expanded into virtual space with the advent and increasing use of computer networks. First used to connect remote defense industry computers throughout the country in the late 1970s, the Internet has now expanded to include educational, government, and personal computers through a web of phone lines and data centers nationally and internationally. Over the last decade, computer use has greatly expanded in health care settings. Most professional health care workers now have at least some access to a computer. SDSs must now consider cyberspace in the mix of environments of learning.

Access to the Internet allows people to search for information at any time. This instant access to information and training is a powerful learning tool. Internet-based training multiplies learning opportunities and places control in the learner's hands.

Many large organizations have created and use an "intranet" for information and education. Intranets use web-based technology to connect employees to a wide pool of information on their computers through an organization's web server (Masie, 1997). Unlike the Internet, which can be accessed by anyone with the proper equipment, an intranet is accessible only by organization employees. Organizations use them to build a knowledge, performance, and learning network.

Little documentation has been done regarding the use of intranets by health care organizations, but the potential applications are numerous. Several examples of corporate training and development uses are cited by Cohen (1997). Hewlett-Packard has used an intranet to post lab exercises after a broadcast program. Trainees review material as needed and hold discussions through intranet chat rooms. Digital Corp. used an intranet to provide learning services to employees throughout the world. Intranet applications expand the environment of learning by increasing the possibilities for collaborative efforts throughout an organization. Information is instantly available and does not have to await a class schedule or the arrival of an instructor.

The following examples suggest uses for intranets in health care facilities:

- SDSs can use intranets to facilitate "just-in-time learning" for health care providers on all shifts.
- Institutional policy changes and revisions can be broadcast.
- In-service education through the multimedia advantages of an intranet can provide immediate reinforcement at the time needed.
- Search engines can assist in providing standard drug information when needed.
- Administrative tasks can be streamlined with course calenders and registration mechanisms available by intranet.

The possibilities seem endless. SDSs are encouraged to advocate for intranet mechanisms and play an active part in guiding the creation of this new environment of learning in their facility.

"Extranets" are another technology-based expansion of the environment of learning. An extranet connects two or more organizations through web-based technology. Extranets have been developed to allow instant ordering capabilities between a purchaser and a supplier. This decreases written or voice ordering, thereby streamlining the process. Although not fully developed in the health care industry, extranets have the potential to link health care providers along the care continuum, reducing the workload involved in maintaining patient files and exchanging ever-changing patient information. Extranets can provide consistent education to care providers in the prehospital and home care or rehabilitation settings.

CREATING AN ENVIRONMENT THAT PROMOTES LEARNING: CLASSROOM LEVEL

The classroom environment is an artificial environment created by the instructor to facilitate learning. There are many opportunities to manipulate the physical, psychological, mental, and social aspects of the environment.

Physical Environment of Learning

Maslow (1968) established a hierarchy that identifies physical needs as a primary motivator, a requirement that must be met for the person to move to higher levels of self-actualization. Physical comfort is an important consideration in classroom learning. The physical environment should encourage learning by being comfortable and supporting the work of the educator (Finkel, 1997).

Safety should be considered when choosing a location for a program, particularly a program held at another facility. Consider the availability of parking and its location, the lighting, and the walkways into the building. A participant who had difficulty finding a parking space or locating the meeting room can become distracted and unable to concentrate early in the program. Poor lighting or hazardous walkways can cause participants to leave a program early, particularly during the shorter winter days. The facility should be handicapped-accessible.

The physical amenities of the classroom also create an environment conducive to learning. A relaxing environment reduces fatigue and increases concentration. Chairs should be ergonomic, with good back support and padding. Uncomfortable chairs can lead participants to fidget, move frequently, stand in the back of the room, or sit on the floor. Participants should have ample elbow room and writing surfaces. Furnishings should be in good repair to minimize injury.

Physical comfort is enhanced and distractions are minimized by having ample, convenient restrooms. Waiting in a restroom line during a short break with a bladder expanded by morning coffee can decrease the participant's satisfaction level and increase his or her distraction.

The room arrangement does much to create an environment of learning. Make sure participants in all areas of the room can see the screen; depending on the content, learning and application may be directly related to the ability to see the visuals. Placing seating too far from the screen or blocking the visual field by other participants or room support poles will inhibit learning.

The arrangement of chairs can greatly affect the outcome of a learning experience. The location and arrangement of chairs set the stage for teacher–learner and learner–learner interaction. Standard seating choices and their impact are presented in Table 12-1.

Replacement bulbs for audiovisual equipment should be immediately available to decrease downtime. Even in smaller classrooms, a microphone or sound system should be considered so that speakers with soft voices can be heard by all, particularly in rooms with less-than-optimal acoustics.

The learning environment is enhanced by the appropriate use of handouts. Note-taking increases the retention of content, and handouts enhance note-taking by organizing the task for the participant. Having the material already organized allows the participant to pay attention to the presentation while jotting down notes that come to mind during the presentation.

Proper lighting also enhances the learning environment. Strong, glaring light can be tiring to the eyes in a long program. Dim lights can also be a problem. If the room is darkened for audiovisuals, make sure the learners can still see for note-taking.

Sound can be a distracting factor and should be reduced at every opportunity. Random noises from air conditioners, buzzing fluorescent lights, and chatter from adjacent rooms or corridors should be minimized. Music can have an effect on the learning environment and could be used as a prelude to the class. Think of how music sets the mood in movies; the same principle can be applied to set a mood for the learning experience. Music can be relaxing, motivational, calming, or spirit-lifting (Finkel, 1997).

Psychological Environment of Learning

Learning is enhanced by a psychologically safe environment. SDSs have many opportunities to create a psychologically safe environment of learning through their teacher–learner

TABLE 12-1

STANDARD CHAIR ARRANGEMENTS AND THE LEARNING ENVIRONMENT IMPACT

Arrangement	Description	Impact
Theater	Chairs arranged in rows facing the speaker. No tables provided. Usually arranged with a middle aisle.	Maximum number of participants in a room. Discourages note taking. Teacher–participant interaction possible. Participant–participant interaction discouraged.
Schoolroom	Chairs arranged in rows behind long tables. All chairs face the speaker.	Maximizes note taking. Teacher–participant interaction possible. Participant–participant interaction difficult but can be accommodated.
Banquet	Chairs arranged around round tables.	Maximizes interaction of participants. Teacher–participant interaction may be difficult because some participants do not face the presenter.
Hollow square	Chairs arranged around the outside of a square of tables. Instructor usually sits with participants along one side of the square.	Maximal teacher–learner interaction. Encourages participant interaction. Minimizes the number of participants in a program.
U-shaped	A hollow square with one side removed. Instructor usually stands at the open side.	Maximal teacher–participant interaction because instructor can travel into the U to meet the participants. Encourages participant interaction. Minimizes number of participants.

interactions. Rogers (1969) postulated that learning in the context of a humanistic relationship is more significant and influential than other options. A humanistic relationship is characterized by genuineness, trust, honesty, empathy, respect, self-disclosure, and positive regard. It is student-centered rather than teacher-centered. This relationship is characterized by the humanistic interactions between the learner and the teacher, providing a framework for sharing the responsibility for learning. The positive regard given to the learner by the educator through genuine, honest communication creates a safe psychological environment of mutual trust. The learner can see the teacher as a facilitator rather than just an imparter of knowledge and an evaluator. Self-disclosure in the teacher–learner relationship allows the SDS to model appropriate learning behaviors by showing that learning is continuous. Interaction and dialogue within a helping relationship move the learner toward goal attainment. The humanistic teacher–learner relationship provides a psychologically safe learning environment.

The psychological environment of learning can be enhanced through the use of Freire's (1970) "liberating" teaching philosophy. While running a literacy program for slum residents and peasants in Brazil, Freire found that the social and emotional situations in the participants' lives could not be divorced from their learning experience. He found that education could transform the lives of the learners through the interaction of the teacher and learner. Education involves the experiences, cultural expectations, and life pressures of the learners. Freire proposed using an approach in which the educator and the participant are both learners. Both use investigation to discover together the answers to posed problems. During this colearning process, the implications of previous life experiences, cultural backgrounds, and current pressures are explored. The outcome is that the learner becomes liberated and empowered.

The feminist process proposed by Wheeler and Chinn (1989) is an interactive process based in part on Freire's work. This process encourages empowerment of learners and seeks to move the teacher–learner relationship away from a patriarchal model. This feminist process encourages a learning environment of "PEACE":

- Praxis
- Empowerment
- Awareness
- Consensus
- Evolvement.

Praxis involves the interaction of theory with practice. Praxis is experienced when practitioners actively apply theory to the clinical situations around them. Reflective action takes place as practitioners take time to reflect on the interplay of theory and practice. Freire (1972) described this as a dance in which theory and practice influence each other. Instructors have opportunities to engage staff members in praxis in the classroom. Case studies and role playing can be used to help staff reflect on their practice and thoughtfully consider theoretical applications.

Empowerment in the feminist process involves the reduction in the classroom of hegemony, the process by which the status quo of power is maintained and retained. Hegemony is reinforced through the traditional teacher–student relationship. In a hegemonic, "disempowering" environment, the teacher is the powerful, all-knowing imparter of knowledge and the participant is a blank slate to be filled with new knowledge "owned" by the teacher. The learning environment is enhanced when efforts are made to acknowledge the combined knowledge of the learners. SDSs can encourage participants to bring their personal knowledge to the learning experience and can emphasize their own role as colearner in the experience.

Awareness of self and others in the learning environment involves tuning in to the moments of learning. Engaging participants in learning experiences that lead to greater self-knowledge and self-understanding enhances the learning experience.

Using the feminist process, the SDS can gain group *consensus* regarding directions the class will pursue. Some subject areas, particularly those heavily cognitive in nature, do not lend themselves to this approach. However, group consensus can be gained regarding the beginning points of information where participants have a background in the area. Learner consensus can guide discussions for application of classroom objectives in situations involving content such as ethical or legal situations, patient care dilemmas, or critical thinking.

Evolvement, the final element of the feminist process, involves a commitment to growth and change. Evolvement is a conscious and deliberate commitment by the instructor and participants to grow through the experiences in the classroom. The SDS can verbalize and serve as a role model for such commitment to growth. Including instructional elements such as journal-writing and storytelling allows participants to reflect on their personal professional practice, thereby enhancing their personal growth.

Incorporating humanistic, liberating, and feminist process principles in the classroom can enhance the psychological environment for learning. SDSs should consider incorporating these principles in their educational practice.

Mental Environment of Learning

A learner's set—his or her mental approach to the learning situation (De Tornyay & Thompson, 1987)—must be considered in any classroom environment. Set encompasses the elements of arousal, expectancy, and incentive.

Participants in staff development programs frequently attend by mandate or requirement of the employer. SDSs face the challenge of overcoming learners' lack of interest and motivating them to become actively involved in the learning experience. Arousal to the learning experience can be created by an environment that initiates and maintains the learner's interest in the subject. Participant arousal can be enhanced by providing opportunities to discover information. This involves the careful preparation of questions, cases, and exercises that allow the learners to investigate propositions, create connections between facts, and discover personal meaning for the content presented.

Expectancy allows participants to understand the direction the class is heading and their part in the journey. Expectancy is assisted through course structure. SDSs can help meet expectancy needs and create set by providing a course syllabus, course goals and objectives, and an overview of the program at the beginning of the class. Promotional materials that clearly state the course content, level of program, and expected outcomes prepare learners to participate. This decreases frustration and eliminates potential attendance by those for whom the course is not intended. A well-structured learning experience that advertises its objectives before the experience creates a framework for learning. Presenting the objectives and an outline of the material early in the program and allotting time for learners to evaluate the objectives at the completion brings to full circle the expectancy principle.

Building incentive into a classroom experience also helps create a positive set. For some programs, incentive might be the accomplishment of certification or recertification. For others, incentive might be the ability to move up in a career ladder system. Incentive may be as simple as establishing the relevance of the course material to the work experience of the participants. This can create a desire for information to be applied in the practice setting. Case studies and suggestions for practical uses, sprinkled throughout the presentation, can increase the incentive factor.

Social Environment of Learning

Consider the social environment of learning when preparing a program. As noted above, women learn best in a supportive environment that emphasizes community (Gallos, 1995). Opportunities for participants to connect with others early in the program will encourage cohesiveness of learning purpose. In the breaks and meal periods during the program, the SDS can encourage discussion of the implications of the course content. Participants then have an opportunity to integrate the learning experience with their work and life experiences.

Fostering the social environment of learning during classroom experiences can also help create an organizational climate of community and continuous learning. The artificial environment of a classroom can help decrease barriers along organizational lines when participants return to their work settings. Misperceptions harbored among professional groups can dissipate when key figures within these groups have shared a meal or break and discovered similarities in their views and experiences.

CREATING AN ENVIRONMENT THAT PROMOTES LEARNING: UNIT LEVEL

The SDS as an Instrument of Learning

SDSs, in their role as clinical resources, help staff members to learn continuously in their clinical practice. Whether coordinating preceptor relationships, providing follow-up services after the initiation of new clinical products, or investigating a patient care issue, the SDS interacts with patients, staff, and family members at the unit level. An attitude of open, positive regard encourages a learning relationship. In a nonthreatening environment, staff members are more willing to identify their learning needs and seek assistance. SDSs must cultivate a trusting relationship with staff to encourage a learning environment.

Many of the principles that shape the psychological, social, and mental environment of learning at the classroom level are applicable at the unit level in direct clinical teaching. Unlike the structured classroom educational experience, however, unit-level education focuses on application to the clinical situation. SDSs can frame clinical situations into a learning context. Principles taught in the classroom can be applied clinically. For example, education can continue on the unit after a basic dysrhythmia class when the SDS regularly performs clinical rounds, discussing with staff members their patients' dysrhythmias. Ask questions regarding treatment protocols, and make connections between outcomes and treatment choices. This can help achieve a more holistic view of the significance of various dysrhythmias to the expected patient outcomes. Encourage staff members to seek new levels of understanding regarding cardiac function and treatment modalities.

SDSs have opportunities to engage staff members in praxis at the unit level. Case discussions, walking rounds, and critical incident debriefings can be used to help staff members reflect on their practice and thoughtfully consider theoretical applications.

Social Learning

Bandura (1969) developed a social-cognitive theory that postulates an interaction of the learner and the environment that places emphasis on the social context of learning. Learning occurs as persons "abstract information from the behavior of others, make decisions about which behavior to adopt, and later enact the selected behaviors" (Gredler, 1992, p. 302). This theory has major implications for the creation of a learning environment at the unit level.

SDSs can influence the social milieu on the clinical unit to encourage learning. By their direct involvement in the care provided on the clinical unit, they can model critical thinking, caring behaviors, and expert clinical skills. Clinicians can learn new behaviors in a natural setting. When they enact these new behaviors, they learn through the effects of their own actions.

Modeling cues can be provided for learners through the SDS's interaction at the unit level. These cues, provided to the learner during activity, prompt the learner toward enacting appropriate behavior and thereby learning. For example, an SDS may assist in a clinical procedure with a novice nurse. The nurse sees the SDS gowning and gloving to begin the procedure, and so does the same. The SDS is observed making eye contact with the patient, engaging the patient in conversation, and keeping the patient informed of the progress of the procedure. The novice nurse, observing this modeling cue, is encouraged to do the same. After the procedure, the SDS can reinforce these behaviors by affirming them during a debriefing conversation.

Mentoring

The mentorship process provides another avenue for the creation of a learning environment at the unit level. SDSs are often seasoned clinical professionals practicing at the expert level. They have often accomplished professional milestones such as public speaking, publication, and advanced studies. Through a mentor–protégé relationship, SDSs can provide support and encouragement for the development of staff members.

A mentorship relationship is a voluntary relationship based on trust, compatibility, mutuality, and personal attraction (Fuszard, 1989). SDSs may enter into a formal or informal mentorship relationship with staff members who exhibit an interest and aptitude to advance professionally. In the role of mentor, the SDS acts as a role model for professional behavior. In the clinical setting, this may include modeling professional communication with patients, family, coworkers, and other health care providers. Other examples include exhibiting critical thinking and problem-solving skills in the face of a clinical challenge, or time management skills and prioritizing during a crisis situation.

As a mentor, the SDS serves as an encouragement and support system. The specialist may support the protégé in risk-taking activities such as suggesting a new treatment regimen to a hostile physician, or broaching the subject of organ donation with a distraught family member. This encouragement and support can extend to professional activities such as enrolling in graduate school or preparing a manuscript for publication.

The SDS mentor may provide counseling and moral support during difficult times. This may include initiating some debriefing activities after an unexpected emergency situation, or helping staff members to assimilate new staffing patterns into their clinical practice. Through framing difficulties as challenges, a mentor can help staff members rise above the difficulty and learn from it.

Finally, the SDS can fulfill a mentorship role by encouraging staff members to serve on organizational committees and task forces. Mentoring clinical staff in these roles provides opportunities for these people to effect change. Staff members gain a new understanding of the process of change in an organization and can better support organizational decisions.

DOMAINS OF LEARNING: EFFECT ON ENVIRONMENT

Rinne (1987) provided an effective framework for discussing the domains of learning in the context of health care. Figure 12-1 illustrates this framework, which places caring, or the art of nursing, in the affective learning domain. The cognitive and psychomotor domains make up coordinating, or the science of nursing. SDSs can consider the environment of learning based on the dominant domain of learning involved in the educational experience in question.

Determining the primary domain of learning and choosing appropriate teaching methods to match that domain will enhance the learning environment in staff development programs. Table 12-2 presents possible teaching method choices for the cognitive, psychomotor, and affective learning domains.

Cognitive Domain

The cognitive learning domain was first described by Bloom (1956). Cognitive processes involve knowledge acquisition and the development of intellectual skills (Reilly & Oermann, 1990). This domain is comfortably traveled by SDSs and represents the vast majority of learning experiences planned in health care staff development departments. Continuing

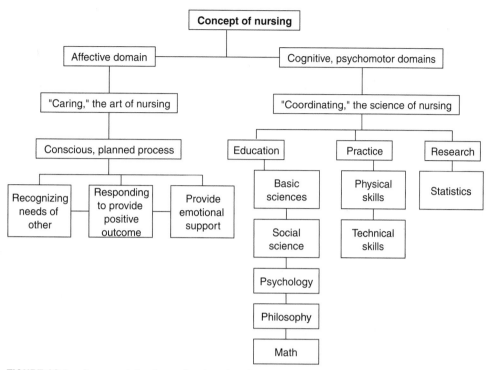

FIGURE 12-1. Framework for discussing domains of learning in context of health care. Rinne, C. (1987). The affective domain: Equal opportunity in nursing education? *The Journal of Continuing Education in Nursing, 18*(2), 40–43.

education programs such as a basic dysrhythmia course, pharmacology, ventilator management, or emergency procedures review fall primarily in this domain.

Cognitive learning is enhanced by an ordered learning environment that allows for maximal mental processing. Teaching techniques such as outlining, repetition, quizzes, and questioning are helpful. Provide the participants with thorough, well-organized notes. Offering examples and applications helps the participants categorize and connect new knowledge with previously mastered information.

Understanding is the focus of learning in the cognitive domain, and from understanding the learner can advance to application. Information can also be manipulated through analysis and synthesis.

Information-processing theory provides a possible framework for constructing a learning environment in the cognitive domain. This theory seeks to describe the methods people use to acquire and remember information and solve problems. Research in this area focuses on determining the nature of the human memory system and the ways knowledge is represented and stored (Gredler, 1992). Several teaching strategies have emerged from the ongoing development of information-processing theory to encourage a learning environment in the cognitive domain:

- Advance organizers
- Acronyms
- Mnemonics
- Imagery formation.

TABLE 12-2

SELECTED TEACHING METHODS FOR THE ENHANCEMENT OF THE LEARNING ENVIRONMENT WITHIN DOMAINS OF LEARNING

Domain	Teaching Methods
Cognitive	Lecture Discussion Examples Outlines Quizzing and questioning Advance organizers Acronyms Mnemonics Imagery formation
Psychomotor	Sequencing of subskills Demonstration Lab skills practice Clinical practice
Affective	Case studies Discussion Simulation gaming Role play

Advance organizers provide a schema for mentally organizing the new information to be presented. These organizers can create logical relations between elements within a new area of knowledge (*e.g.*, the relations within the cardiac pharmacology categories) or connect new information to previously understood concepts (*e.g.*, the relation of ventilator mechanisms to pulmonary physiology) (Mayer, 1979). Advance organizers can be as simple as creating an outline of key elements into which learners can collect more detailed information. In this way, the instructor creates a mental "filing system" for the student, complete with file drawers, file folders, and paper clips.

Acronyms are words made up of the first letter or syllable of a series of words or concepts that need to be remembered. An example of an acronym used earlier in this chapter is the use of the word PEACE to remember the five elements of the feminist process.

Mnemonics associate easily forgotten routine data with easily remembered sounds or images. The use of rhyming words and melody makes it easier. Many remember the number of days in months by reciting, "30 days hath September..." Another example is the common spelling rule, "i before e except after c..." A mnemonic variation is the keyword method, which links an unknown word to a known word through a picture to assist in memory and recall. Gredler (1992) gave an example that could be used to remember the Spanish word for egg, "huevo," pronounced "wave-o." The learner could imagine an egg surfing the crest of a large wave. SDSs can incorporate this technique when a large group of unfamiliar terms, such as in medical terminology classes, must be memorized.

Image formation encourages learners to create visual or auditory cues to help remember information. The more elaborate and absurd the visual image, the more memorable the information. Some encourage adding hand or body movements to to the visual and auditory cues.

Psychomotor Domain

Educational content within the psychomotor domain requires neuromuscular coordination. These neuromuscular activities fall within three general areas (Pollard & Green, 1995):

- Manual skills: eye–arm coordination; CPR training, bedmaking, creating a sterile field
- Gross motor skills: large muscle and body movement; performing range-of-motion exercises, turning and moving patients
- Fine motor skills: delicate, precision movements; cannulating a vein, placing a gastrointestinal tube, inserting a urinary catheter.

Gagne's conditions of learning (1985) provide a framework for creating a learning environment for the psychomotor domain. This model was initially developed to encourage rapid skill mastery for the armed forces during World War II. Gagne identified five varieties of learning:

- Verbal information
- Intellectual skills
- Cognitive strategies
- Motor skills
- Attitudes.

Motor skills acquisition will be the focus of this discussion. An underlying principle of this learning model is that complex skills are learned by building on previous learning. Simple learning tasks are sequenced to produce a complex skill. Learning takes place as the learner's internal state interacts with stimuli from the environment. The events of instruction make up the external conditions, or environment, of learning.

Gagne identified three requirements for the development of motor skills: smoothness of action, precision, and timing. The events of learning should take into consideration these three aspects. In motor skill acquisition, a set of different actions is executed in a sequential fashion; this is referred to as a procedure.

When creating a learning environment for teaching a clinical procedure, first construct a step-by-step list of the actions that make up the skill. Identify any decision points in the sequence. Once this is accomplished, the external conditions of learning can be established in the teaching plan. To prepare the participant for learning, first demonstrate the skill, initiating recall of the linear progression of subskills. Next, encourage mental rehearsal for the skill sequence. Mental rehearsal is followed by psychomotor rehearsal of the sequence steps, with corrective feedback. This rehearsal is repeated as necessary for the learner to begin to acquire the smoothness of action, precision, and timing required for basic proficiency with the skill. The final component that allows transfer of learning is an opportunity to perform the skill in situations that progress toward the unassisted clinical setting.

An intravenous cannulation skill session following these principles would run as follows:

1. The SDS reviews and demonstrates the basic technique, with special emphasis on decision-making areas such as site selection and cannula size.
2. Participants mentally rehearse the sequence, visualizing the performance steps.
3. Participants demonstrate the skill sequence using a simulation model, with corrective feedback from the instructor.
4. Participants practice the skill sequence on lab partners, again with corrective feedback.
5. As the participant is ready to transfer the learning into the clinical setting, protective experiences are created, such as supervised intravenous cannulation of patients in the preoperative holding area.
6. Supervised experiences continue until the skill is performed proficiently without assistance. Less-than-optimal smoothness, precision, and timing may continue for some time but will improve over time with continued skill use.

Affective Domain

"Effective nursing practice depends as much on the humanity of the nurse as it does on the nurse's knowledge and technical skill" (Curtin & Flaherty, 1982). This statement remains relevant, perhaps even more so, more than a decade later. Nurses and other clinical care providers grapple daily with ethical, moral, and legal dilemmas. They are confronted with pain and human suffering. They must assist others in dealing effectively with death and disability. They are called on to provide emotional, physical, and psychological support to others as part of their professional life.

Nursing and other health care disciplines are value-laden professions that have long histories of values-based practice. Nightingale's *Notes on Nursing* (Carroll, 1992) established a moral imperative for the nursing profession. Sobriety, honesty, and chasteness were established as the defining characteristics of a nurse. The ANA's *Code for Nurses*, first published in 1926, identified ethical behavior toward patients, other health care practitioners, and society. The Patient's Bill of Rights and Patient Self-Determination Act, like the Code for Nurses, are embedded with values of human dignity, truth, justice, and freedom. Other codes and statements illustrate the value-laden nature of health care professions.

The SDS is frequently faced with the challenge of developing an affective learning experience to help clinical staff deal with health care situations requiring empathetic, values-based care. Creating an appropriate environment for learning is crucial to the success of education based in the affective domain. Affective learning involves feeling, being, and finding meaning. Setting the climate of the learning experience will determine the likelihood that participants will take risks and involve themselves in the learning experience. Participants are more willing to take risks if they perceive a climate of acceptance within the group. When working with a group in which the participants are unfamiliar with each other, spend time in doing preliminary warm-up exercises or ice-breakers (Schoenly, 1994). Help create a desirable climate by modeling desired behaviors (Tanner, 1990). Reilly (1982) suggested that mutual respect, support, and freedom create an atmosphere conducive to affective learning. Developing a trusting relationship between the SDS and the learners allows for an open exchange of feelings, values, and attitudes, thereby creating a learning environment conducive to growing and changing. Ground rules that value openness and risk-taking should be established early in the program.

$\bigcirc$ ISPLAY 12-1

Elements of an Affective Learning Environment

Instructor role-modeling
Warm-up/ice breakers
Comfortable, safe environment
Trusting relationship
Minimized "power-over" relationship

As noted above, a safe and comfortable physical environment is important. In a classroom setting, this might involve arranging chairs in a circle or U shape to allow interaction and conversation. Minimize the "power-over" nature of the instructor position. Avoid standing and lecturing in front of the group; instead, sit among the participants. The key elements of an affective learning environment are summarized in Display 12-1.

SUMMARY

SDSs have the unique opportunity to move a health care organization forward by creating an environment of learning at every level in the organization. An environment of continuous learning allows the organization to remain flexible and keep pace with rapid changes in the external and internal environment. Understanding the importance of the health care context and the predominance of women in the health care field can help the specialist create a learning environment. Applying learning theory to practice, the SDS can be a positive force at the organizational, classroom, and unit levels. Incorporating learning principles specific to the cognitive, psychomotor, and affective domains will enhance success.

Setting the Stage for Learning

LORRAINE ANDERSON

Orientation to the bone marrow transplant (BMT) unit at the University of Minnesota Hospital and Clinic includes 1 day of the theory and principles of BMT followed by a day for application of theory to clinical practice. We set the stage at the outset of orientation to create a learning environment for the second day as an interactive one. We explained to the learners the components and expectations of orientation and how to prepare. We gave them each a notebook with objectives, outlines, and handouts for each learning activity to decrease their anxiety and improve their motivation to learn.

Before the learners arrived for the interactive

day, I prepared the room and the environment. I arranged the tables in a square so that everyone could see each other. This would encourage discussion and allow me to see each learner. It would also allow for a clear view of audiovisual presentations and free movement by instructors and learners. The learning environment was further enhanced by displaying supportive learning materials in the room so that learners could review them during breaks. Blackboards were cleaned and ready for use, and clutter was minimized. I was attempting to increase the potential for curiosity, exploration, and self-discovery.

I greeted the participants as they arrived with

a sense of openness and approachability. This exchange proved useful throughout the day. The group members introduced each other and stated their backgrounds and past experiences.

Because a substantial amount of information about BMT was new for most learners, I tried to use the initial activity on the second day to respond to questions from the first day's presentation. Many staff members expressed concern about the vast amount of information needed to care for these patients. I reassured them that the interactive nature of this day's content and their mentor experience would provide ample opportunity for practice and inquiry. Giving the learners a chance to ask these questions and express their concerns allowed them to set aside the distractions they had brought to class. This strategy also accommodated latecomers.

The first topic for the day was the medications common to BMT patients. I used a combination of matching games and discussion. For medications likely to be familiar to them, the matching games provided a brief review and resolved misperceptions. We devoted most of the discussion to medications new to the learners and implications for use with BMT patients. Staff members commented that the review was helpful because it challenged their recall of information they thought they might not remember. Providing the complete picture of medication administration prepared them for the next learning activity.

We moved on to an IV management workshop. The workshop included case studies to practice priority-setting relevant to IV, medication, and blood product administration. I used two levels of case studies because there were experienced and inexperienced nurses present. The first case study was easier and provided short scenarios with questions related to a sample medication administration record. I had copied a patient's medication administration record and, after obliterating confidential patient information, used it to provide learners with typical situations they would encounter. Each nurse answered the questions, and then the group shared answers. This exercise provided an opportunity to discuss assumptions and rationales for differing ways to handle the scenario. There was a possibility for more than one correct answer to questions, as in the real world of BMT.

The second case study focused on more complex infusion procedures over a 24-hour time span. Learners were divided into three groups to represent the three sections of the case study or three shifts of work (day, evening, night). They were grouped according to experience levels, the most difficult section or shift to the more experienced staff and the easier shift to less experienced staff. Each group was provided with clear instructions, BMT unit assignment sheets, the medication administration record, and the Kardex containing IV and blood product information, as well as shift-specific details that affected the prioritizing decisions. Learners used resources from the previous medication discussion. Each group worked through the schedule for administration of medications and blood products as well as IV fluid management for their shift. The groups then reported back to the large group with the schedule and rationale for their shift scenario. This was another opportunity to identify alternative approaches to scheduling and prioritization; again, there was more than one right way to schedule the medications.

IV and medication administration is one of the most threatening aspects of BMT care delivery. This small-group activity enhanced retention and promoted confidence in the learners. According to the evaluations, the real-world application was most beneficial to the learners. The use of a case study approach provided flexibility for me, too, because it can be used with any group size. It offered an opportunity for higher-order reasoning such as analyzing, forming judgments, and critical thinking, and it encouraged free-flowing discussion. Time was required for debriefing and reflection.

My role became one of helper, listener, and monitor. Discussions wandered, and I needed to refocus the groups occasionally. Some experienced staff shared "war stories." This is common with small-group work, but I knew that talking also clarifies thinking.

A skills lab was part of the IV workshop to practice using a multichannel pump for IV administration and to learn the techniques for administering bone marrow and blood products. Standard IV set-ups were also demonstrated, with an opportunity for practice. This hands-on simulation promoted learner participation and increased retention. The learners paced themselves according to their needs and practiced general or specific skills. They were learning both from me and from those in class who had used the pumps or IV set-ups previously.

The next activity examined nurses' role in BMT care delivery, including routines for 24-hour coverage, issues of death and dying, working in a research setting, and coping strategies for self-preservation and professional growth. This was accomplished with dialogue, a self-learning packet, and group discussion. Learners clarified their thoughts, read with a purpose, and reflected on others' thoughts.

A BMT crossword puzzle served as a sum-mary and provided learners with an opportunity to review key points from the 2 days of orientation. It prompted clarification and instilled confidence as the nurses were able to recall specific content. After 2 information-packed days, learners used this time to exchange knowledge while having fun.

Using the elements of active learning—talking and listening, reading, writing and reflecting—was a successful strategy. It allowed learners to engage in the learning process, remain self-directed, collaborate with their colleagues, and reflect critically throughout BMT orientation.

REFERENCES

ANA. (1985). *Code for nurses with interpretive statements.* Kansas City, MO: Author.

Bandura, A. (1969). *Principles of behavior modification.* New York: Holt, Reinhart & Winston.

Belenky, M., Clinchy, B., Goldberger, N., & Tarule, J. (1986). *Women's ways of knowing: The development of self, voice, and mind.* New York: Basic Books.

Bloom, B. (1956). *Taxonomy of educational objectives—Handbook I.* New York: David McKay.

Burrus, D. (1993). *Technotrends: 24 technologies that will revolutionize our lives.* New York: Harper Business.

Calvert, G., Mobley, S., & Marshall, L. (1994). Grasping the learning organization. *Training and Development, 48*(6), 38–43.

Carroll, D. P. (Ed.). (1992). *Notes on nursing: What it is, and what it is not.* [Commemorative edition]. Philadelphia: J. B. Lippincott.

Cohen, S. (1997). Intranets uncovered. *Training and Development, 51*(2), 48–50.

Curtin, L., & Flaherty, M. J. (1982). *Nursing ethics: Theories and pragmatics.* New York: Brady.

De Tornyay, R., & Thompson, M. A. (1987). *Strategies for teaching nursing* (3d ed.). New York: Wiley.

Finkel, C. L. (1997). Meeting facilities that foster learning. *Training and Development, 51*(7), 36–41.

Freire, P. (1970). *Pedagogy of the oppressed.* New York: Seabury.

Freire, P. (1972). *Cultural action for freedom.* Harmondsworth: Penguin.

Fuszard, B. (1989). *Innovative teaching strategies in nursing.* Rockville, MD: Aspen.

Gagne, R. M. (1985). *The conditions of learning* (4th ed.). New York: Holt, Rinehart, & Winston.

Gallos, J. V. (1995). Gender and silence: Implications of women's ways of knowing. *College Teaching, 43*(3), 101–105.

Gilligan, C. (1977). In a different voice: Women's conception of self and of morality. *Harvard Educational Review, 47*(7), 481–517.

Gredler, M. E. (1992). *Learning and instruction: Theory into practice* (2d ed.). New York: Macmillan.

Marsick, V. J., & Watkins, K. E. (1996). Adult educators and the challenge of the learning organization. *Adult Learning, 7*(4), 18–20.

Masie, E. (1997). Seizing your intranet. *Training & Development, 51*(2), 51–52.

Maslow, A. H. (1968). *Toward a psychology of being* (2nd ed.). New York: Van Nostrand-Reinhold.

Mayer, R. E. (1979). Can advance organizers influence meaningful learning? *Review of Educational Research, 49*(2), 271–281.

Pollard, M., & Green, P.H. (1995). Domains of learning. In Avillion, A. (Ed.). *Core curriculum for nursing staff development.* Pensacola, FL: National Nursing Staff Development Organization, pp. 23–32.

Reilly, D. E. (1982). *Teaching and evaluating the affective domain in nursing programs.* Thorofare, NJ: Slack.

Reilly, D. E., & Oermann, M. H. (1990). *Behavioral objectives: Evaluation in nursing* (3rd ed.). New York: National League for Nursing.

Rinne, C. (1987). The affective domain: Equal opportunity in nursing education? *The Journal of Continuing Education in Nursing, 18*(2), 40–43.

Rogers, C. (1969). *Freedom to learn.* Columbus, OH: Merrill.

Schoenly, L. (1994). Teaching in the affective domain. *Journal of Continuing Education in Nursing, 25*(5), 209–212.

Senge, P. (1990). *The fifth discipline.* Boston: Currency Doubleday.

Tanner, C. A. (1990). Caring as a value in nursing education. *Nursing Outlook, 38,* 70–72.

Tudge, C. (1991). *Global ecology.* New York: Oxford University Press.

U.S. Government. (1996). *Statistical abstract of the United States: The national data book.* Washington DC: U.S. Government Printing Office.

Wheeler, C. E., & Chinn, P. L. (1989). *Peace and power: A handbook of feminist process* (2nd ed.). New York: National League for Nursing.

13

Quality Management: A Staff Development Tradition

DONNA GLOE

In recent years, there has been a major quality movement in the United States. It has become important to assess the services being delivered to evaluate quality. One of the major questions is, "What is quality?" Lawrence Holpp (1993) gave several definitions of quality in health care:

1. Quality is continuous process improvement focusing on incremental change over a period of time, with the emphasis on continual improvement—improvement in the way employees perform their jobs to create greater efficiency and cost-effectiveness, produce greater learning, and apply their skills in health care.
2. Quality is outstanding service. Providing education that important, necessary, and easily assimilated into day-to-day practice enhances patient care. Such education will help employees in working smarter rather than harder.
3. Quality is cost control and resource utilization. Education departments are often the first target of cost reductions. By showing money, time, or resource savings and patient benefit, clinical staff development specialists (SDSs) can assure themselves a place in the health care organization.
4. Quality is doing the right things right the first time. Quality is accomplished by putting customers first when considering changes and by making decisions based on data rather than gut feelings.

As the Joint Commission on Accreditation of Healthcare Organizations (JCAHO, 1993) stated:

> High-quality care means that the clinical management of patients, residents, or clients is efficacious and appropriate, and that it is available when needed, delivered in a timely fashion, respectful and caring from the recipient's perspective, effective, safe, efficient, and coordinated over time and across practitioners and settings. (p. A1)

This chapter presents an introduction to quality in staff development. Customer satisfaction themes are becoming more important, so knowing what customers' desires and preferences are is necessary if SDSs are to provide worthwhile services and remain a vital part of the health care institution. The items key to customer satisfaction are presented in this chapter. Suggestions on creating a positive image for the staff development department are presented, as well as hints on how to tie staff development goals to the organization's goals. Political positioning of the staff development department is a key factor in success. This chapter discusses the major components of political positioning, such as internal and external marketing, designing a practice manual, and showcasing the staff development department's programs and accomplishments. Sample forms are included, as well as information on forming partnerships, accrediting mechanisms, and integrating staff development practice into the changing health care paradigm.

SDSs must actively put the term "quality" into operation to apply the concept to their improvement activities. Clinical staff development and continuing education lend themselves to being identified as a process, one that is constantly evolving. Its evolution is driven by changes in the health care environment, changes in technology, and changes in the principles and methods of adult education.

Each SDS is also evolving. As he or she travels along the novice to expert continuum, his or her planning, delivery, and evaluation of educational offerings will change and progress. It is the nature of education to change, improve, and develop. Several models can be used to assist the evolution of staff development programs. Three that will be discussed here are total quality management (TQM), continuous quality improvement (CQI), and performance improvement. A fundamental shift is required from the old premise of management to the new approach, a shift from hierarchical and individualistic thinking to a system and customer philosophy. Contrary to popular belief, it is not a shift from individualistic thinking to team thinking, although teams and teamwork are important (Scholtes, 1995). Quality must become the responsibility of everyone in the organization.

THE UMBRELLA OF QUALITY

Health care professionals have always tried to give the best or highest-quality patient care possible. But what does that mean? What can patients expect when they receive services from a provider? SDSs have also tried to deliver their best when providing services. But again, what does that mean? What can the organization and the learner expect from the education program, and how does it affect patient care? Philip Crosby (1989) defined quality as conformance to requirements, not "goodness." The evaluation of educational activities, the annual evaluation of the SDS's performance, and the establishment of annual goals and objectives all represent efforts toward improvement of education (Jeska & Fischer, 1996).

Avedis Donabedian is considered the founder of the field of health care quality assurance (Berwick, 1989). He and others who have followed him believe that the quest for quality should be a continuous search for small opportunities to reduce waste, rework, and unnecessary complexity. All schools of thought share one basic approach: that scientific thinking is required at all levels of the organization in the continuous improvement of the processes through which work is done (Berwick et al., 1991).

Berwick differentiated the current approaches to quality management from past quality assurance practices. He described the old practice as the "theory of bad apples," one that relied on inspection. He designated the new approach as the "theory of continuous improvement" and described current efforts to understand and revise systems based on data. He also emphasized the importance of involving all workers in the process.

Several quality leaders have emerged. The works of Shewhart (1931), Deming (1986), Crosby (1989), and Juran (1988) are often cited in the quality management literature, and their principles guide most quality improvement efforts. Crosby is best known for his belief in "zero defects." He summarized quality management in one word: prevention. Intermountain Health Care of Salt Lake City, UT, one of the pioneers of TQM in health care, defined quality through the eyes of the patient: "Quality is defined through customer expectations and evaluated through explicit measures of customer satisfaction" (Weber, 1991, p. 57).

Deming and Juran were successful in Japan before their principles were accepted in the United States. Deming was a statistician and used the work of Shewhart in bringing Japanese industry into the 20th century after World War II. He advocated employee participation in decision making and believed that management should break down the barriers that prevent employees from doing their jobs, thus encouraging them to work smarter, not harder. Juran was the first to deal with the broader issues of quality, such as organization, communication, and structure of functions. He also recommended the use of statistical process control, but not as the sole determinant of quality measurement.

TOTAL QUALITY MANAGEMENT/CONTINUOUS QUALITY MANAGEMENT

TQM has become a watchword in contemporary business. It is a way of serving customers. The tenets of TQM include decentralization and participative management; decisions are made where the work is done and by the people who do the work. Workers know best what they require to make their jobs productive and to produce quality products or to deliver quality services. As applied to education, the learners must be involved in planning.

Often TQM and CQI are used interchangeably. They both embrace the belief that the employee is interested in doing the best job possible and the system or process is what impedes the worker in meeting the organization's goals and the personal goal of pride in performance. TQM began in business, has spread to the service industry, and is usually considered a plan or process to manage quality. CQI has developed as an offshoot of TQM, emphasizing the continuous process improvement portion as the goal of TQM. CQI is rapidly becoming a plan as well as the goal of a plan.

The customer is the focus of the TQM/CQI philosophy. Finding out what the customer wants and delivering what the customer wants is the central theme. The service that meets customers' needs provides income to the supplier, be it an education department or a manufacturer. Quality is freedom from waste, trouble, and failure. One should meet and even exceed customers' needs so that they will be pleased with the service and will return. Quality is not a program, but a philosophy and a way of life.

Leadership is an essential component of the philosophy of TQM/CQI. It requires:

- A people-oriented leadership style
- Cooperation and collaboration on all fronts
- Win-win relationships
- Total commitment by the executive leadership
- A long-range plan focusing on the achievement of high-quality services for every customer of the organization.

Leadership will put each health care worker in the business of providing quality service for customers, shouldering the responsibility for patient care.

Long-term commitment to this philosophy will achieve continuous improvement of productivity and services to the consumer. It requires a future focus, a commitment to innovation, and support of education as a valuable resource to the worker who needs to adapt in the changing health care environment.

Education can be viewed as a service business within the organization. The three elements of staff education as a service business—the customer, the instructors, and the system—represent the major domains of an education service. The customer is typically identified as the learner, but managers, physicians, and patients who depend on the competence of the staff are also customers. There may be multiple types and levels of instructors in the department.

TQM requires strong lines of communication throughout a department and an organization to create a network of organization-wide quality improvement. Work is viewed as a process and part of a larger system rather than isolated in departments. The department that endorses TQM is customer-driven, with continuous improvement of service as the goal of everyone in the department. The department is managed by data, so benchmarking is a critical aspect of CQI. The staff development department must know where it started to identify any progress made. By benchmarking, the department can describe where it is and can measure its progress toward higher levels of quality.

The team approach is used because it greatly reduces the traditional barriers to communication and understanding of other roles. Teams bring together staff members from all facets of the process under study because no single person is in a position to view the whole process. The team can develop a common understanding of the process and plan improvements. By combining perspectives, the plan for improvement will benefit everyone, not just solve one department's problem.

The most logical way to improve the process is to use the honesty and creativity of the people doing the work. Deming used the work of Alfredo Pareto, an Italian economist, in finding that 80% to 85% of the problems encountered are with the system or process of work; only 15% to 20% are with the workers. Thus, the greatest gain can be made by improving the process. Deming's theory of management includes 14 points, and SDSs can apply these 14 points to their own practice (Display 13-1).

Quality and education are lifelong pursuits that focus on the identification and resolution of problems or deficiencies (Katz, 1996). In both processes, it is important to take advantage of opportunities for growth and development. Both can have a significant impact on the performance of the person and the organization, and both require adaptability.

Several models provide a framework to organize quality improvement efforts. One model is the ANA's *Standards for Nursing Professional Development: Continuing Education and Staff Development* (1994):

1. Administration: Administration of the provider unit is consistent with the organization's mission, philosophy, purpose, and goals. The organizational structure facilitates the provision of learning activities for nurses.

DISPLAY 13-1

Quality Management Philosophy for Staff Development Based on Deming's 14 Points

Based on the Deming principles of quality management, the staff development department is committed to strive constantly (Point 5) toward improvement of services (Points 1 and 2). Within this new philosophy, we will monitor and evaluate our processes (Point 3) and work toward the efficient use of resources for the best-quality program (Point 4). Continued learning activities will be designed to help personnel learn to do their jobs and develop professionally (Point 6). Staff development specialists will help employees learn how to learn (Point 8) and assist with intradepartmental and interdepartmental team building (Point 9). Staff development specialists will help personnel develop professional pride and assist with the removal of system barriers to quality patient care (Point 12). To that end, this department will provide a vigorous staff development program (Points 13 and 14).

Source: Kelly Thomas Associates, Alexandria, VA. Reproduced with permission.

2. Human Resources: Qualified administrative, educational, and support personnel are responsible for achieving the goals of the provider unit.
3. Material Resources and Facilities: Material resources and facilities are adequate to achieve the goals and implement the functions of the provider unit.
4. Educational Design: Principles of education and adult learning are used to design educational activities.
5. Records and Reports: The provider unit establishes and maintains a record-keeping and report system.
6. Professional Practice: The professional development educator role is practiced in a manner that enhances learners' competence to provide quality health care and enhance their contributions to the profession.

Appendix A lists the standards with corresponding criteria.

The standards and criteria provided in this document are highly flexible and can be used in any educational setting. Each standard is designed to be independent of the others, so each can be used separately or in combination. The frequency and intensity of use must be driven by the needs of the education department.

One of the components on which TQM/CQI rests is that evaluation mechanisms should be integrated into the learning experience. Kirkpatrick's (1994) four levels of evaluation have proven to be a useful framework to cover all aspects of evaluation:

- Level 1, Reaction: the participant's reaction to the program and appraisal of the various components of the program.
- Level 2, Learning: the participant's knowledge or skills acquisition on the day of the program. It measures only the learning of the content presented in the program. Tests are most often used in this evaluation.
- Level 3, Behavior: the assessment and measurement of the transfer of learning presented in the program. It shows a change in behavior.
- Level 4, Results: the measurement of the results of the program in relation to the organization's goals.

Each level measures different items, ranging from knowledge of the subject to values. The evaluator who has a categorization system such as this and who understands relationships can analyze the evaluation task more efficiently and can make better decisions based on data. Level 1 is the easiest evaluation to accomplish and requires the least amount of resources. With levels 2, 3, and 4, there is an increasing difficulty and a greater expenditure of resources. Level 4 requires the greatest effort and the most resources to measure.

Those involved in educational programs—coordinators, instructors, program participants, and administrators—all benefit from evaluation. Administrators are interested in the summary of quality, results, and value of the total program, and this can be derived from evaluation data. Adult instructors and coordinators are interested in evaluation data that can help them enhance programs and increase professional competence. In today's world of limited funding, evaluation data can enable SDSs to obtain the greatest value for investments in education (Steele, 1989).

Pine and Tingley (1993) conducted a study tying a team-building course with performance of teams that repair manufacturing machines in an effort to tie the training to business outcomes. An experimental group took the 2-day team-building course, and a control group did not. All four of Kirkpatrick's evaluation levels were successfully tied to performance in some manner:

- Level 1: Those who participated in the training rated it highly.
- Level 2: A test showed that the participants' knowledge of team-building concepts improved after completing the course.

- Level 3: Behaviors related to skills and knowledge used on the job improved.
- Level 4: Job response time and job completion time improved in the experimental group, resulting in a cost savings per job.

Thus, it is worth the effort to tie training directly to the business results that management is emphasizing.

PERFORMANCE IMPROVEMENT

Performance improvement is a term that has evolved in the TQM/CQI movement. One of the key concepts is continuous improvement. Each institution must define what it means by quality health care. JCAHO has suggested using a performance improvement framework as a cycle beginning with design and progressing through measurement, assessment, and improvement steps. Health care organizations seeking accreditation must produce evidence that these components are in place. JCAHO presented a model for monitoring and evaluation in its 1992 publication *Examples of Quality Improvement in a Hospital Setting*. This model contains 10 interrelated steps: steps 1 through 5 operate in a linear fashion and steps 6 through 10 in a circular fashion in a continual check system (Display 13-2).

This publication also presented the Hospital Corporation of America's model of FOCUS-PDCA as an example of CQI. Based on Shewhart's (1931) and Deming's (1986) work in quality improvement, FOCUS-PDCA is an acronym for a method of continuous improvement:

- Find an opportunity (process) to improve.
- Organize a team.
- Clarify knowledge of the current process.
- Understand the sources of variation.
- Select a process improvement.
- Plan.
- Do.
- Check.
- Act.

Both models involve the assessment, selection, measurement, and evaluation of a process or aspect of care. Measurement provides the mechanisms to determine whether improvement is achieved and what opportunities exist for further improvement (Jeska & Fischer, 1996). The basic concept is that this cycle is an ongoing process with no beginning and no end, resulting in continuous performance improvement. This cycle is applicable to persons, departments, and the organization as a whole.

Benchmarking

Benchmarking was defined by David T. Kearns (1987) of Xerox Corp. as a continuous measurement of products, services, and practice, comparing performance against the toughest competitors or institutions recognized as leaders in their field. An organization compares itself to another organization that is considered by expert opinion or standards to be of high quality and to deliver excellent, cost-effective products or services. Benchmarking is one of the best ways to identify improvements that can make a significant difference to an organization.

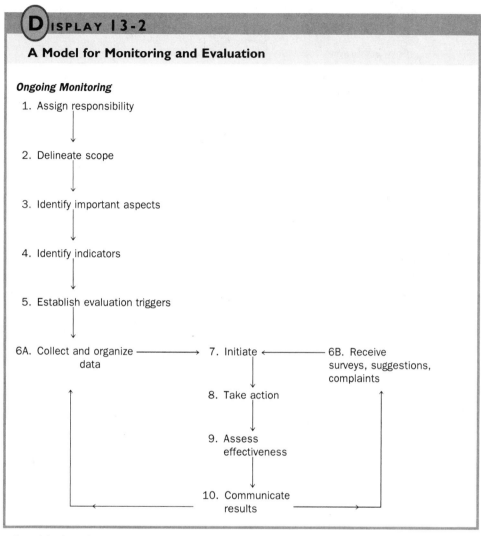

DISPLAY 13-2

A Model for Monitoring and Evaluation

Ongoing Monitoring

1. Assign responsibility

2. Delineate scope

3. Identify important aspects

4. Identify indicators

5. Establish evaluation triggers

6A. Collect and organize data ⟶ 7. Initiate ⟵ 6B. Receive surveys, suggestions, complaints

8. Take action

9. Assess effectiveness

10. Communicate results

From Joint Commission on Accreditation of Healthcare Organizations (1993). Reprinted with permission.

Benchmarking can be performed in one of three ways:

1. With a primary competitor: probably the most difficult, because competitors are unlikely to provide a wealth of factual information
2. Internally: comparing similar activities performed by different divisions of a large organization
3. Against "world-class" performers: Often, these companies are recognized by awards they have received in the quality arena. Part of the responsibility of receiving an award is to share the mechanisms by which changes within the organization were achieved.

Benchmarking should not be limited to organizations that are in the same business. It can be very beneficial, once the activity or problem is identified, to compare functions

---

DISPLAY 13-3

Key Guidelines for Benchmarking

- Benchmarking alone will not tell what customers actually want. The customer must be asked.
- Benchmarking is of benefit only if the improvement actions are implemented.
- Always seek to find out how a company has improved its performance. This normally comes from the people, not the management (who will tell how much performance has improved but not necessarily how).
- Always clearly identify specific key areas of interest and stay focused on them.
- Plan thoroughly in advance to make sure none of the key elements are missed.
- Remember that improvements are continuous and benchmarks go out of date quickly.
- Always remain honest and thoroughly professional.

Griffin, P. (February 12, 1996). *Benchmarking*. Electronic text retrieved from the Quality Network World Wide Web site.

with an organization that provides different services. Peter Griffin (1996) developed key guidelines for benchmarking; these are outlined in Display 13-3.

Once the education department understands where it stands in relation to other similar departments, the department can set its own goals based on its level of performance within these parameters. When the baseline data are gathered and benchmarking has been done, then the department can define and prioritize the improvements it wants to make.

Quality improvement is a matter of improving systems within organizations. Examples of system improvement are greater efficiency, the elimination of redundant or unnecessary steps in a process, or better buying strategies to lower costs. Improvements can mean streamlining, greater efficacy, and better resource utilization. By improving the system, the level of performance within the system can be improved.

As each institution defines quality, the result across the health care profession will be a related but diverse group of definitions and applications of the concept of quality. This makes it difficult to compare quality across the health care profession. In an effort to assess and report quality, the concept of performance seems to stand out. Because quality is essentially what the institution determines it to be—the concept is not uniformly defined—many have turned to performance as a concept that is more concrete. Performance can be assessed and evaluated by comparing it to established standards or benchmarks. Thus, a logical approach to quality from a personal and organizational standpoint is to compare oneself or itself to established national standards or benchmarks. The performance of persons in an organization and the organization as a whole is compared to implicit standards and measured against standards, against itself, and against benchmarks to determine improvement.

The ability to perform can be measured. JCAHO (1994) defined two dimensions of performance: doing the right thing, and doing the right thing well. "Doing the right thing," in terms of education, involves efficacy and appropriateness. The efficacy of the education process is assessed in relation to the learner's educational needs and involves measuring the degree to which the education accomplishes the desired learning outcome. The appropriateness of a specific education program is the degree to which the education is relevant to the learner's needs, given the current state of knowledge. "Doing the right thing well" has seven components:

- *Availability* of a program to the learner who needs it: the degree to which appropriate educational intervention is available to meet the learner's needs

- *Timeliness* with which a needed program is provided: the degree to which the education is provided to the learner at the most beneficial or important time
- *Effectiveness* with which services are provided: the degree to which the education intervention is provided with the best teaching strategy, given the current state of knowledge, to achieve the desired educational outcome for the learner
- *Continuity* of the services provided to the learner with respect to other services provided over time: the degree to which the education is coordinated among educators, among departments, and across time
- *Safety* to the learner: the degree to which the risk of the education and the risk in the learning environment are reduced for the learner as well as the instructor
- *Efficiency* with which education is provided: the relation between the learning outcomes and the resources used to deliver the education
- *Respect and caring* with which education services are provided: the degree to which the learner is involved in his or her own learning decision, and the degree to which those providing education services do so with sensitivity and respect for each learner's needs, expectations, and individual differences (JCAHO, 1994).

Performance measurement should encompass all the components of a position description and the roles and responsibilities attached to that position. Acquisition and mastery of skills and knowledge and the application of these factors represent a continuous process for health care providers. The foundation of performance measurement would include determining the measure of compliance with defined processes and standards established by the organization or society as a whole. Measurement is a definitive process for determining the level of performance of the existing processes against the standards. This is an integral part of any quality improvement program. Organizational quality can be the measurement of aggregate performance to demonstrate quality and value as compared to standards. The development of indicators allows the measurement of performance, both on an individual and an organization level. Once the current performance level is determined, it can be benchmarked against standards or the performance of other SDSs or departments viewed as excellent. After this comparison is complete, individual and departmental goals can be written and a plan put into place to reach those goals. This begins the performance improvement cycle. Performance improvement means implementing the improvement plan and reaching the goals written for the educators and the department.

Performance improvement can be broken down into two major categories: organizational and personal. Both are needed to make health care more efficient and of higher quality. Organizational performance improvement is based on a value system from which the vision and goals of the organization are developed. From the organization's vision and goals, each department and employee can identify tasks that support and push the institution toward meeting those goals. Organizational performance improvement is determined by benchmarking against similar organizations, setting goals based on these baseline data, and moving the employees toward those goals. The JCAHO (1992) model provides a systematic approach to this improvement.

Organizational improvement or improvement in patient care is accomplished by employees within the organization. Without giving employees the knowledge and motivation to do the best job they can, the organization cannot improve its overall performance. Organizational performance improvement thus depends on personal performance improvement.

Staff development departments must be cognizant of the values and goals of the organization and must be committed to providing educational products that can help employees find ways to meet those goals. Peter Senge et al. (1994) wrote that superior performance of employees and organizations depends on their ability to learn, and that the organization's ability to learn is directly related to the quality of services the organization renders. Senge and his colleagues at MIT Sloan School of Management stated that everyone is born with an innate curiosity and desire to know and to love, but the institutions in our culture have been oriented toward controlling rather than learning. Thus, the very creativity that would spur workers to the process of lifelong learning is stifled. Lifelong learning is a major building block of performance improvement. Without knowledge about the organization, as well as their own tasks, employees cannot make the contributions they are capable of making. This requires dramatic learning efforts, both for the employees, who must learn to act in the interest of the whole enterprise, and the whole organization as well.

Personal performance improvement means being the best one can be, obtaining the knowledge and skills needed to be an expert in one's field or job description, and performing optimally. Performance improvement is a component beyond competence development. Competency means a person has the knowledge needed to perform a job and the skills to apply that knowledge. Performance improvement means being a lifelong learner. Being a lifelong learner is a never-ending developmental path. Performance improvement means always looking for ways to develop and use knowledge. Performance improvement is a continual striving, on a personal and organizational level, to be the best. It means following a lifelong journey of honing and developing talents in which one's perceptual capacity develops and one learns new ways of looking at the world.

An example of organizational performance improvement is the atrial fibrillation project initiated by a surgical stepdown unit at a Midwestern hospital. The nursing staff noted a delay in treatment for patients who experienced atrial fibrillation after open-heart surgery and formed a team to look at the issue. The team tracked the onset of atrial fibrillation, the time of initial treatment (physician contacted, treatment ordered, treatment began), the risk of complications, the length of stay, and, indirectly, costs and patient satisfaction (patients had to stay longer in the hospital). The team discovered that patients who began having asymptomatic atrial fibrillation during the day received treatment sooner than patients who experienced the onset at night. In the latter case, the physician was notified of the onset of asymptomatic atrial fibrillation early the next morning. By delaying notification of the rhythm change, treatment was delayed and the length of stay and cost increased. The team proposed a written treatment protocol that could be initiated by the RN as soon as the patient experienced a sustained atrial fibrillation, along with notification of the physician that the protocol had been initiated. The results were impressive. Treatment was initiated sooner for both nocturnal atrial fibrillation and atrial fibrillation onset during the day. There was a decreased length of stay for the night onset of atrial fibrillation by 1 to 2 days, resulting in decreased costs.

These nurses identified an issue and a mechanism by which to improve a system of treatment. The result was an improvement in the performance of the system as measured by length of stay, complication rate, and cost, as well as patient satisfaction (organizational performance improvement). In this case, the performance improvement of the organization hinged on the performance of the nurses. Suppose these nurses could not read or interpret cardiac rhythms; without that knowledge, they could not have identified atrial fibrillation. The improvement in atrial fibrillation treatment hinged on the nurses' ability to interpret cardiac rhythms, so each nurse had to learn and practice rhythm interpretation (personal performance improvement). Another aspect of their goal of personal improvement was recognizing the delay in treatment and linking it to increased length of stay, increased cost, and increased complications, all things the organization had targeted for improvement.

Personal performance improvement extends beyond competence and helps employees achieve proficiency and expertise. It is a matter of continually moving along the continuum toward expert. Even at the expert level, still looking for ways to improve patient care is part of performance improvement. It is a matter of personal pride; it is striving to do the best job possible each and every day.

Performance improvement is a result of continuous quality improvement. By becoming more proficient and knowledgeable in one's profession or job, personal performance improves. In turn, as personal performance improves, employees discover and implement ways to improve organizational performance. This cascade of events results in higher-quality patient care and greater satisfaction with the organization as a health care provider.

The departments that are more adaptable to pressures and opportunities will be those that survive and thrive in health care today and tomorrow. Indeed, flexibility may be more important than vision in the modern health care industry. Strategic advantage goes to the education department that:

- Knows its customers
- Knows what its customers want before they know or can articulate it
- Responds to what the customer wants
- Customizes to fit the customer's needs.

By doing something new or better, the department creates its own market rather than competing in the old one. The staff development department must plan for the learner who does not yet exist. This requires becoming familiar with the likely future, basing decisions on data and trends. The SDS must provide programs to help clinicians learn the tools they need to develop their competence as well as travel along the continuum to expert practitioner.

PROGRAMS TO ACHIEVE COMPETENCE DEVELOPMENT

Clinical Ladder Program

Clinical ladder programs are developed to reward nurses and other professionals consistently for their professional expertise and contributions. Although many clinical ladders include leadership ladders, most recognize the bedside nurse or caregiver. According to Day and Scidmore, the purpose of a clinical ladder is "to recognize achievement and to promote professional growth" (1995, p. 805). Glenn and Smith (1995) described the purpose of clinical ladders as keeping expert nurses and their continuing excellence at the bedside. Participation in clinical ladder programs is usually voluntary.

Clinical ladders usually consist of several levels and a point system used to score achievements. A point system is easy to monitor and apply because the categories and their points are well defined. A point system can consist of many categories, such as:

- Leadership (committee chair, charge nurse)
- Education (degrees, academic hours, continuing education credits)
- Research and publication (local, regional, and national)
- Teaching
- Membership in a professional organization
- Community volunteer activity
- Certification in a specialty
- Positive peer reviews
- Completion of role development or leadership classes
- Tenure
- Nursing experience.

Monetary awards are based on the levels of achievement; each level requires a certain number of points. The monetary reward may be a bonus that must be re-earned each year or an increase in salary.

Clinical ladder programs vary from organization to organization. Kelly (1992) stated that there are four elements in most programs: expectations, competencies, evaluation, and documentation.

Performance expectations differentiate the levels of competence in practice. As Benner (1982) wrote, a novice practitioner does not function at the same level as an expert. Practice development is a result of both knowledge and experience. Levels of practice differentiate performance expectations among nurses and provide a ladder of progression as advanced competencies are acquired.

Performance expectations include a variety of competencies. These competencies are in the categories of nursing process, education, leadership, and research. Performance expectations pertaining to the nursing process include advanced clinical knowledge and skills, care planning, patient care management, and clinical judgment and decision making. Educational performance expectations are related to the provision of patient, staff, and student education as well as activities related to one's ongoing professional growth and development. Performance expectations related to leadership include activities associated with formal or informal leadership in a unit, the organization, or the community (e.g., responsibility for developing projects, participation in activities that support unit goals, committee work, problem solving, working with groups). Research performance activities include competencies related to systematic analysis of clinical problems, participation in CQI activities, and operationalizing nursing practice from a research base.

The formalized evaluation process includes self-evaluation as well as management evaluation. Many clinical ladder programs also include peer evaluation and a review process conducted by an external body, such as a committee or review panel, as part of the advancement process.

The fourth component of clinical ladder programs is the requirement for written documentation of competencies, activities, or individual accomplishments that reflect an identified level of practice. Documentation may be in the form of a professional portfolio, summaries of specific activities, or written materials that illustrate the nurse's ability to perform specific competencies, such as developing patient care plans or education plans.

In many health care organizations, clinical ladder programs are the responsibility of the staff development department. Linking the clinical ladder activities to staff development is consistent with the department's goal of developing competence within the nursing staff. SDSs are the ideal people to provide resources to the organization that promote the ongoing professional development of nursing staff. The development and implementation of the clinical ladder program should involve SDSs. By helping to create and refine these programs, they can assist in defining basic, intermediate, and advanced competencies associated with the different levels of practice. As experts in education, they can identify knowledge competencies as well as the time frame and experience that nursing staff will need to advance from one level to another.

Kelly (1992) stated that the goal of a clinical ladder program is to reward the accomplishments and achievements of the clinical nurse. By establishing meaningful performance criteria, accompanied by realistic time frames, the clinical ladder program has meaning to the nursing staff, management, and patients. The SDS can help develop a clinical ladder program that is meaningful but realistic. Without the input of the SDS, the clinical ladder program may be developed by staff who may lack knowledge and experience; this sets the program up for failure and reduces the professional growth it was intended to achieve.

Kelly (1992) wrote that the implementation of a clinical ladder program has several implications for educational program development. The first step is to provide an educational offering that explains the program and what roles various staff members have in its operation. This should be undertaken before the program implementation. Educational programs must also be planned and in place before the program implementation. These programs must cover three areas:

- Education relevant to the design of the clinical ladder program
- Education to develop advanced practice competencies
- Education that provides an opportunity for professional development.

Educational programs in a clinical ladder program design include those areas of knowledge and skill required by the staff to support the components of the program. For example, if peer evaluation is an element of the program, education should be provided for those who have little or no experience conducting formal evaluations. The nurse manager's role may shift from one of appraising performance to one of performance management. This change must be supported by education concerning skills in coaching, goal setting, and aligning advanced practice competencies with the unit goals. Staff nurses who wish to participate in the clinical ladder program may need to develop skills in writing a curriculum vitae or developing a professional portfolio that documents their professional accomplishments.

The SDS must also provide programs to promote nurses' ongoing professional development. These activities encompass a wide range of areas, such as:

- Developing a clinical protocol
- Developing an in-service offering
- Organizing a journal club
- Giving a presentation
- Developing patient education materials
- Conducting a research study
- Leading a team.

Professional development programs provide a golden opportunity for the SDS to share his or her expertise with other nurses. There are many types of professional development activities besides formal education programs. Spending a working sabbatical in the staff development department or quality resources department to complete a project, mentoring a staff nurse, offering an individual consultation to a learner, or organizing small-group learning experiences are all effective strategies that can be used to support the professional development of the nursing staff.

By maintaining responsibility for the ongoing management of the clinical ladder program, SDSs take on the additional role of counseling and advising nurses who wish to pursue clinical advancement options. Career counseling, assessment of performance competencies, and helping nurses establish plans to enhance their advancement are additional support services that are needed to implement a clinical advancement program successfully.

Team or Committee Development

Each team or committee needs certain skills and education:

1. Honesty: For the team to initiate change, the current reality must be articulated openly and honestly. The team must bring to the table what is really happening, not what its members wish were happening.

2. Principles of effective meetings: Ways to organize and move the meeting along are valuable tools to enhance the productivity of the team. Being aware of the time and monetary resources used in meetings helps make members more productive. Tools that can be used by teams to run more effective meetings include:

Assigning roles (*e.g.*, timekeeper, recorder, meeting leader)

Establishing ground rules for the conduct of the meeting

Setting procedures to follow during each meeting

Following a written agenda, with assigned times for each item; the time spent on each item can be negotiated, but the meeting cannot run beyond an established time

3. Team building: Activities such as courtesy, improving communication, becoming better able to perform everyday work tasks together, and building strong relationships will enhance the team's productivity. Devoting a short amount of time in each meeting, particularly at the beginning, to team building, getting to know one another, and identifying communication styles enhances the team's cohesiveness, and generally the more cohesive the team, the more productive it is. A literature search will provide a wide variety of sources for team-building exercises.

4. An environment that promotes learning: Teams that practice dialogue and skillful discussion build a shared understanding and thus become more effective problem-solvers. Team learning goes beyond team-building skills; it inspires more fundamental changes, with enduring applications that will ripple through the organization. Team learning is challenging intellectually, emotionally, socially, and spiritually. It is a process of learning how to learn collectively (Senge et al., 1994).

Unit or Group Development

The same principles for team or committee development can be applied to unit or group development. One goal of unit development is to encourage thinking toward improvement of patient care. Thinking is best developed through practice and is best practiced in a supportive environment. Often, managers try to teach people to think by attacking their ideas before they have had a chance to develop them as fully as they wish; this type of management is counterproductive.

Staff development departments can lead the way by rewarding thought and creativity whenever they are found. To encourage people to think for themselves at work, get out of their way. Rather than managers telling employees what to do, managers can learn to ask them what they think should be done. Creating a culture that encourages people to think for themselves is a challenge and a skill that must be learned. Some people can be spurred on by rejection to greater persistence and effort, but rejection causes most people to shut down their creativity.

A learning organization provides continual permission and incentive for everyone in the organization to think well and to benefit from the thinking of others. Encouraging a move from managing to coaching may be helpful. This means helping employees to solve problems and think creatively about their work and how it is done. The philosophy of coaching involves the following:

- Leadership pulls together people with diverse backgrounds.
- Employees are encouraged to be responsible and to continue to achieve.
- Employees are treated as full partners and contributors in a department.

- Employees are encouraged to answer questions for themselves (within reasonable limits) rather than being given answers.
- Management assumes that employees are intelligent, thinking people who can contribute greatly to the organization.

Coaching means paying attention to people, believing in them, caring about them, and involving them in the decisions related to their work. Coaching is enabling others to act, building on their strengths, encouraging them, and providing learning opportunities to enable them to strengthen their weaknesses and build on their strengths.

CUSTOMER SATISFACTION

Customer Needs

Customers approach a service organization because they want or need something, but often what they really want goes beyond the obvious. Psychologists have studied and debated for years what customers really want, and after much study 11 basic customers' needs have emerged. When even one of these needs is not met, customers are likely to feel distressed and critical. Understanding these 11 needs will help interpret customers' complaints and handle them with compassion and positive action (Leebov, 1990).

1. Learners want control over their lives. People often feel out of control, helpless, and at the mercy of others. To counteract this feeling, the SDS should help learners feel they are active participants in the decisions that affect them. Learners must feel they are not being taken advantage of, manipulated, or deceived. They must feel that their consent is required and that their feelings and opinions matter. They need to feel that they are active and intelligent partners in their own education.
2. Learners want to achieve goals and need to feel that whatever they learn is moving them toward a goal. They want to know that the SDS's actions serve an important purpose that will bring them satisfaction and achieve the desired results of more knowledge and greater skill.
3. Learners want to preserve their self-esteem. Learners like to feel good about themselves no matter what they are doing. They want to think of themselves as intelligent, wise, and competent and want to be treated with courtesy, dignity, and respect.
4. Learners want to be treated fairly. Fairness is one of a person's strongest drives. Learners want to feel they are receiving the same attention, the same degree of quality, and the same level of treatment as everyone else.
5. Learners want a friendly reception. Learners come to the SDS hoping and expecting to like and trust him or her. They like friendly, warm, and caring relationships, and they want interactions with the SDS to be as pleasant as possible.
6. Learners want to know what's going on and why. Information must be given in a way that learners can understand.
7. Learners have a strong need to feel safe and secure. They want to feel physically safe coming to and leaving programs and do not like unpleasant surprises.
8. Learners want approval, acceptance, and recognition. They want to feel that they are recognized as individuals who are important to the SDS, not just

nameless faces. Learners need to feel welcome and affirmed and need to be praised for participating in their own education.

9. Learners want to feel important. They want those who interact with them to recognize their importance and not to ignore them or treat them as bothersome interruptions. They expect full and prompt attention and proper consideration.

10. Learners want to be appreciated. They deserve to know that their time, energy, and trust are valued and appreciated.

11. Learners want to have a sense of belonging. They want to feel that they are insiders with a stake in the organization's success. The SDS should greet learners by name, talk with them, respond to their complaints fully, and acknowledge their loyalty.

Learners consciously or unconsciously bring these basic needs into every interaction with the staff development department. Learners come to the staff development department for education services, but for learners to be completely satisfied, the services provided should fulfill all these needs.

Specific Organizational Goals

The values, vision, and strategic initiatives of the organization are an integral part of any staff development program. The department must set aside time to develop a vision and goals that fit with the values and vision of the organization. The staff development department and its members must have a vision of where they want to go so they can anticipate what they need to learn to get there. This requires a broad strategy for reaching their goal to know whether their learning is moving the organization toward its vision. SDSs must develop measurable mechanisms to contribute to the strategic initiatives of the organization. The staff development department should develop goals that assist the organization in its movement toward its strategic initiatives.

Image Making and Changing

The staff development department must focus on service. If it is seen as a department that provides only orientation and the "mandatories," its image needs a makeover. Instead, the department must be known for its creativity, flexibility, and skill to meet the competence needs of the organization. Traditionally, hospital-based nursing education departments have focused on nursing orientation, in-service education, and continuing education, but the focus now is broader. Staff development departments must provide for the competence assessment and development demands of the entire cadre of clinical care providers. That may mean all departments within a hospital or health care system, including clinic personnel, physicians, and others who are a part of an integrated health system. Staff development departments today must cater to customers and establish programs that please and satisfy customers so they keep returning; they are compelled to develop customer loyalty. The department must provide an integrated system of education, not just single classes.

Cosponsoring Programs With Other Departments

Eliminating departmental barriers enhances communication and relationships within the organization. SDSs should take advantage of experts in the institution. By using them for content and education design, the staff development department can offer programs of higher quality and greater usefulness to the participants. At St. John's Health Systems

(Springfield, Missouri), for instance, the Department of Continuing Education joined the Quality Resources Department to plan CQI training for the system. Using experts in quality management and educational design and presentation, this group put together a series of programs on CQI that changed the way the system does business in health care. The culture in this institution is moving toward a CQI philosophy, the language of CQI is being spoken, and enthusiasm has been created for the model. Many of the participants noted how the team overcame departmental barriers to produce an effective training program.

CQI TRAINING PROGRAMS

Design

The design of a CQI training program varies from institution to institution. Some institutions have hired consultants to advise on the design of the program or to provide the training. The institution and the staff development department must take into consideration the cost of hiring a consultant; also, consultants will probably be unfamiliar with the culture and environment of the institution. Another mechanism for designing a CQI training program is to train SDSs to develop a customized training program in-house. Some institutions have charged the members of the staff development department with developing the training programs using the resources available to them. This provides an opportunity for the SDS to be creative and to form a multidepartmental team for CQI education and development. Ideally, the CQI training is developed in conjunction with the quality resources department within the institution to gain a realistic view of the potential for improvement and the data for those improvements. Collaborating with the quality resources department provides for a team relationship between departments, which presents a valuable role model for the participants in the training program.

Another collaborating body is the executive leadership group, which is the driving force behind such a quality movement. These leaders must be involved in the development of training for support and also for providing the necessary resources.

The following are some recommendations for beginning a quality improvement program:

1. *Train the executives and upper-level management first.* This group must support the initiative and has the power to allocate resources to the initiative.
2. *Choose a champion* for the program. This may be a physician who is compensated for assuming this role. This person must be willing to commit his or her time and energy to propel the program forward and must be able to negotiate with the executive group for resource allocation. This person must also have credibility with the members of the organization to be effective.
3. *Establish a quality council* or a similar group to oversee the program development and roll-out. This council should include executives, upper managers, and physicians.
4. *Tie the training to the survival of the organization* in the minds of those being trained. If the employees understand that the success of the organization at least partially rests on this initiative, they will also understand that the future of their jobs hinges on the success of CQI, and they will be much more willing to master the material presented.

The program can be minimal or extensive, depending on the resources available. Display 13-4 lists topics that should be included in a CQI education program.

DISPLAY 13-4

Topics for a CQI Education Program

A. Principles of Quality Improvement as Applied to Health Care
   1. W. Edwards Deming
   2. Avedis Donabedian
   3. Philip Crosby
   4. Joseph Juran
   5. Donald Berwick
B. Principles of team formation
   1. Composition of teams
   2. Team roles
   3. Team responsibilities
C. Team building
   1. Stages of team growth
   2. Activities to promote team formation
      a. Brainstorming
      b. Team-building activities
D. Productive meetings
   1. Tools for productive meetings
      a. Agendas
      b. Ground rules
      c. Team roles
      d. Meeting evaluations
   2. Consensus building
   3. Tools for consensus building
      a. Multivoting
      b. Nominal group technique
E. Building an improvement plan
   1. Performance improvement model
   2. Tools for performance improvement
      a. Flow chart
      b. Opportunity statement
      c. Cause-and-effect diagram
      d. Run chart
      e. Pareto chart
      f. Control chart
F. Data collection
   1. Principles of data collection
   2. Design of data collection tools
   3. Operational definitions
   4. Conducting pilot studies
   5. Research design
G. Conflict resolution

Source: Kelly Thomas Associates, Alexandria, VA. Reproduced with permission.

Targets

Using a benchmarking process, the staff development department can learn what opportunities exist for improvement. These opportunities can then become targets of the CQI process. Another mechanism for discovering targets for the CQI process may be customer satisfaction surveys. By asking the customers of educational programs to describe their level of satisfaction with components of the program, opportunities for improvement (targets) can be identified. Customer satisfaction can be measured through focus groups, questionnaires, reaction evaluation forms, or interviews. The staff development department should use a standardized method of measuring customer satisfaction and should update it periodically.

Outcomes

Outcomes are the results of CQI efforts. In the atrial fibrillation example, two outcomes could be identified. First, the staff development outcome was the competence and continuously developed expertise of the nursing staff in interpreting and treating cardiac rhythms. The second outcome was the more timely treatment of patients with atrial fibrillation; this resulted in the outcomes of decreased length of stay, decreased cost, decreased chance of complications, and increased patient satisfaction.

POSITIONING THE STAFF DEVELOPMENT DEPARTMENT

Leadership in the staff development department is a key factor in the political positioning of the department in the organization. Through effective leadership, systems problems, performance problems, and knowledge deficits can be identified and addressed (Jeska & Fischer, 1996). Actions can be targeted to the appropriate issues among the right groups.

The leaders of the staff development department are critical to getting SDSs involved in all aspects of the organization. Excellent leaders get the attention of team members through the strength of their vision and their ability to communicate. They create a focus for the team, set clear expectations, and instill self-confidence in others. They create trust and shared vision within the department and the organization. They are accountable, predictable, reliable, and persistent; they "walk the talk" (DeGraff et al., 1996). Effective leaders accept people as they are, focus on the present, treat friends and strangers courteously, and trust others in the face of risk, and they can do without the constant approval of others. This type of leader is recognized in the organization as a valuable asset and is used to the fullest. This kind of leadership makes the department an active, valuable asset to the organization and secures its position.

The staff development department must be visible and on the cutting edge of changes happening in the organization. It must be willing to embrace any task remotely connected to education. The department must be constantly alert for opportunities throughout the organization. For example, if the pharmacy is purchasing a new software program, the staff development department should volunteer to coordinate the training on this new software. Watching for such opportunities takes effort and means keeping in touch with key players. When the SDS initiates activities to improve the educational environment, he or she is contributing to organizational performance improvement efforts.

Internal Marketing

The importance of internal marketing of staff development programs cannot be overlooked or minimized. Health care providers represent the core of the customers for any staff development program based within the institution. The programs developed by the staff development department must be tightly linked to the organization's values, goals, and objectives. SDSs look at the genuine needs of the organization and focus on its mission and goals. This builds internal credibility for the program. Programs are a result of careful

---

DISPLAY 13-5

Elements in a Staff Development Specialist's Repertoire

- Work with the manager to meet perceived and actual needs.
- Obtain frequent feedback to ensure that needs are adequately addressed.
- Involve learners early in the program development.
- Remain enthusiastic about the potential effects of the program.
- Continue to talk about the benefits to the unit and staff as a result of participation.

Source: Kelly Thomas Associates, Alexandria, VA. Reproduced with permission.

planning and deliberate intervention based on identified needs within the organization. SDSs must work in harmony with organizational goals and objectives and the direction the organization is moving. They should be aware of what services are being phased out and what new services are being planned for the organization and should expend their energies accordingly.

Successful SDSs keep in tune with the pulse of the organization. The SDS is in contact with many people throughout the organization and can identify needs as expressed by staff. Successful SDSs build coalitions among key players to keep the staff in tune with the objectives, goals, and direction of the organization. Working with these coalitions, the SDS can help determine the educational programs presented. Kelly (1992) described several elements that make up the repertoire of the SDS; these are listed in Display 13-5.

According to principles of adult learning and internal marketing, customer involvement is essential to all elements of the planning process. This involvement can directly affect the success of the program. The learner who has "ownership" of the program ensures support for the program and is committed to its success.

The same principles used in external marketing can be used for internal marketing of staff development programs. Informational flyers are more commonly used for internal marketing, and space may be limited. Use appealing language, layout, and colors.

External Marketing

Direct mail is the most common form of external marketing used by SDSs. Because direct mail pieces send many messages, the SDS should consider carefully what messages will be included in any promotional piece sent from the department and the organization. Direct mail pieces should promote the organization and the staff development program. The message communicated is important. Marketing specialists within the institution or consultants can help develop materials that will promote the organization and the program to be advertised.

SDSs can also use their own expertise as recipients of direct mail in the design of promotional materials. Collecting direct mail pieces can trigger ideas for design, layout, and message. Look for style and design differences and similarities. Notice which are the most attractive. A graphic artist can help adapt the most attractive ideas for the department. Looking at these promotional materials will also spark ideas that can be developed in graphic form.

Many health care organizations have an identifying logo that may be required for use on all materials released from the organization. Other items that may be standard for promotional materials may be color, awards the institution has received, or specific wording describing the institution.

> ### Ⓓ ISPLAY 13-6
>
> **Minimum Information for a Brochure or Promotional Piece**
>
> - Title
> - Date, time, location of the event
> - Program description
> - Objective
> - Target audience
> - Program schedule
> - Faculty
> - Registration information
> - Contact hour information
> - Cancellation/refund policy
> - Phone number for additional information

Once a design is developed for direct mail and other promotional pieces, it should be used consistently in all pieces. This will promote recognition of the staff development programs in the market. If all brochures, flyers, and catalogs look similar, name recognition will follow. The design can also be incorporated into conference folders, name tags, and other conference handouts.

The copy in the brochure is very important. Bear in mind who the prospective learner is. Everything in the brochure should focus on the benefits of the program to the learner. The copy should be written in the second or third person and should use familiar language. The program titles and their descriptions must be consistent with the institution's image. The titles should be clearly stated and should describe the programs in a few words. The cover of the brochure must be eye-catching and should boldly display the name of the sponsoring institution. Display 13-6 lists the minimal information that should be included in the brochure or promotional piece. Other elements that may be included are short faculty biographies, E-mail addresses, fax numbers, the program coordinator's name, and a short description of each program topic.

Getting started on brochure design can be the toughest obstacle. If possible, modify a piece that has been successful in the past. Keep the participant of the program in mind and design the brochure to interest him or her. Address the potential participant in a professional, personal tone. Match the language of the brochure to the language of the participant.

Bulletin boards can be used to highlight the benefits of attending the program. Questions that will be answered during the program might be listed.

POLICIES AND PRACTICES

Practice Manual

A practice manual for the staff development department contains the policies and practices that have been proven successful. It can include guidelines for program development, program administration policies, record-keeping policies, a departmental orientation program, and other items consistently used by the SDS. The manual may include resources for the SDS as well as information about the staff development practice in the organization.

Attendance

The staff development department needs a standardized mechanism for recording and tracking attendance at its programs. Records of program attendance are important in meeting standards of an accrediting body and employee recertification requirements. Several mechanisms can be used for attendance tracking. A sign-in sheet that includes the program name, hours of credit, and the category of the program can be used. Another method is computerized; each participant fills out a card, which can be entered or scanned into a computer, or the participant can scan his or her identification badge directly into a preset program code.

Cancellation

Developing a standardized cancellation policy is necessary to control the cost of programs. To obtain numbers for food orders and printed material, an accurate count of attendance is necessary. The department should set a cancellation policy that will allow time to adjust food orders and material printing. Participants must cancel if they cannot attend. Usually cancellation 2 to 10 days before the program allows sufficient time to make any adjustments necessary.

Records and Reports

Maintaining records and generating reports are part of the responsibility of the staff development department. Finding a mechanism that works for the size of the institution and the department is a challenge. Mechanisms for recording and reporting education opportunities and attendance vary. For some institutions, a filing system is adequate. For larger institutions, computerized record-keeping software can make this responsibility more manageable.

Program File

Staff development departments use a program file to organize their programs and to keep records of the planning, implementation, and evaluation of their offerings. The program file contains vital information about the programs, such as the source of need, planning process, faculty, credentials of faculty, agenda, objectives, evaluation summary, responsible SDS, syllabus, outlines, attendance roster, faculty critique summary, and possibly a postprogram critique.

Employee Transcripts

Some staff development departments are charged with maintaining employee transcripts or education records. A variety of computer programs can be used to automate this record-keeping process and provide reports (*e.g.*, individual education records, department education records, program attendance records). The Ed-U-Keep Co. offers Ed-U-Keep 2000, *American Journal of Nursing* offers AJN Target, and Business Management Solutions offers the Hospital Education Tracking program. These are examples of software programs used to maintain health care education records.

Faculty File

A faculty file lists faculty members, area of expertise, qualifications and credentials, evaluations or reactions to their presentations, and contact information. It can serve as a valuable resource when searching for speakers.

Annual Report

An annual report is a collection of the work of the entire department each year. It should summarize the programs presented over the last year. By including cost information—especially cost reduction information—and the outcomes and impact of programs, the staff development department can use this report to show executive leadership the value of the programs and the department. This can provide valuable evidence for keeping successful programs and dropping those with low impact or poor outcomes. It also can be used as a data tool for improvement activities.

Contact Hours

To maintain their certification or license, many health care workers are required to accrue continuing education contact hours. Offering contact hours approved by an accrediting body provides an added incentive for attending the program. Education can be made more attractive to participants if continuing education units or credits are attached to the programs. Formal contact hours require an application process, which is designed to ensure that the program meets the guidelines established by the granting agency; this guarantees the relevance and quality of the program. Using the ANA standards as a guide, each state nursing society and other training societies provide mechanisms by which an institution or a single event can be credited with continuing education hours.

The following are the forms filed for one continuing education course, "Humor in Healthcare," given in Missouri in May 1995. These standards can be used to ensure that American Nurses Credentialing Center (ANCC) standards for educational programs are met and are similar to other training and education standards published.

1. Application for offering approval (Display 13-7). This introduces the program and gives the cost for approval, the time frame for seeking approval, and the offering approval duration.
2. Application for sponsor of offering (Display 13-8). To ensure that the continuing education credits are meaningful and to guarantee consistency and high-quality programs, a form like this must be filed with the state nursing association to provide nursing continuing education credits for a program.
3. Offering documentation form (Display 13-9). This provides information about the objectives, content, time frame, faculty, and teaching methods.
4. Biographical data form (Display 13-10). This outlines the qualifications of the program faculty.
5. Program evaluation form (Display 13-11). This elicits the reaction of the participants to all aspects of the program.
6. Certificate of attendance (Display 13-12). This is awarded to the participants at the close of the program. The participants must attend the majority of the program to receive the certificate, and it must contain the elements outlined by the accrediting body.

(text continues on page 331)

DISPLAY 13-7

Missouri Nurses Association (P.O. Box 105228, 1904 Bubba Lane, Jefferson City, MO 65110-5228) Application for Offering Approval

In order for your application to be reviewed, four (4) copies of the following information must be submitted to the Missouri Nurses Association office **at least 45 calendar days prior to the offering date** accompanied by the appropriate application fee. Applications submitted later than the 45 day deadline will *not* be reviewed. This form must accompany each completed application. Please refer to "Continuing Education Excellence in Missouri, 3rd ed.," for additional guidance in completing this application. **Offering approval is for *two years*.**

Application fee is enclosed in the amount of:
  _X_ $50.00 (Sponsors located in state of Missouri)
  ___ $65.00 (Sponsors whose headquarters are located outside the state of Missouri)

Sponsoring agency: Nurses' Recognition Committee
Person submitting the application: Donna Gloe
Person to notify of Approval: Donna Gloe   Tel: 417-885-0000 or 417-859-0000
Address: Rt. 8 Box 4   City: Anywhere   State: MO   Zip: 00000
Offering title: Humor in Healthcare
Date(s) to be offered: May 8, 1998   Time: 12:30 p.m. to 5:00 p.m.
Number of times to be offered: once
Place: St. John's Regional Health Center   City: Springfield   County: Greene   State: Missouri
Registration fee: $25.00

Criteria for Approval

1. Submit the biographical data on the form provided, which specifies the education and professional qualifications for the person administratively responsible for planning and producing the offering.
2. Submit a list of the planning committee and biographical data on the form provided for each member that specifies:
   a. Educational preparation;
   b. Professional qualifications related to content and/or planning continuing education.

Note: If no RNs are on the planning committee the application will not be reviewed.

3. Describe the target audience.
4. Describe how the need for this offering was assessed.
5. Describe how learner input was considered in such areas as location and scheduling. Please submit information related to the following criteria on: (6) *objectives,* (7) *content,* (8) *time frame,* (9) *faculty,* and (10) *teaching methods* using the format of the Offering Documentation form.
6. State the objectives in operational/behavioral terms.
7. Provide a brief description (or outline) of the content to be presented for each topic area. Indicate which offering objective(s) is related to each topic area.
8. State the time period for each topic or content area.
9. List the faculty person or presenter for each topic or content area.
10. List the teaching method used by each presenter for each topic or content area.
11. Submit the biographical data on the form provided, which identifies education and professional qualifications related to content for each faculty person or presenter.
12. Describe how faculty take part in planning their presentations.
13. Describe the method used to evaluate the offering. Submit a copy of the learner evaluation instrument.

D ISPLAY 13-7 (Continued)

14. Describe the physical facilities in relation to: a) accommodation to teaching methods; b) environmental comfort; c) target audience accessibility.
15. Submit a sample of the verification form/certificate awarded to the participants. The verification must include:
    a. Successful completion of the offering.
    b. Number of contact hours awarded.
    c. The provider of the offering.
    d. Title, date, city, and state of offering.
    e. MONA approval number.
    f. Appropriate statement of approval, which identifies the ANCC-accredited organization that has approved the offering for contact hour credit.
16. Describe the system for record filing, storage, retrieval, retention, security, and confidentiality of all records, especially participant records. Submit a written statement of the commitment to maintain for a minimum of five (5) years records for each offering that include the essential information listed in the guidelines.
17. Is the offering coprovided? Yes ___ No _X_
    If yes, submit a copy of the written coprovidership agreement.

Source: Missouri Nurses Association. Reprinted with permission.

D ISPLAY 13-8

Missouri Nurses Association Application for Sponsor of Offering

Humor in Healthcare
Monday, May 8, 1995
1:00 p.m.–4:00 p.m.

1. Person administratively responsible:
   Donna Gloe, BSN, MEd, RN, C, CCRN (Biographical Data Form Attached)
2. Planning committee:
   The planning committee for the offering consisted of 2 persons chosen from the larger Nurses' Recognition Planning Committee. The Nurses' Recognition Planning Committee is a regional group of nurses who annually plan an afternoon educational offering and a recognition dinner for nurses in the southwest Missouri region.
   Pat Clutter, BSN, MEd, RN, CEN (Biographical Data Form Attached)
   Donna Gloe, BSN, MEd, RN, C, CCRN, Chair
3. Target Audience
   The target audience for this offering will be nurses from all specialty fields. This subject is diverse enough to interest all.
4. Needs Assessment
   The use of the right amount and type of humor in certain circumstances can help to defuse an escalating negative situation and in some instances help to build and support a positive nurse/patient relationship. Also humor has been shown to have a positive impact on the physiological healing of patients.
   A second aspect of humor in healthcare relates to today's health care arena in which the level of tension and stress has risen for our nurses related to future job responsibilities and even job security. Humor can help reduce stress and hopefully help deal with burn-out, which often affects nurses.

(continued)

DISPLAY 13-8 (Continued)

Discussion with nurses on the Nurses' Recognition Planning Committee which included 10 nurses representing specialty areas including emergency trauma center, surgical intensive care unit, continuing education, orthopedics, mental health, oncology, hematology, school of nursing, and pharmaceutics concurred with these thoughts. Positive feedback was given regarding this potential topic. Humor has been successfully presented at national and state programs. Since there has not been an opportunity to present humor in the southwest Missouri geographic area, it was agreed it was a timely topic that would be positively received.

5. Location and scheduling.

The location and type of presentation (afternoon seminar, dinner) was also discussed informally with nurses on the planning committee. They agreed that combining a social event with a learning opportunity was a good idea. We are attempting to bring nurses together away from their places of employment to foster collegiality, celebrate nursing, and provide a neutral ground for networking, collaboration, etc.

6–10. See offering documentation form.

11. See biographical data forms.

12. The planning committee planned this offering in cooperation with the speaker through personal contact and telephone conversation. Once the topic was determined and objectives written, the speaker identified appropriate content for the presentation. After the presentation, the speaker will receive a copy of the evaluation summary for this presentation.

13. See evaluation form.

14. The facility has a large auditorium with full audiovisual capabilities. The atmosphere is comfortable and very conducive to learning. The location that was chosen was centrally located and the only room available for the anticipated attendance. The location is on a main thoroughfare with good parking and is handicapped accessible.

15. Participants will receive a certificate with the appropriate information provided. See certificate of attendance.

16. Records will be maintained by the Nurses' Recognition Committee secretary, who is currently the Assistant Nursing Director of the Surgical Intensive Care Unit (SICU), in a locked file cabinet accessible only to the secretary in the SICU office. The records will be accessible to the secretary, the committee chair, and the present and future planning committee members with approval of the chair or secretary. An agreement has been made with SICU to maintain the records from year to year even though the elected secretary may change. Retrieval of records can occur by contacting any member of the committee who would refer the seeker to the current chair or secretary. These records will be kept for 5 years and will include the following information:

   a. Title of offerings
   b. Name and title of planning committee
   c. Planning committee information
   d. Planning committee biographical data form
   e. Presenter biographical data form
   f. Objectives, content, time frames, and teaching method of offering
   g. Evaluation tool used
   h. Description of target audience
   i. Methodology used to determine offering need
   j. Participant names and addresses and contact hours awarded
   k. Number of contact hours awarded for offering
   l. Evaluation summary

Source: Missouri Nurses Association. Reprinted with permission.

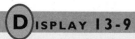

Offering Documentation Form

Title of Offering: Humor in Healthcare

Objectives	Content (Topics)	Time Frame	Faculty	Teaching Methods
List objectives in operational/behavior terms.	List each topic area to be covered and provide a description or outline of the content to be presented.	State the time frame for each topic area.	List the faculty person or presenter for each topic.	Describe the teaching method(s) used for each.
	I. Do you mean there is stress in nursing?	180 minutes	Denise Schorp, RN	Lecture Class participation Handouts Slides

List two benefits of stress.	A. Benefits of stress
	  1. Develop strength
	  2. Opportunity for growth
	  3. Enhances physical condition			

List two hazards of stress.	B. Hazards of stress
	  1. Physical illness
	  2. Decreased coping
	  3. Increased risk of substance abuse			

Describe how you can better handle stress using humor.	C. How to handle stress
	  1. Handling stress positively
	    a. Share good humor
	    b. Share good events
	    c. Avoid gossip
	  2. Handling stress negatively
	    a. Share gossip
	    b. Share negative events			

Describe how sharing humor with coworkers can enhance communication	II. Do you mean there is something to laugh about in nursing? A. Physiology of laughter B. What is your HQ (humor quotient)? C. Using your HQ to enhance communication			
List the five "S's" of humor.	III. The Five "S's" of humor A. See humor B. Share humor C. Search for humor D. Save humor E. Savor humor			

(continued)

DISPLAY 13-9 (Continued)

Describe how using humor can ease change.	IV. Are you a Bee or a Buzzard? A. How do you use humor? B. How can you learn to better use humor?			

Differentiate between positive and negative humor.	V. Do you mean there are different types of humor?
	A. Visual
	  1. Positive
	  2. Negative
	B. Verbal
	  1. Positive
	  2. Negative
	C. Shared inference
	  1. Positive
	  2. Negative			

Define black humor.	D. Black humor E. 1. Negative humor vs. black humor			

Source: Missouri Nurses Assocation. Reprinted with permission.

DISPLAY 13-10

Missouri Nurses Association Biographical Data Form

Instructions: Make as many photocopies of this form as necessary to provide information required to document adherence to the criteria. Information for each person must be **typed** on this form. **Do not attach any additional material**.

___X___ Person Administratively Responsible

_____ Planning Committee Member

_____ Instructional Staff

Name: Donna Gloe, BSN, MEd, RN, C, CCRN _____
(Name and Degrees)

Preferred mailing address:

Rt. 8 Box 4 _____
(Number and Street)

Anywhere, MO 0000 _____
(City, States, Zip Code)

Telephone: 000-000-0000 _____

(continued)

DISPLAY 13-10 (Continued)

Present Position
(title and description): <u>Education Coordinator</u>
<u>Primary responsibility is to identify and meet the education needs of an assigned employee population</u>
<u>through needs assessment, planning, development, and evaluation of appropriate learning experiences.</u>
<u>Serves as a team member to provide quality education that supports the goals of the Health Center, the</u>
<u>Philosophy of the Sisters of Mercy, and the Employee Code of Conduct.</u>

Education (include basic preparation through highest degree held):

Degree	Institution (Name, City, State)	Major Area of Study	Year Degree Awarded
1. <u>RN</u>	St. John's School of Nursing Springfield, MO	Nursing	1983
2. <u>BSN</u>	Southwest Baptist University Springfield, MO	Nursing	1991
3. <u>BA</u>	University of Missouri Columbia, MO	Psychology	1973
4. <u>MEd</u>	Lincoln University Jefferson City, MO	Guidance and Counseling	1977
5. Doctoral Candidate	Nova Southeastern University	Health Care Education	Projected Graduation 1996

Use the space below to briefly describe your professional experience or areas of expertise (including publications) that contribute to this continuing education activity.

Critical care nurse in Surgical Intensive Care for 9 years. Developed Open-Heart Patient Teaching Video for preoperative teaching. Currently maintain PRN status as a staff nurse in the PTCA and SICU units. Formerly adjunct faculty with Southwest Baptist University, Nursing Department, Springfield Center for 2 years.

Published numerous articles in <u>THE PRISM</u>, St. John's Nursing newsletter. Also published in <u>Critical Care Nurse</u>, <u>Heart and Lung</u>, <u>Journal of Nursing Staff Development</u>. Editor of <u>THE PRISM</u> 1991 to present.

Coordinator and faculty for Foundations of Critical Care Course, ACLS Instructor, BLS Instructor-Trainer, and Preceptor Worship Coordinator. Taught various topics including Adult Teaching/Learning Principles, Cardiac Tamponade, Peripheral Vascular Disease, Ethics in Critical Care, Cardiomyopathy, Hemodynamics, Code Blue Protocol, and semester course on pathophysiology.

Source: Missouri Nurses Association. Reprinted with permission.

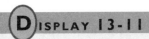

Evaluation Form: Humor In Healthcare

Speaker: <u>Denise Schorp, RN, MEd.</u>   Date: <u>May 8, 1995</u>

Your candid and complete responses are important so that we can continue to provide quality continuing education activities. Please circle the number beside each statement that best reflects the extent of your agreement. Thank you.

Content	Agree		Disagree	
1. The content was related to my practice.	4	3	2	1
2. The content extended my knowledge of the topic.	4	3	2	1
3. The content was relevant to the objectives.				
a. List two benefits of stress.	4	3	2	1
b. List two hazards of stress.	4	3	2	1
c. Describe how you can better handle stress using humor.	4	3	2	1
d. Describe how sharing humor with co-workers can enhance communication.	4	3	2	1
e. List the five "S's" of humor.	4	3	2	1
f. Describe how using humor can ease change.	4	3	2	1
g. Differentiate between positive and negative humor.	4	3	2	1
h. Define black humor.	4	3	2	1

Teaching Methods				
1. The teaching material was well organized.	4	3	2	1
2. Overall, effective teaching methods (lecture, handouts, audiovisual aids) were utilized.	4	3	2	1
3. The handout materials provided are likely to be used as a future reference.	4	3	2	1

Setting				
1. The room was conducive to learning.	4	3	2	1
2. The program site was physically accessible.	4	3	2	1

Learner Benefits				
1. My thinking about the topic is more focused.	4	3	2	1
2. I gained new insight relevant to my profession.	4	3	2	1
3. I will be able to use the information presented in my practice/work setting.	4	3	2	1

Faculty Effectiveness				
1. The presentation was clear and to the point.	4	3	2	1
2. The presenter demonstrated knowledge and expertise of the topic.	4	3	2	1
3. The presenter was responsive to participant concerns.	4	3	2	1

List the major strengths and weaknesses of this program:

Strengths	Weaknesses

Comments:

What topics would you like to have presented in the future?

Source: Missouri Nurses Association. Reprinted with permission.

Sample Certificate Awarded to Participants With All Information Required By Approval Body

CERTIFICATE OF

ATTENDANCE

Awarded to

(Name of Participant)

For successful completion of

Humor in Healthcare

Presented by

Nurses' Recognition Committee
Of Southwest Missouri

May 8, 1998

This program has been approved for 3.6 contact hours of education credit by the Missouri Nurses Association which is accredited as an approver of continuing education in nursing by the American Nurses' Credentialing Center's Commission on Accreditation
MONA Number 597-SO-640

Source: Missouri Nurses Association. Used with permission.

ACCREDITING MECHANISMS

Various organizations provide recognition of professional achievement. This recognition comes in the form of certification and validates the knowledge and expertise of practitioners. Certification assures customers that providers have have achieved a level of excellence in their specialty.

American Nurses Credentialing Center

The ANA established its certification program in 1973 to provide "tangible recognition of professional achievement in a defined functional or clinical area of nursing" (ANCC, 1996, p. 1). The ANCC bases its credentialing programs on the standards set by the ANA Congress for Nursing Practice. Goals of the ANCC include promoting and enhancing public health by certifying nurses and accrediting organizations using ANA standards of nursing practice, nursing services, and continuing education. Primary responsibility for ANCC certification and recertification programs rests with the boards on certification, whose members are volunteers nominated by their peers.

In 1974, the ANA established a voluntary system for accreditation and approval of continuing education in nursing. The system is based on a peer review process in which nurses review and approve educational activities using national standards and criteria. This process recognizes the capacity of an organization to approve or provide quality educational activities in nursing over an extended period of time. There are two categories of accreditation: accreditation as an approver of continuing education in nursing, and accreditation as a provider of continuing education in nursing. The accreditation is for a 6-year period; each accreditation period is independent of all other accreditation periods. At the end of the accreditation period, if the organization wishes to continue its status, it must submit a new application. This application documents the adherence to all appropriate criteria and policies of the ANCC (ANCC, 1996).

International Association for Continuing Education and Training

The International Association for Continuing Education and Training (IACET) is a non-profit association of training and education organizations and professionals who are devoted to the consistent use of the continuing education unit. It is committed to improving the quality and effectiveness of continuing education, training, and human resources development. This organization has been instrumental in the development of continuing education and training around the world. It promotes improvement in continuing education and training by recognizing organizations that undergo a peer review of their practices and make a commitment to adhering to IACET criteria and guidelines. IACET promotes and conducts research on effective practices in education. It values and promotes high-quality, research-based continuing education and training programs that help establish standards as the benchmark for quality program delivery.

Other Professional Groups

Other professional groups also provide certification or professional recognition programs within training and education. For instance, the American Association of Critical Care Nurses has been instrumental in the continuous improvement of critical care nursing.

The ANA has a recognition mechanism to acknowledge "magnet hospitals," those that create a work environment that recognizes and rewards professional nursing and whose nursing services provide quality patient care through nursing excellence. The objectives of the magnet hospital recognition program are:

- To recognize nursing services that build programs of excellence in the delivery of nursing care to patients
- To promote the quality of the milieu that supports professional nursing practice
- To provide a vehicle for the dissemination of successful practices and strategies among hospital nursing systems.

The ANCC believes that this program will be of great benefit to nursing systems, as well as to the quality of health care across the country (ANCC, 1996).

SUMMARY

This chapter presented a future-focused view of quality in the staff development specialty. Topics discussed included TQM, CQI, performance improvement, benchmarking, clinical ladder programs, team and unit development, customer satisfaction, marketing, leadership, policies and procedures, record-keeping, and accreditation. Sample program documentation forms were given.

Given the rapidly changing face of health care, SDSs must strive to monitor and improve the quality of the products and services they offer to move the organization forward. SDSs must align their programs with the organization's goals and objectives, creating a positive image for the department in the organization. Staff development practice must be integrated into the organization and seen as a vital part of it.

Improving Quality Through Staff Development

LINDA RISTOW PUETZ

Children's Mercy Hospital in Kansas City, MO, is the only children's hospital in a metropolitan area with a population of 1.5 million. It has a 250-mile-radius rural referral region. Our professional staff must be competent to handle a wide range of life-threatening neonatal and pediatric emergencies. Most of these events involve airway and respiratory problems, in contrast to adult cardiac problems. Prompt airway support and proper use of airway equipment are crucial in managing emergencies in our patient population.

In 1992, the hospital's Code Blue Committee noted a disturbing trend: initial airway interventions by staff were sometimes delayed by inconvenient placement of emergency equipment, or did not meet all defined standards. Two recommendations were made. First, airway intervention equipment (resuscitation bag, mask, and oxygen supply) should be at every bedside, including clinic areas. Second, education was needed on the use of initial airway support and equipment.

The hospital quickly moved to meet the first recommendation. Each clinic and patient room outside critical care had clear plastic, lockable boxes installed on the wall, with easy access to the patient. Each box contained two self-inflating resuscitation bags (450 and 750 mL), five sizes of masks, and oxygen tubing.

To address the second recommendation, the Code Blue chairperson asked the education department to develop a program that would teach proper initial airway support interventions and the use of airway equipment for infants and children. This program was eventually named "Assessment and Management of the Child in Acute Cardiorespiratory Compromise," or CRC for short. The CRC course consisted of formal lecture, a 50-question written test, and demonstration of selected skills on a CPR mannequin, using specific scenarios to prompt critical decisions and expected behaviors. A "train-the-trainer" approach was used to build an instructor base. Decentralized instructors on each nursing service evaluated and certified nursing staff members.

The Code Blue chairperson and the vice president of nursing determined that the CRC course would be mandatory for about 700 RN staff. A massive teaching effort began in 1993. Because critical care staff maintained Pediatric Advanced Life Support certification, managers in those areas chose to update CRC annually. The medical/surgical and clinic managers chose to update CRC certification every 6 months because they used airway support skills less frequently.

For several years after initiation of the CRC program, the Code Blue Committee evaluated initial airway interventions during code events and found they were improved. The committee felt this was due to the CRC course and periodic recertification updates.

To maintain a high-quality CRC program, content, speakers, and evaluators for each course were evaluated by participants. Based on this feedback, the following changes in process and content were made over the next 2 years:

- The written test was shortened and simplified.
- The detailed scenarios were simplified and the number was reduced from 52 to 5.
- CRC was integrated with Basic Life Support (BLS) to reduce redundancy.
- Nursing leadership decided that only RNs who provide direct patient care would maintain the CRC requirement.

Despite these improvements, concerns continued to surface, such as:

- Does the course continue to make a difference in first-responder airway support?
- Does maintaining this requirement show benefits that outweigh the costs?
- Do critical care RNs and advanced practice nurses who use airway interventions in practice frequently and also maintain additional advanced certification need this requirement as well?
- How should the education department respond to these concerns?

We found that we had many opinions on these issues but no data to support our beliefs. Assessment of the CRC program's effectiveness was in order, but how should it be done and how could the information be used? In early 1996, the director of education and the CRC program coordinator decided the best way to collect data about the CRC program's effectiveness was to conduct outcome evaluations in selected patient care areas. Actual airway intervention practice using simulation scenarios and 10 performance criteria from the CRC course would be used as the evaluation standard. The 10 criteria were:

1. States time frame for primary assessment.
2. States three signs of altered level of consciousness.
3. Demonstrates correct head tilt/chin lift maneuver.
4. Demonstrates "look, listen, and feel."

5. Obtains correct size mask and resuscitation bag.
6. Demonstrates correct use of airway equipment.
7. Performs effective ventilations at age-appropriate rate.
8. Demonstrates steps for problem solving.
9. Assesses central pulses.
10. Performs effective chest compressions at age-appropriate rate.

Because all nurses providing direct patient care had both BLS and CRC certification, each should be able to reproduce these skills on request. A form was developed to establish consistent evaluation criteria and to enhance interrater reliability. Four expert evaluators were chosen by the CRC program coordinator.

A sample of eight units and clinics was selected. Representatives of critical care, medical/surgical, clinic, and home care nursing practice were included. Each manager was informed that the education department wanted data about the CRC program. They were told that individual staff evaluations would take no more than 15 minutes each and were asked not to tell their staff that CRC practice would be evaluated. Tentative dates and times were chosen. An hour before we arrived, area workload was assessed to ensure that the timing of the evaluation would not compromise patient care.

Thirty individual evaluations were completed over a 4-week period using the 10 performance criteria in a scenario that matched the clinical practice of the area. The CRC program coordinator collated and analyzed the results. Comments from nurses evaluated were universally positive; they preferred this type of on-site evaluation of actual practice over the classroom format. Analysis of the 10 performance criteria showed inconsistent practice (more than 14% noncompliance) in criteria 3, 4, and 5. At least one of these inconsistencies was noted in every practice area evaluated.

Now supported by data, the education department made three recommendations to nursing leadership and the Code Blue Committee:

- The CRC program continues to be necessary and is effectively targeted.
- Annual CRC certification for all nurses pro-

viding direct patient care is recommended, unless competency is demonstrated by professional credentialing.

- On-site random periodic evaluation of airway support competence should be continued to evaluate actual practice and to assess the continued need for the CRC program.

Nursing leadership and the Code Blue Committee agreed with each recommendation, and all were implemented.

Use of quality improvement in nursing staff development is a powerful tool to ensure that our educational efforts are well targeted and effective, both for new initiatives and mature educational programs.

REFERENCES

American Nurses Association. (1994). *Standards for nursing professional development: Continuing education and staff development*. Washington, D.C.: American Nurses Publishing.

American Nurses Credentialing Center. (1996). *Manual for accreditation as a provider of continuing education in nursing*. Washington, DC: Author.

Benner, P. (1982). From novice to expert. *American Journal of Nursing*, March, 402–407.

Berwick, D. (1989). Sounding board: Continuous improvement as the ideal in health care. *New England Journal of Medicine, 320*(1), 53–36.

Berwick, D. M., Godfrey, A. B., & Roessner, J. (1991). *Curing health care*. San Francisco: Jossey-Bass.

Crosby, P. B. (1989). *Let's talk quality*. New York: McGraw-Hill.

Day, D. S., & Scidmore, C. (1995). A career ladder program designed by perioperative staff nurses. *Journal of the Association of Operating Room Nurses, 62*(5), 805–809.

DeGraff, J., Bogue, E., & Stout, C. (1996). Strategic dislocation: Reconsidering the role of benchmarking in the development of core competencies. *Best Practices and Benchmarking in Healthcare, 1*(2), 75–83.

Deming, W. E. (1986). *Out of the crisis*. Cambridge, MA: MIT Center for Advanced Engineering Study.

Glenn, M. J., & Smith, J. H. (1995). From clinical ladders to a professional recognition program. *Nursing Management, 26*(3), 41–42.

Griffin, P. (1996). Benchmarking. E-text retrieved from the Quality Network World Wide Web site.

Holpp, L. (1993). Eight definitions of quality in healthcare. *Journal for Quality and Participation*, June, 18–26.

Jeska, S. B., & Fischer, K. J. (1996). *Performance improvement in staff development: The next evolution*. Pensacola, FL: National Nursing Staff Development Organization.

Joint Commission on Accreditation of Healthcare Organizations. (1993, Nov/Dec). A framework for improving the performance of healthcare organizations. *Joint Commission Perspectives Insert*, A1–A6.

Joint Commission on Accreditation of Healthcare Organizations. (1994). *An integrated approach to medical staff performance improvement*. Oakbrook Terrace, IL: Joint Commission on Accreditation of Healthcare Organizations.

Joint Commission on Accreditation of Healthcare Organizations. (1992). *Examples of quality improvement in a hospital setting*. Oakbrook Terrace, IL: Joint Commission on Accreditation of Healthcare Organizations.

Juran, J. M. (1988). *Juran on planning quality*. New York: The Free Press.

Katz, J. M. (1996). Designing a quality management program in educational services. In Rodriguez, L., Patton, C. Steismeyer, J. K., & Teikmanis, M. L. (Eds.). *Manual of staff development*. St. Louis: C.V. Mosby.

Kearns, D. T. (1987). *Competitive benchmarking: What it is and what it can do for you*. Stamford, CT: Xerox Corporation.

Kelly, K. J. (1992). *Nursing staff development: Current competence, future focus*. Philadelphia: J. B. Lippincott.

Kirkpatrick, D. L. (1994). *Evaluating training programs: The four levels*. San Francisco: Berrett-Koehler.

Leebov, W. (1990). *Effective complaint handling in health care.* Chicago: American Hospital Publishing.

Pine, J., & Tingley, J. C. (1993). ROI of soft-skills training. *Training,* February, 55–60.

Senge, P. M., Kleiner, A., Robert, C., Ross, R. B., & Smith, B. J. (1994). *The fifth discipline fieldbook.* New York: Currency Doubleday.

Scholtes, P. (1995). A year's worth of learning. E-text retrieved from Scholtes Seminars and Consulting World Wide Web site.

Shewhart, W. A. (1931). *Economic control of quality manufactured product.* New York: Van Nostrand.

Weber, D. O. (1991). Intermountain Health Care is finding out just how well healthcare can be delivered. *Healthcare Forum Journal,* Sept./Oct., 55–59.

14

Operations Management: Administering the Program

DAVID J. MASSELLO

Every professional in the health care field is sensitive to mounting pressures from the unceasing demands of the consumer, the government, and the media for better health care at lower prices. As a result of these contradictory imperatives, the resources of every viable health care organization must be focused on provision of quality care to restore and maintain health, at the most cost-efficient levels of operation. These pressures continually raise the minimum acceptable levels of quality of care while lowering the maximum acceptable cost levels for efficient operations. It falls to the management of operations to meet this unceasing demand for quality, efficiency, results, and productivity.

To be successful, the organization must consider the clinical staff development program, where the most direct, significant, and powerful impact falls. Some organizations understand the relation between education and the organization's ability to realize the outcomes of quality care and cost-efficient operations, but too many act as if they do not.

One outcome that the staff development program and its specialists must deliver is self-evident: increased capability of the people it develops, educates, and trains. Two others may be less evident: to reduce errors (in both number and magnitude) and to manage and reduce variations in process and technique. Achieving these results makes possible further valuable outcomes:

1. Controlled costs. Increased capability decreases the need for rework and increases the proficiency and the speed with which employees can perform their tasks. Reducing errors increases productivity.
2. Increased group cohesiveness. A NASA study of the commercial aviation industry (cited in Cooper et al., 1979) showed a direct relation between increased capability of the persons in a group and the group's ability to work together effectively. This connection between the increase in capability (education) and group cohesiveness is more powerful than other strategies that might raise group cohesiveness. "Guest relations" or communication programs, when used alone rather than in an integrated way, too often fail to deliver the results.
3. Increased employee satisfaction and customer service. The NASA study cited above, and other research in group dynamics, have shown that when group cohesiveness increases, there is a direct impact on employee satisfaction, and then on customer or patient satisfaction.

The connection between efficient staff development and the successful management of the health care organization is a direct one. In one way or another, clinicians touch all parts of the organization. The more capable clinicians are in these contacts, the better able they are to help the organization get the desired results.

CONCEPTS

Four ideas are vital to the successful operation of a staff development program: systematic process, daily practice, system flow, and "mental to automatic."

Systematic Process

Successful staff development departments must employ systematic processes and procedures in the daily operation. About two thirds of the population prefers to operate in a procedural, step-by-step style. Thus, process and procedure, curriculum, leadership intervention, resource management, outcome measurement, and "in-the-trenches" activities must all reflect some structure and organization. Application of systematic processes delivers the desired results. This chapter on operations management will discuss the systematic process and structures needed to organize and manage resources for optimal results.

Daily Practice

When operations management methodologies are applied to staff development, certain elements, when they are in place, will produce the desired results. These elements are resource management, leader interventions, daily work activities that place the clinical staff development specialist (SDS) in the clinical settings where patient care is delivered, and outcome measurement.

Daily practice is where the philosophies of the leaders in operations management meet the detail, emotion, and humanness of day-to-day operations. Daily practice can interweave a conceptual framework and vision with the details of the day-to-day activity that takes place in all clinical and other areas of operations management. For successful outcomes, these details must be discovered and woven into interventions that will develop clinical leaders.

System Flow

Inevitably, the activities of the staff development department have a systems relation with the entire health care organization. This fact should be reflected fully in the operations management philosophy, strategy, daily practice, and behaviors of the SDSs. Departments and people in health care organizations are already connected through the patients they serve. Staff development is not an isolated process but a pervasive one that provides the "glue" to bond the entire organization. The SDS's teaching affects all care providers, and everyone influenced through teaching and other staff development activities go out into the organization and interact as a result of the teacher's influence. It is impossible *not* to influence learners and care providers. A systems relation exists between the skills and the capabilities of clinicians in an education program and the work they do after completing it. The number of people with whom they interact in their day-to-day activities in the organization reveals the importance of an appropriate staff development program.

Mental to Automatic

Ericsson and Charness (1994) described the structure and acquisition of skill with practice and experience that leads to expert practice. "Mental to automatic" is a phrase that describes the rapid mental processing by experts that can appear almost automatic to the novice. Grasping how people acquire the expertise they exhibit in various contexts is a key point to learn on the part of the SDS. Expert behavior is learned, not inborn or genetic. Ericsson and Charness described the elements of belief, strategy, and behavior required to raise capability to an expert level. They pointed out how people operate from their own "theories of the situation" rather than the facts of the situation.

Gardner (1991) reviewed the research on the way children learn and the development of human intelligence and capability. Gardner stated:

> Much of the story of human development must be written in the light of cultural influences in general and of the particular persons, practices, and paraphernalia of one's culture. And chief among these, of course, in any complex culture, will be such educational institutions as apprenticeships or formal schools. (p. 39)

Staff development departments and processes provide a learning environment in which schooling and development can allow expertise to grow. Skills and concepts are taught during the staff development process. These skills and their attendant beliefs, strategies, and behaviors, properly taught, practiced, and used, will become an autonomic expert response to a known set of external stimuli. Expert behavior is acquired through deliberate practice. Further, the cultural environment in which learning and practice take place affects the acquisition and structure of these skills. Given enough exposure to a specific set of stimuli, an autonomic response is developed. That response is a precise pattern, learned and practiced with intention.

If patterns of behavior are developed independently of the structure and precision of the teaching model, the desired results are at significant risk. The random life and work experience, coupled with uncertainty and variation in daily clinical practice, cannot substitute for intentional learning and practice in developing an expert response pattern. Cultural and organizational influence is directly connected to the systems flow and the daily practice concepts described earlier. They are essential elements in the world of operations management.

MAPPING THE OPERATION

In this section, two aspects of operating and managing a staff development department are addressed: managing programs and projects, and managing people. Although some projects managed by staff development departments have distinct start and stop dates and may be projectlike in nature, the management strategies used to operate projects are similar to those used for educational and developmental programs. Managing people is discussed as a separate category to emphasize its overriding importance to the successful operation of a staff development department.

Managing Programs and Projects

The successful management of programs and projects requires consideration of three important ideas: outcomes, time lines, and resource management.

OUTCOMES

It is important to state the expected outcomes in advance and to be able to measure each outcome in sensory-based evidence (outcomes that can be seen, heard, or felt). What participants want and what the organization wants must be considered as well. These wants and the stated outcomes then can be woven together in a tapestry of a successful program. The discovery of sensory-based evidence is discussed later in this chapter.

TIME LINES

It is important to understand the overall time line for the project or program, and multiple time lines must be aligned—those of the leader of staff development, the overall organization, the program participants, and the clinical managers of the areas where potential participants work. There will also be a time line representing the need for the skills to be taught. Few of these time lines are likely to coincide without the intervention of the SDS.

The most important time line is the one that connects the needed outcome to the resources available to accomplish the task. Several ideas to help connect outcomes to resources to develop project and program time lines are shown in Display 14-1. Ask this question: How does the desired completion date of this program compare with the time line constructed for resource availability? The two often differ. The SDS is probably the only person involved who has detailed and systematic knowledge of the project.

At this point, new agreements can be negotiated with the rest of the organization to reallocate and acquire resources and to modify the outcomes and strategies made possible with this information. Display 14-1 shows the impact of resource availability both on a particular program and on all programs. Changes in scheduling for some programs may be necessary; a new program may have to replace one delayed or canceled.

This time line research and subsequent projection is part of the preparation for both fiscal and annual program plans. The approach can also be used to project time lines and

---

ⒹISPLAY 14-1

Resources Needed for Connection to Planned Outcomes

1. People and skills
   a. Leadership and clinical staff development specialists
   b. Participants
   c. Other content instructors
   d. Managers who control schedules of participants
2. Equipment and facilities
3. Program and project completion date (the one staff development wants)
4. Program and project completion date (what others want)

Set a time line for each resource:

1. Availability—calendar time
2. Number of hours/days
   a. Contiguous time
   b. Blocks of time

Discover replacement resources (if substitutions become necessary)

1. Are they under one's own control?
2. Does someone else have them?
3. Will they be available when needed?
4. Is there an agreement to use them?

the needed resources several years into the future, although in today's dynamic health care environment, planning more than 3 years ahead may be wasteful.

GANTT charts or project management software programs are useful to record the time line and the details of a project. There are several such programs. The prime considerations for software are: Is it simple, fast, and easy to use? If so, does it record time frames, people, resources, tasks, and cost information?

RESOURCE MANAGEMENT

The most significant strategy for the successful management of projects is the management of the resources needed to complete the project and achieve the desired results. These resources are people, equipment, and space. With people, the critical elements are their time and energy and their motivation for the work. The following outline of a resource management methodology reflects the in-the-trenches style of leadership and management identified earlier in this chapter. This method of resource management has three important elements: resource inventory, resource requirement and acquisition, and resource allocation.

Resource Inventory

It is important to know what resources are already available. Of all the resources available, which are in use, and to what extent? Determine the time frame for these resources. Which resources in use now will become available at some date in the future? Resources available now may be committed to another project scheduled to start at some future date. Further, resources needed for one's own program may also be needed by someone else for another program. This knowledge enables the creation of systematic, organization-wide relationships and agreements for the use of valuable and often scarce resources. The resource inventory lists the people available and the skills they bring to the staff development program. This inventory should include each person's capability to teach, to perform various office functions, and to interact with others in group management. It notes their communication capabilities, their personal styles, and their previous successes. Display 14-2 shows some points to be considered in compiling an instructor inventory; of course, organizational modifications should be made to fit the circumstances.

Resource Requirement and Acquisition

For each program, a model of the resources required must be created. This model lists the people needed and the skills and capabilities they possess that will help deliver the desired results. It should also include the equipment and the space required by the project. This requirements list must also contain the time line in which the program will operate. It must be prepared carefully to accommodate enough time to perform each of the tasks required in the project.

The completed list of resource requirements is then compared to the resource inventory, and then the inventory list is reviewed against the requirements of the resource model. How is it the same, and how is it different from the model? Each item listed must be written in sensory-based terminology; accuracy and reliability are essential to success.

When complete, this comparison validates the list of resources that must be acquired. This may be nominal or significant. It may be necessary to go outside the organization for some of these resources; others may be located within the organization. It may be necessary to negotiate agreements with other managers to use certain resources. It takes time to acquire resources through negotiations and agreements, so this work must be done well in advance of the announcement of any program. These time lines must be accounted for in the GANTT chart for the program.

DISPLAY 14-2

Resource Inventory for a Potential Instructor

Program Instructor

PROGRAM CAPABILITY—WHAT THIS PERSON CAN TEACH

_____ CPR

_____ IV therapy

_____ Monitor management—Critical care

_____ Fire safety

_____ (Other)

_____

THIS TEACHER'S EXPERIENCE

_____ Program knowledge

_____ Teaching styles

_____ Participant response and feedback

_____ Participant outcomes

_____ Manager response and feedback

_____ Participant capability (after working with this instructor)

_____ (Other)

_____

EDUCATION AND TRAINING

_____ Curriculum content

_____ Teaching process

_____ (Other)

_____

HUMAN SKILLS

_____ Listens

_____ Gives and accepts feedback

_____ (Other)

_____

Resource Allocation

If there is one idea that is consistent in operations management, it is this: there are rarely enough resources for all the work that needs to be done. Thus, the allocation of resources among ongoing projects and along various time lines becomes an important element of success in operations management. It is important to connect this realization with the operational reality that people want results on their own time lines, and they often arrive at these time lines in a completely encapsulated and unsystematic thinking process. Indeed,

TABLE 14-1

MATRIX FOR BUDGET PLANNING

Item	Program A	B	C	D	E	F	G	H	I
Faculty fee									
Faculty travel									
Program site rental									
Catering									
Promotion									
Program materials									
AV rental									
Miscellaneous									
Anticipated registrants									
Projected fee									
Anticipated revenue									
Totals									

From Kelly, K. J. (Ed.). (1992). *Nursing staff development* (1st ed.). Philadelphia: J. B. Lippincott. Used with permission.

the SDS may be the only person in the entire organization who routinely thinks systemically about the allocation, acquisition, and use of the scarce resources required for staff development. This makes it even more important to use the skills of resource allocation in managing projects. Table 14-1 shows a budget planning matrix that can help the SDS plan for required resources.

Resource requirements, acquisition, and allocation are calculated specifically for each project and program, and then systemically for all projects and programs. The manager of each department must fully understand the resource availability and requirements demanded by the desired outcomes. To reach this understanding, all the needs of all the projects and programs must be woven together—all the resource requirements, acquisition strategies and needs, and allocation methodologies for all the programs. This process of resource allocation will contribute to the preparation of an accurate and reliable fiscal operating budget and capital budget for the department.

FLEXIBILITY

Even the best-laid plans are changed, due to such factors as individual decision making, modifications to the amount and type of resources available, time lines that are extended or compressed, the desires of people who have the capability to influence and direct other people, and even the volatility in the health care field. Regardless of the underlying reason for change, flexibility is a requirement for the success of programs. How staff development managers respond to the need or the demand for modification of their plans is an important element of success in operations management.

SIMULATIONS

One of the great characteristics of education and training in the health care field is its emphasis on teaching what to do when the unexpected occurs. In health care, as in aviation, there is a critical need for accuracy and precision. In each profession, human beings are the primary source of errors that lead to adverse outcomes, including death.

No one can predict the future, but we can simulate possible futures. In operations management, it is important to think about what can happen and what actions to take when the original resource management plan must be modified, such as:

- What to do if the people allocated to a program become unavailable
- What to do if space and equipment resources break down or are unavailable
- What to do if the organization changes the staff development department's budget allocation a third of the way through the fiscal year
- What to do if a program fails to produce the results expected during its initial implementation.

Most of us are aware of crisis management strategies, "back-filling" strategies, and damage control. All of these are skills that are developed over time by people who have been caught off-guard by developments that disrupted their best-laid plans. Unfortunately, everyone, to some extent, allows these crisis management strategies to become common or even everyday strategies for operations. Thus, a response to some unforeseen crisis can distract one from returning to the plan when the emergency is over. In the pressure cooker of modern health care operations, there appears to be a never-ending series of demands for change. Frequent use reduces these crisis management skills to expert behavior, and we find ourselves managing daily affairs as though each day were a crisis.

It is vital to the success of managing programs that possible futures be simulated. Display 14-3 is a simple template that can be used to simulate futures for any project. It is apparent from this simulation process that the most significant and most variable resource to be managed is people.

Managing People

In my early days in the health care field, I worked for an administrator whose admitted style of management was intimidation and fear. One of his strategies was to write a subordinate a memorandum the day after he or she left on a 2-week vacation, assigning a task that had to be completed the day before the end of the vacation. On getting back to the office and finding this memorandum, the employee was already late with a task that was a total surprise. When I asked this administrator to explain how he could expect the impossible, he would respond, "I know you couldn't do it; I just wanted to let you know who was in charge."

That occurred in the 1970s; managing people is different today. A leader's style and the behavior he or she uses to interact with others are driven most often by a set of autonomic responses generated from his or her life experience and learning. The response of some people to others at work may actually be more appropriate for a parent–child relationship than for the workplace.

Hogan et al. (1994) cited a study examining the personality measures that influenced the team performance of commercial airline flight crews. This study showed that flight

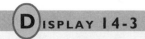

ISPLAY 14-3

Simulation Thinking—Behavioral Management for Leaders

Step 1—Describe the current context within which results are wanted. Describe it fully, so it is an accurate and reliable and consistent presentation of the current situation. In this description it is important to list all the people with whom the leader must interact to get results.

Step 2—In thinking about this context, be mindful of the desired results. List the necessary outcomes you want, and be sure to describe them in sensory-based terminology, so they can be measured. Sensory terminology here means specifically what can be seen, heard, and felt.

Step 3—It is important to understand how you are motivated for this result. What will the sensory-based results listed in Step 2 make possible for you? In the current jargon, you must go ''meta'' to the results to understand your motivation. It must be fully understood as it applies to the business issues, to professional issues, to self-esteem, to ''looking good'' and other vanity issues, to self-worth, and to the results for the organization. By following this procedure, each of these perspectives can be seen as proper, appropriate, accurate, and reliable within any context where results are wanted. They represent the ''theory of the situation'' (NASA, 1979).

Step 4—For the attainment of each result listed in Step 2, there are prerequisite conditions. As the college student finds that passing 101 is a prerequisite to taking 102, one must also understand the prerequisite conditions. List them. For each desired outcome, repeat the question—what are the prerequisites for this result? In this field, prerequisites are the beliefs, capabilities, strategies, behaviors, and environments that must be in place to enable each desired outcome. This process will reveal that the needed information is at hand. Some examples of prerequisites are:

1. Belief that education raises capability and productivity
2. Belief that people are well intended
3. Strategy to connect the teaching program to the business plan of the organization
4. Staff capabilities for particular tasks
5. Behavior that produces the desired patient satisfaction—rapport

Step 5—Step 1 described the context in which results were needed and listed the people with whom you must interact to get results. Now describe those people, as fully as you understand them. This understanding will be accurate and reliable because it is your own view, the leader's ''theory of the situation'' in which all concerned work. Here are examples of these characteristics that will appear in the list of people: happy, angry, sad, motivated, not motivated, lethargic, well educated, poorly educated, lacking in time, having too much time, intelligent, spontaneous, fun to be with, dissatisfied, defensive, afraid, unsure of self.

Step 6—For each of the characteristics listed in Step 5, reflect on what you are like when interacting with someone who has that characteristic. For example, if a student is described as being uninterested and failing to participate, the teacher should ask what he or she is like when interacting with such a student. Be accurate in describing these personal responses. Do this for each characteristic listed, and the result will be a list of your own assets (capabilities, beliefs, behaviors, and strategies) available for the task at hand.

To pursue the example above, a student in class appears uninterested and fails to participate. Create a simulation of possible responses in this context. When interacting with someone who reflects these characteristics, the teacher becomes annoyed and wants to put even more energy into teaching to draw the uninterested student into the process. Now ask this question: When I work with someone who is uninterested and fails to participate and I am annoyed, how does being annoyed help me get the results described in Step 2?

Then ask a further question: When interacting with someone who is uninterested and fails to participate, and I put more energy into my teaching to draw him or her into the process, how does expending more energy help me get the desired results?

Step 7—From the list of capabilities in Step 6, choose those that represent the intelligence, energy, and motivation needed to get results. A powerful pattern of skills, capabilities, and beliefs can now be followed.

This template is used in specific contexts, and it recognizes that human behavior occurs in patterns, within contexts. It can be used for a leader, with other people, and with groups of virtually any size.

Source: Business Performance Institute (1997). Used with permission.

crew performance, defined by the number and severity of errors made by crew members, is correlated with the personality of the captain or leader:

Crews with leaders who were warm, friendly, self-confident, and able to stand up to pressure made the fewest errors. Conversely, crews with captains who were arrogant, hostile, boastful, egotistical, passive-aggressive, or dictatorial made the most errors. (p. 23)

A previous study performed with NASA in 1979 by Cooper et al., cited by Weiner and Nagel (1988), showed that both autocratic and participative leadership strategies, when chosen too often or inappropriately, generated the most numerous and severe errors among crew members.

There are three powerful strategies for managing people that every leader must consider:

1. Developing trust
2. Dealing with resistance
3. Building rapport and relationships with a wide variety of people and in a wide variety of circumstances.

Through these strategies, the leader displays concern for his or her coworkers, their success, their well-being, and their satisfaction.

STRATEGY ONE: DEVELOPING TRUST

Our models for trust in relationships extend back to childhood: parents, grandparents, aunts and uncles, brothers and sisters, or significant other adult influences. Our understanding and knowledge of trust expand as we build relationships with people in grade school and high school and college. We live life together, learning and experiencing a person over 20, 30, or 40 years. In an ever-increasing number of situations, we become able to predict how someone will respond. This predictability expands our capacity to trust, even including behaviors that we may find unacceptable. We can trust someone given to occasional unacceptable behavior, if it is predictable.

In organizations, several important elements for building trust in this manner are missing. The familiarity gained from spending 30 years together is absent; people know each other through only a limited number and type of contacts, which makes it difficult to predict a coworker's actions accurately and reliably. This predictability factor is one of the goals of simulations for the future.

In organizations, trust is built and maintained through three powerful conditions: accuracy, reliability, and consistency. Think about trustworthy people, and it becomes easy to understand how important these conditions are.

Set aside the idea of honesty and focus on the idea of accuracy. Trustworthy associates are accurate in how they present themselves and what they know and believe. They are accurate in their strategy for thinking through an idea. They are accurate in how they approach collecting and analyzing information. Set aside the idea of earth-shaking accuracy that might win a Nobel Prize. The accuracy that we appreciate in people we trust is an accuracy attributable to them personally; it is also a tribute to the way they think, approach their work, and interact with others.

When we think about people we trust, we think of reliability. These people give their word and keep it. We also know those who give their word and don't keep it. Failure to keep one's word is annoying. People do not want to trust those who fail to keep their word, even if we can predict what they will do.

The people we trust are consistent. Each time we interact with them, they present themselves in the same way. In every context of acquaintanceship, we can be confident that they will use the same language strategies, tones of voice, body positions, thinking methodologies, and attitudes. These predictable characteristics we have come to know as consistency.

These three elements—accuracy, reliability, and consistency—are the underpinnings of trust in all relationships. Most leaders usually have little opportunity to choose the people with whom they will work and interact, the people they manage, so one is forced into a multitude of relationships, sometimes with people one dislikes. Leaders, however, must accommodate everyone who works and interacts with him or her to produce the results that the organization requires.

STRATEGY TWO: DEALING WITH RESISTANCE

The second important ingredient in managing people is knowing how to deal with resistance, considered by many the single most powerful and often negative force in the workplace. It is important to understand resistance and to adopt a strategy to use the energy of resistance to get results.

In his book on the therapeutic techniques of Erickson, Haley (1973) spoke of Erickson's strategy for handling resistance. His fundamental approach was one of acceptance: he actually encouraged resistance, understanding the powerful motivation, intellect, and energy that make it possible. By accepting and even encouraging resistance, the attempts to resist become a form of cooperative behavior. When subordinates cooperate, even in their resistance, the leader can begin to channel that motivation, energy, and intellect into new thinking that will produce more appropriate results for the leader, the employees, and the organization.

Resistance is a learned behavior. Children are taught to resist; every child is warned not to talk to strangers or to get into the car with a stranger offering candy. Girls are taught how to resist the unwanted advances of young men who find them particularly attractive. Children are taught to resist drug and alcohol abuse. Churches teach their followers how to hold onto their philosophy, principles, and ethics and morals and to resist those who beckon them down dangerous or inappropriate pathways. This kind of resistance is to be encouraged, and we use our intellect, energy, and motivation to sustain it.

It should come as no surprise to anyone working in an organization that people are powerfully capable of resistance. The leader should be excited and enthusiastic when resistance is encountered, and should even enjoy it; he or she should want to have even more resistance and try to understand it fully. The resister is paying attention, is involved, and is taking part. Once we understand resistance, we can begin to tap the resister's intelligence and energy and can direct the energy and intellect behind it toward more productive outcomes.

STRATEGY THREE: BUILDING RAPPORT AND RELATIONSHIP

A third important consideration for managing people is how to build rapport and relationships. Hogan et al. (1994) described leadership as:

> Persuasion, not domination. A person with power to require others to obey is not necessarily a leader. Rather, leadership is a measure of one's ability to influence and persuade others. There is a causal and definitive link between leadership and team performance. (p. 493)

The authors reported on organizational climate studies from the mid-1950s to 1988. These studies showed that 60% to 75% of all employees in most organizations felt that the worst or most stressful part of their job was dealing with their immediate supervisor.

When we talk about rapport and relationships, we are talking about the management of self—the leader's ability to manage his or her own behavior and focus that behavior toward the desired results. This requires the leader to understand and respect the motiva-

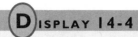

How to Get What You Want

How to Get What You Want has four important steps.

Step 1—Describe what you want in positive terms. When what you want is in negative terms, reframe it to the positive by asking what you want instead. As an example, assume the problem is, "I don't like the attitude of the students in my class." The reframed question would ask what you want instead of the present attitude of the students.

Step 2—When you describe what you want in positive terms, you must specify the evidence that will let you know you have it. This evidence must be stated in sensory-based terminology. Sensory-based evidence can be seen, heard, or felt (and sometimes tasted and smelled). Secondly, you must understand motivation. To understand motivation, ask yourself, "What is important about this idea for me?" When using this template with another individual or group, modify the question: "What is important about this idea for you?" When you get what you want, what will that make possible for you; what will this result do for you?

Step 3 Control—Admittedly, we have very little control over the behavior and activities and thinking processes of other people. Thus, the definition of a leader is one who is influential and persuasive, rather than controlling and directive. Think about the behavior of others as a response to the influence that you as leader and manager have developed through your rapport and relationship, your trust and respect for the resistance offered by these people. In this section of the template, we ask, "Can you get what you want with no one else doing anything or changing anything? Can you act totally independently of all others in the context in which you work and get the results that you want?" When the answer is yes, then you are in a great position to get what you want. The answer, however, is most often no.

To get the results you want, reduce your desired outcome to smaller pieces. As you do so, you will begin to discover actions you can take over which you have complete control.

Example—The desired outcome is that a group of people learn a new skill. This fails the control test. You need other people, over whom you have no control, to do things and to change to realize this outcome.

Consider the steps necessary to enable other people to learn a new skill:
1. Teach the material.
2. Design an effective program.
3. Understand the criteria students have for learning new skills.
4. Students need to study.
5. Students need to practice.

One, two, and three are under your control; four and five are not.

Step 4 Ecology—An ecological assessment is conducted for the desired result. Ask the question, "When I get the result I want, what are the consequences for me and for others? Will I keep the good things I already have?" (This requires an inventory within the context of your work with other people.) Ecology assessments require a systemic understanding—*before* you take action—of the outcome you want, both from your own point of view and from the perspective of those around you in the organization.

Source: Business Performance Institute (1997). Used with permission.

tion, the energy, and the willingness to learn of his or her subordinates. Displays 14-3 and 14-4 are two templates for models of success that can be used to build and maintain rapport, influence, and persuasion with coworkers (Massello, 1995).

When teaching clinical skills, for instance, the desired result is for people to learn the material and then replicate the skills and knowledge in the care of patients. We can measure the evidence for this result from test results. We can witness students' performance in a laboratory environment, and we can listen to them describe the material they have learned. We can observe their interactions with patients as they perform the tasks we have taught them in the classroom. However, we cannot control the learning someone else does. In a teaching environment, learning is a process of influence and motivation as well as instruction. Thus, it is important that these people be motivated to learn what we want to teach them. We need to have a powerful relationship with them.

Ecology is an important consideration in teaching (see Display 14-4). When we get what we want—when people learn the material and can replicate the tasks and ideas they have been taught—we can keep the good things we already have, and so will they. What are the consequences for us and for others when they learn this material and can perform these functions? One of the many aspects of ecology is the interaction between what we want and the self-esteem, self-worth, and motivation of the people around us. Here we must apply the systemic thinking strategies mentioned earlier in this chapter and understand fully the effects on the system of the result we want.

For example, re-engineering projects often involve moving to patient-centered or patient-focused care. In such initiatives, there is often a reduction in the number of RNs who work on a particular nursing floor; unlicensed assistive personnel (UAPs) assume some of these duties, and the remaining RNs must also take on additional tasks. Training is required to accomplish this. What ecology must prevail to ask an RN with a bachelor's degree and 10 years of experience to perform phlebotomy tasks?

Display 14-3 offers a pattern for simulation thinking managers can use to affect staff behavior and bring about desired results. By using it, any leader can simulate the identities, beliefs, strategies, capabilities, behaviors, and environments that can provide or prevent the necessary result. Our colleagues in psychotherapy inform us that human beings operate internally and in parts, and can and do see the same idea through multiple perspectives. Thus, part of me may really enjoy learning new things, but another part may not. A UAP, knowing that others are upset about the re-engineering process being implemented by the hospital, may well be apprehensive about taking the place of an RN. He or she may also be unsure of his or her skills and competency after only 2 weeks of training and practice. A leader may be powerfully motivated and challenged to produce results while also having misgivings about the very ideas he or she feels so motivated about.

This concept must be understood as a normal human condition. The leader must understand fully the impact of any of his or her perspectives (beliefs, capabilities, behaviors). The power of leadership is the ability to know and choose the perspective that delivers the desired result.

HUMAN RESOURCES POLICY AND MANAGING PEOPLE

Managers of people must comply with their organization's human resources policies and procedures, including:

- Job descriptions
- Requirements for new hires and promotions
- Budgets
- Salary and wage administration
- Compliance with job evaluations and disciplinary processes.

Some of the resources available to help managers comply with these requirements are:

- The American Society for Training and Development
- Colleagues in staff development
- Job descriptions from professional societies
- Job descriptions from colleagues
- Professionals in the organization's human resources department.

The first edition of this book (Kelly, 1992) included sample performance standards and development practice manuals for nursing education services. It is an excellent reference for more detailed information.

PRODUCTIVITY

This section examines productivity from two perspectives:

1. Productivity that can be enhanced through the teaching efforts of SDSs
2. Productivity of SDSs.

We will begin with the second and then will return to the first.

How Much

The productivity of SDSs is vital to the success of the organization. Calculate the education, skill set, and competency needs of your organization, and you will begin to understand how much capability the organization needs. What specifically does it need to be capable of, and who in the organization needs this capability? From the perspective of the SDS, the number of people and the amount of time required to train them appropriately far outstrip the resources available for the task. This becomes even more significant in light of the fast-paced time frames that are part of the health care environment today.

The importance of productivity is apparent, but measuring it is another matter entirely. How much time should the SDS spend in the classroom? How much time should be spent making agreements with people whose cooperation is needed? How much time should be allocated to the environment and managing scarce resources? How much time is appropriate to spend in meetings? How much for back-filling and rework? What agreement exists with management as to how productivity will be measured? How is this measurement the same and how it is different from the one applied in staff development?

Here are two ideas to improve personal productivity. First, make agreements—with bosses, with peers, with the managers of departments whose people are to be taught, and with students themselves—about the criteria by which to judge productivity. For example, what will be the outcome if the department teaches 200 people and the organization needs to put 700 through the education programs? It may be quite a significant effort to teach 200 people with the available resources, but in the whole organization 500 people will remain without the skills they need for the organization to achieve the needed results. These agreements must be made in the budget process in preparation for each new fiscal period and as an appropriate, accurate, reliable strategy to the further understanding of productivity.

Second, use the template in Display 14-4. Several months before entering budget negotiations, specify the desired results and how each result is connected to the needs of the organization and its business plan. Calculate accurately how many people need training, what training they need, and how much time will be required in the classroom, in the laboratory, and for on-the-job coaching and mentoring. These needs must be specified for one's own staff and also for the management and staff of the operating departments of the organization.

These calculations can be translated into full-time equivalents for the staff development department and will show the number of people required to fulfill the education obligations for the organization. This process will reveal whether the full-time equivalents actually needed are the same as or different from the budget allocations prescribed for the department.

State of the Art

Improvements in productivity are achieved by stripping away unnecessary behaviors, beliefs, and strategies. Select only those beliefs, behaviors, capabilities, and strategies that can actually produce the desired results.

In clinical practice, pathways are developed that produce successful clinical outcomes. In CPR training, a pattern of behavior is taught and used that delivers the results wanted in the most proficient, cost-effective way possible while maintaining the quality of care and the medical outcome most desirable for the patient. The same methodology can be applied to improving productivity. Here is one way to increase productivity and proficiency, using the template in Display 14-4:

1. Determine the desired outcome. Then complete all four steps of *How To Get What You Want* (see Display 14-4).
2. Determine the skills and resources needed to get the results specified in Step 1. Remember, not every resource is needed in every context to get results; it is easy to commit more resources than necessary to produce a desired result. Practicing skills in a deliberate fashion increases proficiency more quickly than merely performing them. Remember this concept when considering resources and skills. As an employee's proficiency increases and he or she becomes more expert, productivity is enhanced, the number and severity of errors is reduced, rework is diminished, and speed increase.
3. When considering the desired result and the steps already taken to get that result, list the capabilities, strategies, skills, and resources used in that process. Ask this question for each resource in the list: What lets one know that this resource helps attain the result, and specifically how does this resource help do it? Remember, not every resource is required in every context to produce the desired outcome.
4. Assess the department's customers and the managers and staff people it serves, and discover what the department delivers that actually makes it possible for them to get the results they want. Sometimes we place components in a program or a project that we believe are essential but that go unnoticed or are considered frivolous by the customer.
5. In this light, modify the original list of resources and the design you use to get results, and test the new model and pattern.

Productivity Measures

Methods to determine productivity measures for the staff development department are evolving. These formulas are used to demonstrate the quantitative contribution of the staff development program. Most efforts to define productivity begin with a measure of the efficiency with which labor, materials, and goods are converted into goods and services. Linear time standards are often used to express the productivity of SDSs; others use automated systems to accumulate data about staff development productivity. Ulschak (1988) conducted a survey of productivity measures used in hospital training departments and found the following to be most commonly used:

- Achievement of goals and objectives
- Number of participants multiplied by hours in class
- Number of hours per program per instructor
- Set standards based on work units
- Number of programs offered

- Number of contact hours awarded
- Monthly or quarterly reports
- Daily activity logs.

Each of these measures has advantages and disadvantages, but all suffer from a lack of comparison with expected productivity. Kelly (1990) developed a formula that calculated a ratio of expected instructional hours to actual instructional hours given in a calendar year. The expected hours of instruction were calculated based on the number of employees who were expected to accumulate a specified amount of hours each year, and modified with an average attendance. The actual hours of instruction were calculated using program records and modified with an average attendance. Hours of instruction were used rather than contact hours because orientation consumed resources as well. Each year the final figure is compared with the expected figure to determine overall departmental productivity. This formula, used in several organizations during development, is a comprehensive and efficient approach that can be used to determine departmental productivity. Another source that may be useful in some staff development settings is Edwards (1996), who proposed a detailed education allocation system to verify productivity.

The perceived value of staff development to the organization is often subjective. The collection of data and outcomes measures to support this perceived value is an important component of the staff development manager's role.

Productivity is more than just mathematics. Productivity involves detailed in-the-trenches examination of the resources, skills, capabilities, beliefs, identities, and behaviors that we use to produce results. It requires a test of the result itself to ascertain just what resources will produce the outcomes we want in any given context.

BUDGET PLANNING

When difficult financial decisions must be made, education is an easy item to remove from the organization's budget. It usually has the least political impact, and its results in the organization are harder to document and pinpoint. Budgets and budget planning continue to challenge SDSs, and the following information gives perspective and suggestions about this task and process. A framework is presented, followed by practical application of budget basics.

Theoretical Framework

Many theories are available to help the staff development leader manage and administer the department. Classic theories relating to systems, roles, bureaucracies, and leadership have been described, researched, and applied to a variety of health care organizational situations. However, there have been few investigations done to test theories regarding the organization and management of staff development departments. This does not mean theoretical models are not used in practice: to provide the full spectrum of staff development services, some form of organization, task specialization, and decision-making arrangement must exist.

As staff development administrators and department managers become more sophisticated in their designs of programs and departments, more will use organization and management theories. One organizing theory is presented here; others will and should be proposed to meet the continually changing needs of health care organizations.

CRITICAL CONCEPTS OF CONTINGENCY THEORY

To help organizations and in particular clinical personnel accommodate change, it is useful to adopt "open systems" concepts. Contingency theory is a systems theory useful for the staff development administrator.

Classical theorists generally believe there is one best way to organize. Proponents of contingency theory believe that the integration of the environment, technology, and structure of organizations will lead to success, and advocate a variety of structures to meet goals. Woodward (1958), a British researcher, first proposed this theory when she studied the relation between organizational structure and success. She found no relationship between these two concepts during her investigation of English manufacturing firms. She concluded that different technologies imposed different kinds of demands on employees and organizations. Woodward also determined that successful organizations have a structure appropriate to meet these demands. Burns and Stalker (1961) focused on the environment and studied internal management practices and the relation to rates of change in scientific techniques and marketing. They found that each system was appropriate to its own specific set of conditions. Again, a challenge to the "one best way" approach was advanced. Burns and Stalker also suggested that organizational structure depends on the nature of the organizational environment, both internal and external.

Charns and Schaefer (1983) advanced a contingency model for health care organizations. They defined the work of organizations as consisting of two types, direct and managerial, and were among the first to blend these concepts in this way. They divided this direct and managerial work into three elements: structure, coordination, and people. Thus, they modified contingency theory to include people, a feature not specifically addressed by previous authors. In addition, they saw managerial and direct work as organizational work; previous investigators saw management as something done to accomplish work or output. This important distinction is one of the appealing concepts of the Charns and Schaefer model because it recognizes the integration of management work and direct work, rather than management as directing and controlling work. This integration is also consistent with current clinical practice delineations; that is, clinical practice embraces clinical, administrative, and research practitioners, who are all considered to practice and provide health care in various roles.

Charns and Schaefer emphasized environment as the most important element in their framework. In their application of contingency theory to health care, they defined the direct work of organizations as the provision of services to patients. Managerial work includes the strategies and technologies used to accomplish the purposes and objectives of the organization. To extend this concept to staff development, direct work is the provision of services to patients, and staff development work is one managerial strategy used to attain the goal of quality care and the objective of delivering care by competent staff.

This model of contingency theory blends many of the concepts of other contingency theorists and adds new elements that further refine the theory. Contingency theory, although just one of many management theories, seems to have wide appeal. Experience teaches us that there is no single best way to organize a staff development department; various structures meet with success in various organizations. However, the concepts proposed by contingency theory can be applied to the design of staff development services and departments. As departments continue to improve their structure and organization of services, contingency theory can be used to guide that process.

APPLICATION TO STAFF DEVELOPMENT

Charns and Schaefer also proposed a model that illustrates the distinct interaction of all elements (Fig. 14-1). This model of organization and management provides a framework

Charns and Schaefer contingency model
for management

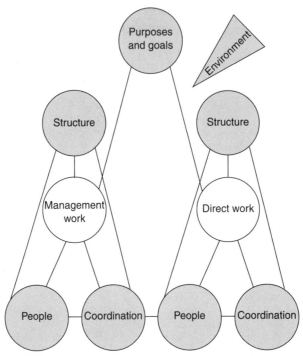

FIGURE 14-1. Contingency model for management. Charns, M.P., & Schaefer, M.J. (1983). Health care organizations: A model for management. Englewood Cliffs, NJ: Prentice-Hall.

for decision making and administration within the staff development department. The administrator may find the following elements and concepts useful when designing or redesigning the structure and organization of the staff development department.

Environment
Administrators consider the organizational environment when determining programs and projects. Elements of the environment include:

- Patients (as clients)
- Consumers of education programs
- Governmental bodies such as the health department
- Regulatory bodies such as the Joint Commission on Accreditation of Healthcare Organizations
- Professional associations and their published standards of practice
- Anticipated or planned changes in services and expectations of departments within the nursing division, particularly those that clearly indicate a need for educational programming to meet identified goals. Most changing organizations would benefit from the use of staff development services to assist with the

changes. This includes changes in competency expectations (*e.g.*, nurses will perform a new procedure) as well as changes in structure and care delivery systems (*e.g.*, nurses must learn how to organize their care within new systems).

Purposes and Goals

The administrator should verify clearly with other nurse administrators their purposes and goals for their assigned areas of responsibility. Only then can the administrator design a staff development program that will address the scope of expected services and the purpose and goals of the educational effort. Successful staff development administrators are those who can link programs intimately with organizational goals and objectives.

Work

Staff development work has been defined as a process that assesses, maintains, and develops nursing competencies. Work associated with this process includes programs such as orientation, in-service education, continuing education, leadership development, skills training, and competency assessment. Several of these work assignments have evolved over the past decade and are frequently designed in response to particular needs of the organization. Past successes with staff development efforts designed to bring about change are more likely to yield creative and flexible responses to organizational needs.

The direct work of staff development is defined as the service delivery mechanisms, such as direct provision of education, coordination, consultation, and collaboration.

Structure

The staff development organizational chart should recognize the talents and skills of SDSs and should be fluid enough to allow for new assignments. The chart should be reviewed and updated regularly. Program reassignments are made based on the changing needs of the organization. Formal communication lines of SDSs to the administrator and clients should also be specified through this structure.

Coordination

The administrator should play a significant role in setting up systems to coordinate activities with the many consumers of staff development services. Structure also dictates who typically is involved in most staff development transactions.

People

Staff development is a service provided for people by people. The skills, abilities, perceptions, motivations, and satisfactions of SDSs should be integrated into their job design to attain high levels of productivity. SDSs also need role development. One of the most important elements of this role development is the ability to remain flexible in the changing environment, with a refined ability to respond to changing needs.

The administrator who uses these elements to refine the staff development program should then define indicators of success. One indicator of success is the positive effect of the staff development program on the organization's accomplishment of purposes and goals. Structure, people, and coordination can be redefined as needed to continue to help the organization effect its mission.

There is some evidence that this theory, or selected elements of it, is already in use by staff development directors. The various structures and forms of staff development programs and departments are indicators that the environment of the organization is already the primary factor in designing staff development programs. Other elements in this model should also be addressed by administrators.

The use of contingency theory as a potential framework for the administration, organization, and design of the staff development program and department will contribute to the success of this effort. Organizations are dynamic, so units such as staff development must maintain a high degree of flexibility and tolerance for ambiguity to contribute to the organization's success. This theory encourages those characteristics.

Basics

Several working presuppositions can be used to guide the preparation of an appropriate and effective budget:

1. Clinical staff development is a powerful intervention. When an employee's capability is increased, errors are reduced, both in number and in magnitude, rework is reduced, and productivity, speed, and proficiency are increased.
2. The audience for a department's budget does not know what its manager knows about its business. The corporate finance people understand numbers, but not the numbers according to the staff development department. Nursing leadership understands the concepts, but not the details of what SDSs do. The staff development budget must be written to satisfy the criteria of those around it—finance personnel, clinical managers, and the managers of the students. These criteria will be congruent in some parts and will disagree in other parts.
3. There is more demand for money in the organization than there is money in the organization to satisfy the demand.

From these presuppositions, two main themes in budget basics may be derived.

First, as simple as it sounds, the department head must be able to multiple, divide, add, and subtract accurately and must learn to extrapolate. Extrapolation is a mathematical process through which small elements of accurate, reliable data are used to project larger data samples. For extrapolation to work properly, those small elements of accurate and reliable data must satisfy the various criteria of one's own department and of everyone who will review and approve its budget.

Second, accurate, reliable, and consistent data are needed. It is hard to find information that is 100% accurate and reliable; whether it is contained in manual records or in computer files, the question of accuracy and completeness can easily be raised. It is important to use live, current information, such as that derived from work sampling, both to calculate the budget and to support and justify it. Current data, collected through direct observation and data logs, make it possible to validate other data bases from which additional information may be drawn—for example, reports generated from data bases collected as a part of normal operations.

In work sampling, observation is important. Observers should be candid and independent of anyone in staff development. Financial personnel should be offered the opportunity to observe, as should nurse managers and other outside observers, while live samples are being gathered. Sample size needs to be considered when using the work sampling methodology. Generally, samples can be taken in 1-week blocks separated by 2 or 3 weeks. Two 1-week data samples should be collected and extrapolated, and then a third sample used to confirm the data collected in the first two. In a staff development context, several classes from one program can be sampled and the findings validated with a third class several weeks later.

When the calculation to annualize or add up and divide by month or trend is performed, the information must be connected to data available through existing data bases. This information makes it possible to validate and challenge any data base. Most data bases in the organization are generated through financial and clinical computer systems. Each places a premium on accuracy and reliability, even when they are not. This gives the administrator even more reason to sample the department's programs and projects.

The information collected in work samples, augmented by observers' comments, includes:

- General information
  - Number of programs offered
  - Number of people trained
  - How the curriculum is connected to the business plan of the organization
- Project-specific information (with observations)
  - Class length (hours, days, weeks)
  - Number of participants
  - Handouts and assigned readings
  - Class structure
    Lesson plan
    Sequence of events
    Teaching style
    Use of laboratory experience
    Mentor or coach process
- In-class activity
  - Participant activity
  - Participant interaction
  - Participant motivation for out-of-class assignments and their completion
- Relation of class time, date, coaching, and leading to proficiency, error rate, and reductions in severity of error.

Testimonials from customers who are managers, participants, and physicians in the organization are an important resource.

There is a valuable advanced step in the budgeting process. Budgeting in organizations eventually becomes a negotiation, and when negotiating any business arrangement, knowing several important pieces of information proves invaluable. First, the administrator must know the criteria that are used by those who will review and approve the budget so that he or she can prepare a budget to satisfy those criteria. Second, the administrator should prepare several simulations of the budget first. The construction of each simulation will present a picture of the department's ability to deliver the results the organization wants.

In negotiation, the staff development manager will be asked a wide variety of questions by people who, generally speaking, are unfamiliar with the department's business. The department manager is the one person in the negotiation who understands the department's business and the numbers in its budget.

There should be at least three simulations in addition to the basic budget. The first simulation must answer the questions: What will happen when more money is allocated than requested? What will happen if the organization asks for even more than the budget projects? A second simulation must answer the question: What if the department is asked to drop one or more planned programs and replace them with other programs that management may find more appropriate and significant? A third simulation must prepare the way to discuss what will happen if the budget is reduced but the hospital still requires the department to produce the same results. The department manager must understand fully how much of a reduction can be accepted while still delivering the results the organization wants.

This information is essential before entering into budget calculations and negotiations. Budget calculations are simple when one has accurate and reliable data. Budget negotiations become even easier when one is prepared, through budget simulations, to discuss a variety of budget forms and structures. Most important of all is to have the budget, the working presuppositions, and the supporting data reflect how the budget request is connected to what other people want and to the important issues of the organization and its business plan for the coming fiscal period.

Resource Allocation Analysis

Three elements are central to resource allocation analysis: cost effectiveness, cost benefit, and outcome measurement. Before we can determine cost effectiveness and benefits, we must first understand what happens when people are taught how to be more capable than they already are.

The outcome of staff development is competence. The goal is to increase the capability of the people taught. When their capability is increased, their confidence and group cohesiveness are expanded. They are given more resiliency and more stamina. Their errors are reduced both in number and in severity. When the number of mistakes and the severity of mistakes are reduced, people spend less time doing the work over again. When they spend less time doing the work over again, they deliver more productivity from the same number of full-time equivalents. Should volumes drop in the department, then more productivity can be achieved from fewer full-time equivalents. When volumes increase, the department has the capacity to expand its service.

We want to measure the results of teaching people to be more capable. In terms of the reasons for adequate funding of staff development, these ideas can be classified in the following categories:

1. The government or a regulatory body demands that we teach certain skills—for instance, fire safety or CPR, where certification must be re-established annually.
2. We teach skills people already know with the goal of bringing their proficiency and capability to a high enough level to produce a known, clinical outcome that is appropriate for patient satisfaction, that satisfies standards of care, and that is fiscally responsible.
3. We teach people new skills that allow them to perform appropriately and properly in the organization, to meet the demands of new clinical standards, and to support new programs and initiatives.

The first category, mandated education, includes a wide variety of items. This type of education uses some portion of the staff development budget and the resources that are allocated to staff development activity. It is important to document how much of the budget is dedicated to mandated programs.

The second category, teaching people skills they already have, is the most significant contributor to reducing error rates in the organization. A good example is starting an IV. It is said in some quarters of clinical medicine that an RN must start at least 60 IVs per month to maintain proficiency. Whatever the true number, the idea is very powerful. When an RN takes more time than is appropriate and necessary to start an IV, there is a systemic operational impact, affecting the rest of the nurse's work and the work of everybody else on that shift and the following shifts, where this impact will be noted and must be managed.

The third category, teaching people new skills, must be connected directly to the business plan of the organization. These new skills should be associated with revenue streams and marketing initiatives, both new and existing, and customer service and satisfaction—results that are important to the overall success of the organization.

One must measure the outcome of teaching people skills. For each of these categories, the outcomes must be specified. Each outcome must be accompanied by sensory-based evidence through which we can know that the teaching has been delivered and learning has been accomplished. Observation and work-sampling methodologies satisfy the demand for supporting evidence. Each one demonstrates that these reaffirmed and new behaviors acquired through the learning process have reduced the number of errors and raised proficiency. However many data are gathered from reports and computers, it is the in-the-trenches observation of the results of the department's teaching efforts that ultimately will satisfy the organization's demand for cost effectiveness, cost benefit, and measurement of outcomes.

The staff development manager is responsible for using resources efficiently and effectively within a plan or framework. Decisions about which resources to allot for which program can be difficult; the manager must consider financial and personnel management processes as well as ethical and legal issues. The systematic budgeting process used by the organization will help prepare the manager for this role. Budget preparation requires a classification of costs into categories such as:

- Salaries and benefits
- Personnel travel and incidentals
- Tuition and registration fees
- Office supplies
- Program materials and supplies
- Printing, graphics, and reproduction
- Faculty fees and honoraria
- Faculty travel, lodging, and incidentals
- Equipment expense allocation
- Equipment rental
- Equipment maintenance
- Miscellaneous.

Reviewing these categories and determining the budget for each line item are the first steps to resource allocation analysis. At periodic (often monthly) intervals, the manager should analyze budget reports to determine if expenses are consistent with allocated resources. Each line item should be evaluated to determine if it is adequately funded, efficiently spent, and appropriately used. Experience will help the manager gain confidence with projecting costs for new programs with no track record of expenses. Using expense records from a similar program is helpful.

The manager should be realistic about resource allocation and analysis. The highest expense related to any staff development effort is the loss of patient care hours related to learner time. Analyses of any staff development offering will consistently show that 80% to 98% of the cost of the staff development experience is learner salary. Paying attention to this fact will do more to contribute to the efficiency of the operation than any other detail. The time spent by staff in a staff development activity must be tightly planned; time must be used well. In addition, using measurable outcomes to demonstrate outcomes of learning will contribute to the efficiency of the staff development department.

Advanced resource allocation analysis techniques, such as cost-benefit analysis and cost-effectiveness analysis, may be required by some organizations. One formula that has proven worthy was developed by Del Bueno (1980). This formula requires the assignment of a value for the actual outcome or effectiveness of the program, which is then related to the associated costs. To calculate the costs, the usual expenses related to supplies and equipment are determined. The cost of the learner salary is also calculated, and a value is assigned to the final costs. This formula illustrates the high cost of learner salary and

---

D ISPLAY 14-5

Cost Effectiveness Analysis Worksheet

Costs

Learner salaries   _____

Instructor salary   _____

Development time/salary   _____

Materials   _____

Facilities   _____

Evaluation/assessment of learning   _____

Cost per participant hour (total costs/# participants)   _____

Calculate (or estimate) average learner salary   _____

Convert to cost value such as   _____
       1 = average learner salary + $20
       2 = average learner salary + $15
       3 = average learner salary + $10
       4 = average learner salary + $5
       5 = average learner salary + $1

Effectiveness

Select an effectiveness value based on actual evaluation method and
data such as   _____
       1 = evidence that participants were present in room
       2 = evidence that participants learned in class (written or performance tests, direct
          observation, expressed change in attitude or thinking)
       3 = evidence that majority of participants transferred learning to work setting as noted
          through planned direct observation
       4 = evidence that majority of participants transferred learning to work setting noted by
          quality monitoring activity
       5 = evidence that majority of participants transferred learning to work setting noted
          through data collected by unobtrusive evaluation measures

Compare cost value to effectiveness value   _____
       1:1 = poor use of scarce resources, no outcomes
       3:3 = good use of scarce resources, classroom outcomes
       5:5 = ask for a raise! (can get to this data with planning)

Address your findings in your continuous improvement plans and reports!

Source: Karen Kelly-Thomas, 1997. Used with permission.
Modified from formula developed by Dorothy del Bueno, 1980.

---

gives insight about how a manager can achieve a more cost-effective operation: by reducing the costs (learner time) or raising expected outcomes. Managers who recognize the high cost of lost patient care hours will make concerted efforts to use time spent in staff development activities efficiently. Raising the outcome measurement to ensure learning is one way to accomplish this task. Cost-benefit analysis techniques have also been described to assist staff development managers. These strategies are less common but may have some value for the manager attempting to determine additional benefits of staff development activities for the organization and patient care.

There is no single, correct, and simple efficiency analysis formula. Many formulas are used, each with its strengths and limitations, biases, and assumptions. Some are reasonable, some are comprehensive, still others seem superficial, and others are quite unbelievable. Disparity exists between the definitions as well. In general, the broad definitions provided by Rossi and Freeman (1990) are the most useful:

COST-BENEFIT ANALYSIS   Requires the economic efficiency of a program expressed as the relation between costs and outcomes, usually expressed in monetary terms

COST-EFFECTIVENESS ANALYSIS   Measures the efficacy of a program in achieving given intervention outcomes in relation to program costs, usually expressed as cost per unit of outcomes achieved.

Managers should select programs for resource allocation analysis. This analysis yields data useful in the continuing management of the overall program. Display 14-5 shows one time-tested and updated cost-effectiveness formula that demonstrates a cost-to-outcome ratio. This is a useful formula for budget planning and evaluation.

SUMMARY

Milton Erickson, the father of modern hypnotherapy, is regarded as one of the most innovative and powerful change agents of our time. He stated quite simply, "You can pretend something long enough and you'll get good at it." In aviation, pilots, copilots, and flight engineers spend time in flight simulators every 6 months reaffirming their existing skills and learning new techniques. They must perform appropriately or they will be unable to fly. Experts in all fields acquire their capabilities through deliberate practice, and we measure the success of their efforts by direct observation of their skills.

It is time for staff development departments to use effective and efficient models, to stretch their influence, and to recognize the systemic, organization-wide impact that their efforts have. "Give a man a fish and you feed him for a day," goes the ancient Chinese proverb. "Teach a man to fish and you feed him for a lifetime." An organization that stops teaching, or teaches inappropriately, is threatening its very existence.

The practice of health care arose in compassionate response to human suffering and disease. It was centuries before the scientific revolution introduced a time of unending change in medicine, nursing, and other caring professions. The development of hospitals was not a climax but a point on a curve in the rise of the modern health care organization. A cot, a towel, a prayer, and perhaps a bowl of chicken soup were no longer enough. Advanced training, clinical specialization, staff development practices. resource allocation, competition for adequate budget share, and data bases: this progression from historical nursing to operations management is still evolving.

This is why SDSs must work continuously to teach people in their organization new skills as well as to reaffirm the skills they already have, to produce the results the department wants and the organization must have. And it is why operations management must be continuously recognized as an essential element of the staff development program. In the modern world, they are inseparable. Operations management is the connection between the department's programs and the people and the business plan of the entire organization. Mastering it, and keeping fully attuned to its continuing evolution, will make the staff development leader more capable and successful than he or she already is.

The Evolution of Organization and Staff Development in a University Medical Center

DORI TAYLOR SULLIVAN

The last decade has been a time of tumultuous change for both the health care industry as a whole and the SDSs who strive to meet the learning needs of their organizations and to ensure the achievement of the organization's mission and goals. The following case study describes the evolution of a staff development department in a university medical center setting.

In 1985, the Department of Nursing Education and Research was created at John Dempsey Hospital, the acute care hospital of the University of Connecticut Health Center. The major impetus for creating the new department was twofold: first, the need to establish and ensure compliance with educational standards for nurses throughout the hospital, and second the recognition of the growing importance of nursing professional development, particularly related to the use of scientific research as a basis for practice. The Department of Nursing Education and Research was initially staffed with three full-time equivalents: a director, a nursing education specialist, and an education coordinator. A nursing quality specialist was added shortly thereafter. The director became a member of the executive nursing council; the nursing education specialist joined the clinical nurse specialist forum. Clinical nurse specialists were expected to spend about 30% of their efforts in staff development and reported to the Department of Nursing Education and Research in a matrix structure.

During the 6 years of its existence, the department surpassed its stated goals. Some of the accomplishments of that period include:

- Development and implementation of a research-based nursing standards model that received national exposure
- Standardization of educational requirements for professional nurses, including the development of a clinical ladder that called for continuing education hours and demonstration of research utilization competencies
- Creation of a management development program for nursing and other medical center leaders
- Coordination of the nursing department quality assurance program
- Establishment of a nursing research committee to foster nursing research activities and increase staff nurse knowledge of research
- Evolution of a reputation for excellence in educational knowledge and internal consulting skills to help staff and leaders with problem solving.

In 1991, the department's responsibilities expanded to include the entire hospital staff. Hospital administrators clearly recognized the value and results produced by the education staff and wanted to provide this support throughout the hospital. It also became more difficult to justify why only nurses were entitled to educational support! Additional factors in favor of the expansion were the beginning emphasis on competence assessment and the rumored focus of the JCAHO on areas other than nursing.

Although it was a time of great excitement and opportunity, the greatly broadened scope of service responsibilities created a mini-crisis: the department had to rethink its mission, priorities, and values related to staff development. Early on, the lesson of how much learning would be required was evident. Each department and discipline had its own ways of approaching staff education and development, and any hint that "nursing" was being imposed on them was a giant *faux pas*! Most importantly, there was a greater urgency to determine the necessary resources, decide how best to deploy them, and demonstrate the outcomes that were achieved. The use of key operations management principles and practices was essential to optimize the department functions. Notable achievements during this time were:

- Development of a hospital-wide competency assessment system that included department orientation, competency demonstration, and performance evaluation
- Consultation provided to every department manager regarding his or her area's performance and staff education needs
- Expanded continuing education opportunities for all staff
- Involvement with and support of the overall plan for improving organizational performance.

In early 1994 the department again expanded to include the office practices of faculty physicians, and in late 1994 a final change was made: the Department of Organization and Staff Development (OSD) was created and expected to serve the needs of the entire medical center—including the clinical areas previously mentioned, the medical and dental school staffs, and personnel within the central administrative services, such as public safety, facilities management, research administration, and more. Staffing in OSD now consists of eight full-time equivalents, including an assistant vice president who is part of the medical center administration. OSD has one focus on the more traditional elements of staff education such as orientation, in-service, and continuing education. In addition, new responsibilities—quality improvement and work redesign activities, organizational development, and culture change to support achievement of the organization's goals—were included in the department's charge.

Our department grew dramatically and became an integral and highly visible contributor to the medical center, and some of the lessons we learned are applicable to any staff development department. No matter how excellent the educational quality is, SDSs and their departments must still manage and validate their use of resources in exemplary fashion, and must be willing to demonstrate their contributions and effectiveness.

The elements of our department's success can be divided into structure, process, and outcome domains.

The structural factors relate to the membership of the education administrator in high-level management groups and the ability to focus on organizational needs and goals rather than other, more traditional needs. The importance of the relationships and credibility that develop from ongoing interaction with key administrators and clinical leaders cannot be overestimated. This is the best opportunity to show how education and development activities can promote achievement of organizational goals. The ability to embrace change and flexibility without compromising core values greatly enhances this credibility.

Process factors relate specifically to operations management. The analysis of the work to be done and the establishment of strategic goals organize the work of the department and clearly articulate to the rest of the organization what staff development is charged with providing. It is key to assess the relative amount of resources being invested in various activities, because there is often a mismatch between stated priorities and how time is spent. Efficient systems for routine work must be in place to create the time needed for high-priority areas.

The mapping of staff development work involves stating the scope of operations and how they can best be organized. Project assessment and management skills go hand-in-hand with staff productivity measures to ensure that realistic, equitable assignments are made and that projects are completed on time and within budget. Increasingly, staff development administrators are asked to track resource use and allocation and report that information to various entities in the organization, whether by cost center, department, or other categorization system. This is similar to the "billable hours" calculated in various professions.

Finally, SDSs must model continuous improvement by constantly and aggressively assessing customer needs and satisfaction, calculating and presenting cost-benefit analyses of key educational activities, and revising services to respond to organizational needs.

The staff development administrator should ponder the following points:

- Consider the structure and organization of the staff development department. Does it enhance the department's effectiveness and ability to determine and respond to learning needs?

● What is the nature and quality of the department's relationships with key administrators? How can these relationships be enhanced?

● How does the department promote and model the ability to embrace change and increase flexibility for increased organizational success?

● Are the mission, role, and goals of the department clearly articulated? Are they consistent with key customer requirements?

● To what extend does the department determine and report on resource use related to important projects? Do these reports include SDS productivity and the use of supplies and equipment for learning? Is the cost of evaluating learning included?

● What is the department's track record on completing projects and responsibilities effectively, on time, and within budget? How can this be further improved?

Answering these questions will serve the manager well as change continues in our turbulent health care system.

REFERENCES

Burns, T., & Stalker, G. (1961). *The management of innovation.* London: Tavistock.

Charns, M. P., & Schaefer, M. J. (1983). *Health care organizations: A model for management.* Englewood Cliffs, NJ: Prentice-Hall.

Cooper, G. E., White, M. D., & Lauber, J. D. (1979). *Resource management on the flight desk.* (NASA Conference Publication #2120; NTIS No. N80-22083). Moffett Field, CA: NASA Ames Research Center.

Del Bueno, D., & Kelly, K. J. (1980). How cost-effective is your staff development program? *Journal of Nursing Administration, 10*(4), 31–36.

Edwards, G. B. (1996). Surviving the ax: Developing an education and allocation system to verify productivity and resource consumption. *Journal of Nursing Staff Development, 12*(2), 59–65.

Ericsson, K. A., & Charness, N. (1994). Expert performance: Its structure and acquisition. *American Psychologist, 49,* 725–747.

Gardner, H. (1991). *The unschooled mind: How children think & how schools should teach.* New York: Basic Books.

Haley, J. (1973). *Uncommon therapy: The therapeutic techniques of Milton H. Erickson, M.D.* New York: W. W. Norton & Co.

Hogan, R., Curphy, G. J., & Hogan, J. (1994). What we know about leadership: Effectiveness and personality. *American Psychologist, 49,* 493–504.

Kelly, K. J. (1990). A productivity measure for nursing staff development. *Journal of Nursing Staff Development, 6*(2), 65–70.

Kelly, J. K. (Ed.). (1992). *Nursing staff development: Current competence, future focus.* Philadelphia: J. B. Lippincott.

Massello, D. J. (1995). *Creating great leaders.* Highland Park, IL: Business Professional Institute.

Rossi, P. H., & Freeman, H. E. (1990). *Evaluation: A systematic approach* (4th ed.). Beverly Hills, CA: Sage.

Ulschak, F. (1988). *Creating the future of healthcare education.* Chicago: American Hospital Association.

Weiner, E. L., & Nagel, D. C. (1988). *Human factors in aviation.* San Diego: Academic Press.

Woodward, J. (1958). *Management and technology.* London: Her Majesty's Stationery Office.

15

Future Forecast: Leading the Journey

KAREN J. KELLY-THOMAS

I was running in the mountains recently and thinking about this chapter and the opportunity to say something. Perhaps it was my running, but I kept returning to the theme of clinical staff development and leadership as a sustained effort. As I dwelled on thoughts about health care, nursing, leadership, and staff development, many experiences were streaming through my head. As I tried to hold onto a few, particularly the stories that might be useful and help me write this last chapter, I found myself gasping at times and gliding at others.

You see, as much as I love the idea of story and what story can do for us, it still takes a sustained effort to develop ideas into real experiences, experiences into stories, and stories into the written word. Sometimes clinical staff development requires sustained effort, and other times it flows. It is my intent in this last chapter to generate ideas in the reader by offering information and thoughts about creating a practice, inquiring and investigating, leading, and strategic thinking. It is my sustained hope that you will try them as you go about the business of clinical staff development. Love what you do and do what you love!

CREATING A CLINICAL STAFF DEVELOPMENT PRACTICE

What does it mean to have a practice? It can be anything you want it to be in some settings, but in general, clinical staff development practice has certain common characteristics. Those characteristics are the ones that connect so many clinicians together. The characteristics are the ones that, when having conversations with other clinicians, cause you both to start the "phenomenological nodding" that Munhall spoke about so eloquently in her text *Revisioning Phenomenology* (1994). Munhall described the frequent experience of nodding and how it serves to confirm, validate, and improve the rigor of a belief or idea. When other people start nodding when you are talking, you are gaining validation and they are confirming similar thoughts. This doesn't quite mean that we should all go around nodding continuously like the spring-mounted dogs in the back windows of cars. The nodding is meaningful and can serve to connect you with another clinician who shares a concern about patient care. If you find yourself nodding as you read parts of this chapter, you are confirming your own beliefs and values. This is not to say that this text is the sum total or the best way to go about doing clinical staff development, but it is to say that there are commonalities among clinicians engaged in staff development. Here are four of those common characteristics.

The primary characteristic of clinical staff development is the connection provided by the patient. The person requiring health promotion, health maintenance, or health restoration services looks to the health care provider to behave in a coordinated and helpful way. Unfortunately, complex systems sometimes prevent that from happening. At other times, individual care providers are remiss in their skill level or their use of that skill in daily practice.

The second characteristic that connects clinicians creating a staff development practice is their commitment to quality. This is usually evident in the manner in which they go about their clinical practice. They are helpers, helping improve systems and people for improved care. A caring stance, attention to detail, and diligence about the care provided are all evident in their daily practice.

A third characteristic is optimism about the future. Despite some evidence to the contrary, clinical staff development specialists (SDSs) creating a practice do so within a personal value system that views the optimistic possibilities of the future rather than the doldrums of today. A spirit of inquiry and the intent to do good are part of this characteristic.

Finally, a fourth characteristic shared by those creating a clinical staff development practice is the manner in which they lead. Leadership styles fall into the categories that support the notions of altruism and compassion. Others may perceive these clinicians as unconventional, individualistic, and opinionated about how things should be. It is this idea of what should be or can be that often drives the SDS.

Leading

There are many more characteristics shared by SDSs who are creating a staff development practice every day. One of them is leading, using a variety of styles and strategies. The leading performance patterns of SDSs are documented throughout this text and in professional journals such as the *Journal of Nursing Staff Development, Training and Development*, and others. Conversations about clinical staff development surround us. Tannen (1990), in her works about conversations among men and women, addresses the different words, different worlds, asymmetries, and cross-purposes expressed during conversations. She advises us to live with the asymmetry and open lines of communication. She uses the example of a couple walking down the street, illustrating their comfortable but asymmetric movement by describing how one's arm is on the other's shoulder and the other's arm is around the waist. Despite this asymmetry, their movement is comfortable and effective for communication. This does not mean that all SDSs should walk down the halls of their health care facilities arm in arm, but it demonstrates the different but complementary stances possible by people with a common goal. That common goal is quality patient care.

Leading toward that common goal is carried out through the competence assessment and development activities of SDSs. Notice that leading, as it is used here and later, does not mean holding a certain position within a hierarchical structure. Instead, it means using one's influence, through the credibility one has gained, to improve care, caregivers, and the systems of care where patients seek service.

Haller's (1998) recent proposal about the difference between management and leadership is clear and can be applied to all SDSs, regardless of their formal roles and titles in various health care organizations. She wrote:

> Leadership implies effective use of influence that is independent of one's position in an organization. Management implies formal authority and power based on one's position in the organizational structure. (p. 405)

SDSs hold so many different titles that management-like titles have inherent managerial tasks such as staffing and budget preparation and control. It is in the boundless leadership opportunities present today in health care organizations that SDSs can shine.

Guiding

To guide, as a term to describe how SDSs create their practice, means to counsel, mentor, and teach. Sharing the assumption of a common goal—that is, improved care for patients—the SDS engages people and groups in competence assessment and development activities. Guiding in staff development practice is not about required learning, mandatory classes, and dreary procedure-driven tasks. Rather, it is about the continued improvement of a system of assessment and development activities that will guide people and groups toward the envisioned care for patients.

Porter-O'Grady (1995) suggested considering the following three realities when creating new systems of health care. They are relevant to SDSs as they create new systems of staff development.

1. "The continuum of care will define the activities in health care for at least the next two decades. A capitated noninstitutional model for health care delivery that seeks the health of the subscriber is the linchpin of any emerging system" (p. 408). SDSs will be challenged to provide assessment and development services to clinicians who work in various settings that are all part of a system. Virtual education and distance learning will become more of a reality for care providers and consumers. "Telehealth," and the requisite critical thinking, interpersonal, and technical skills, will be part of the staff development curriculum.
2. "Information is becoming increasingly important to the successful operation of a continuum-based health care system. Computerized clinical data base approaches will be essential to documenting and validating clinical approaches, quality outcomes, and cost variables that can result in good management. Value will depend on the level of information available, its quality, and its accuracy" (p. 409). SDSs will find opportunities to help many learn new ways of thinking about clinical data and records. CPR (cardiopulmonary resuscitation) will be supplemented by CPR (computerized patient record)! Resuscitation skill training will still be part of the staff development curriculum, of course, but so will training about data bases and the use of computerized clinical data sets to help people and groups assess and develop competencies to improve that information and the care that it represents. SDSs will have usable data sets about organizational, group, and individual competence that will add value to quality care.
3. "Physicians will be partners in the process in new ways. There will be a close systems association requiring different relationships and behavior between physicians and other players in the health system" (p. 410). As full-fledged players in the health care system, SDSs will focus on building these relationships among and between groups to accomplish commonly identified clinical outcomes. The role of the SDS may vary from being responsible for developing an evidence-based critical path to leading the team to define new clinical outcomes based on new technology.

These realities can serve as guideposts for SDSs creating a staff development practice in the health care system of today.

I often think about the guidance provided by so many who came before us. Schorr and Zimmerman (1988) discussed this mentoring stance in their book *Making Choices, Taking Chances*. This book is about two leaders who helped 47 other leaders tell their story. These leaders were surprised when they were identified as such, but given the opportunity to reflect on their choices, all realized that they took chances to accomplish tasks and goals that were important to them. They all spoke of their hard work and their sustained effort. It took time and love to develop their practice, and that development turned them into leaders.

Seizing this same opportunity when thinking about this chapter, I enjoyed reflecting about nurse leaders who have influenced me, mentored me, guided me, and advised me. My first head nurse in the emergency department of St. Elizabeth Hospital in Elizabeth, NJ, gave me gentle, good guidance as I tried to be a good new graduate in 1970. I was a closet hippie then. I had been taught well by the nurses and sisters of Holy Name Hospital School of Nursing, so when I went to work, my braid was under my cap and my granny glasses made me look very nurselike. Mrs. Majeski, my head nurse, was a Polish immigrant who had to work hard to learn a new language and continue work that she loved. For her, nursing was also a sustained effort. She taught me well.

Joanne Johnson was my charge nurse and another nurse leader who influenced my thinking and my way of being a nurse and a leader. She was a beautiful, tall woman who also wore granny glasses. Her hair was an Afro that made a statement about who she was. It was her elegance that impressed me the most; the way she moved among the patients in that busy inner-city emergency department in the early 1970s was a thing of beauty. I learned much about organizing and taking care of priorities from Joanne, and I also learned about compassion from her. Joanne's sustained effort was in showing me how to nurse through her expert mentoring. It has left a lasting impression on me.

Frances Louden is another nurse leader who mentored me as a very young, new nurse manager. As a 23-year-old head nurse, I was quite impressed with myself. Mrs. Louden mentored me and gave me opportunities that taught me about being a good head nurse. I'm not sure if I was Mrs. Louden's sustained effort, but I am sure that I gave her, as my supervisor at a 950-bed tertiary care hospital center in Washington, DC, a few memorable moments. One I recall had to do with a conversation I had with a lab tech about some needed blood work. I remember saying to the tech, "I'm the head nurse on this unit and you better do what I'm telling you to do!" Mrs. Louden's leadership emerged as she counseled me, "Now, Karen, tell me what you said..." Those days of ignorant bliss make me smile now, although I still hear them on occasion when I visit clinical settings.

There were nurse leaders in my many years of school that have left lasting impressions on me. I still hear Mrs. Christanovich and Miss Marshall in my head. I will forever be grateful to Dr. Carrie Lenburg for her leadership of the Regent's College degree program. In 1975, when I was looking for a BSN, Dr. Lenburg was leading the effort to develop a competency-based education program for nurses like me who were willing to put their money where their mouth was and engage in systematic competence assessment to validate requirements for a baccalaureate. She believed adults could sustain the effort to meet the requirements of a baccalaureate degree, and had the tests and test results to prove it. Carrie's sustained effort was in the accreditation process as she had to answer questions about the program, a university without walls, like, "Where's the library?"

The nurse leader who gave me the opportunity to do staff development also comes to mind during this reflection about mentoring and staff development. Sara Carnes promoted me to the staff development role in a small community hospital in rural Loudoun County, VA. To me, the "promotion" meant day work with most weekends off and a bit more control over my schedule. As the mother of a 2-year-old daughter, this seemed very appealing at that time. Little did I know that this would begin a 20-year career for me and the beginning of a life's work. During some very difficult times and with limited resources (like me!), Sara sustained the effort to develop the kind of nursing care given to patients in that hospital. She worked hard, her hours were long, and she usually took work home with her. Despite having a husband and small son, she modeled guiding leadership for me as she pursued quality care for patients.

Dorothy del Bueno was the first staff development leader who taught me. Through pragmatic, funny, but always clear thinking statements, she solved many problems that we were having in staff development. Although the practice and discipline of nursing staff development was evolving, we were still immature. Dorothy helped me, and I believe many of us, recognize that the sustained effort required to position ourselves for success was worth it. She strongly advocated a no-nonsense business-like approach, and said we would be successful through alignment with organizational goals and use of good evaluation strategies. She was always irreverent in her presentations: I'll never forget her references to the "Sisters of the Sniveling Poor" and "Bucket of Blood Hospital."

Belinda Puetz is another nurse leader who has influenced me and taught me much. I've learned about quality and taste from Belinda. As our relationship developed and we became friends, I learned about how to live a good life, work hard, and enjoy the trips required to do work that is loved. She also taught me how to maintain relationships with people who are important to me. As she and her husband Werner continue to care for their 91- and 96-year-old mothers (or "muzzas," as they are fondly known to many), I have had the privilege of learning from Belinda about grace in life and work.

Stewardship

As I reflect about guiding and creating a clinical staff development practice, the theme of sustained effort continues. It is also evident in Block's work (1993). His "stewarding" notion of leading and guiding is appealing in today's turbulent health care environment. Block used the metaphor of stewarding in organizations to explain his view of how leaders should lead today. He compared leading an organization to stewardship, defined as holding something in trust for another. Block further defined stewardship as:

> [T]he willingness to be accountable for the well-being of the larger organization by operating in service, rather than in control, of those around us. Stated simply, it is accountability without control or compliance. (p. xx)

Block challenges us to deepen our commitment to service and to seek the experience of authentic service, which has the following characteristics:

- There is a balance of power.
- The primary commitment is to the larger community.
- Each person joins in defining purpose and deciding what kind of culture the organization will become.
- There is a balanced and equitable distribution of rewards.

These highly virtuous ideas are not new to most health care providers; most are drawn to the caring professions because they want to be of service to others. Block suggested that we replace leadership with stewardship and choose partnership over patriarchy, adventure over safety, and service over self-interest. SDSs will find Block's case studies and advice helpful in their everyday stressful environment that shows little evidence of the above attributes. This work about stewardship may also help SDSs who are helping others learn about the interrelationship skills required to achieve quality outcomes in our complex environments. This notion of stewardship can also be applied when creating a staff development practice. Stewarding your own development and helping others develop is the core of this work. SDSs will find the idea of stewarding useful in creating a vision for staff development in organizations today.

Drucker (1989) cited new realities in government, politics, economics, business, society, and the world. He blamed the American hospital for its crisis because it failed to take political responsibility, and with it leadership, in controlling costs and the quality of health care. Drucker confronted the societal aspect of health and the fact that health has never been a priority among the very poor.

Despite its best intentions, the American hospital system does not serve society well by, for instance, setting up inner-city clinics without addressing the larger social context of those clinics. The health care system's dependence on government and tax money for financing must change in a pluralist society. Government's main task in the future will be to set limits and standards for the greater good. Drucker predicted that in our knowledge-based and information-overloaded society, we will return to home-based care; hospitals will be used for complex surgery or health crises, and mental health services will be provided primarily on an outpatient basis. Some SDSs have already experienced these shifts and transformations; some were assigned to make them happen. Drucker's view of health care in the context of the world will serve the SDS well. His work about knowledge-based workers has spawned a whole new area of study, referred to as "building a knowledge-based culture."

Tecker et al. (1997) proposed a decision-making system and operational model for use in organizations interested in building a culture of knowledge. To build a knowledge-based culture, we are advised to consider elements of knowledge-based decision making, the organizational culture that supports these efforts, and the changes in governance or structure needed to move forward to a competitive, successful future. Using such elements as sensitivity, foresight, insight, and consideration of ethical implications, Tecker et al. challenge us to create systems for exchanging information and insights in a style of decision making that requires competencies and strategies to achieve identified outcomes. This work can be useful to the SDS who is in the midst of significant organizational "right-sizing." Use of the principles and techniques suggested will help SDSs move through the white-water turbulence that is considered the daily reality of today's health care systems.

RESEARCH IN CLINICAL STAFF DEVELOPMENT

Any self-respecting group of professionals will advocate for more research about its beliefs, practice theories, means, and methods of operationalizing stated principles, concepts, and ideas. Clinical staff development is like many other disciplines in this respect. Adapting a stance of inquiry is natural for SDSs.

The discipline of clinical staff development can be considered within the five learning disciplines described by Senge et al. (1994). Within a framework of lore and learning, these authors provided a guidebook to help us learn while treading the fertile ground of organizational life. Driven by a vision of collective experience and imagination, they implore us to create learning organizations by exchanging information, cultivating conversations among people, and generating communities of commitment. This lofty-sounding notion has its practical aspects, many of which are provided by the writers as they model their vision of a learning organization. The five lifelong programs of study and practice, called disciplines, are the core of a learning organization. They are familiar to many of us and are presented here to reinforce a basis for inquiry into an evolving field.

The learning disciplines or programs of study and experience are:

- *Personal mastery*: learning to expand our personal capacity to create the results we most desire, and creating an organizational environment that encourages all its members to develop themselves toward the goals and purposes they choose
- *Mental models*: reflecting on, continually clarifying, and improving our internal pictures of the world, and seeing how they shape our actions and decisions
- *Shared vision*: building a sense of commitment in a group by developing shared images of the future we seek to create and the principles and guiding practices by which we hope to get there
- *Team learning*: transforming conversational and collective thinking skills so that groups of people can reliably develop intelligence and ability greater than the sum of the individual members' talents
- *Systems thinking*: a way of thinking about, and a language for describing and understanding, the forces and interrelationships that shape the barrier of systems. This discipline helps us see how to change systems more effectively and to act more in tune with the larger processes of the natural and economic worlds.

According to these philosophers, to practice a discipline is to be a lifelong learner on a never-ending developmental path. This belief system and the value of inquiry can be of benefit to the SDS who is interested in investigating specific aspects of staff development practice or the whole. Many of those who share the discipline of staff development already exchange information through journals and associations, cultivate conversations among others who share the common interest of clinical staff development, and generate communities of commitment through shared projects, programs, and quests toward understanding.

State of the Art and Science

The state of the art and science of clinical staff development is found in many marvelous sources. Journals abound with case studies, anecdotal data, proposals, frameworks, theories, and experiments. There are even some randomized controlled trials, considered by many to be the gold standard of scientific research. This entire text attempts to provide an evidence base for novice SDSs and refers to the past and present work of many.

As mentioned in Chapter 3 and other sections of this book, there is a continued need for sound thinking and intellectual discourse to support the shared belief of clinical staff development as a discipline within health care. Few would argue that learning, competence assessment, and competence development need to take place in an organized and systematic manner. Tests that yield similar or better outcomes of competence must continue to inform those who are committed to helping society through this field of practice.

The Research Committee of the National Nursing Staff Development Organization has pledged to evaluate and provide information about outcomes in staff development. It is time for this group to join other similar groups with common interests in clinical staff development outcomes and broaden the discourse. Through these conversations, practical advice and counsel can be offered to those who do not understand the value of clinical staff development or need to learn more about its methods. These findings must also be disseminated through more than the discipline's journals and meetings; publishing and presenting at a variety of venues is essential to achieving a common understanding.

It seems fitting that this research committee would identify staff development outcomes as a priority. Although outcomes are of interest to any discipline or clinical practice setting, the need to identify means, methods, and modes of measuring clinical staff development has never been more prevalent. The health care work force is the foundation of the American health care system; it is the talent, intellectual capacity, and commitment to care embodied in many health care providers. The assessment and development of work force competence underlie that capability.

Continued Need

Few would argue with the notion that more research is better. Others argue that certain kinds of research are best suited for certain kinds of questions or problems. Still others disagree about the best scientific method to solve health care work force problems. I will argue that there is a place at the table of health for all of the caring professions and their members. This sounds like a somewhat limitless work force, but in fact it is discrete. According to data from the National Center for Health Statistics (1997), there were 3,049,213 active licensed health care workers in the United States in 1994. That translates to 1,173 physicians, nurses, dentists, optometrists, pharmacists, and podiatrists per 100,000 population, or 1.2 health care workers for each 100 persons. As a very large group of people committed to health and the care of it, we should be healthier. We continue to focus on illness rather than health promotion and health maintenance.

The Pew Commission Report of the Taskforce on Health Care Workforce Regulation (Finocchio et al., 1995) proposed that "the changes in and the transformation of the American health care delivery and financing structures have highlighted the roles that America's 10.5 million health care practitioners (including assistive personnel) play in the cost, quality, and accessibility of health care" (p. vi). As a result, the education, training, and distribution of the health care work force have received increased attention. The task force found that the health care work force is out of step with today's health care needs and expectations. The regulatory systems that have served the public and the professions well in the past are now "criticized for increasing costs, restricting managerial and professional flexibility, limiting access to care, and having an equivocal relationship to quality" (p. vi). Fifty separate state systems have created complex procedures that are absurd. Regulatory bodies are thought to be largely unaccountable to the public they serve. Perhaps Safriet (1994) said it best when he wrote:

> Since health and illness are for the most part biologically and physically based, with some psychological and emotional components, it is not at all clear why licensure laws, that is, proxies for competency, should vary according to political boundaries rather than competency domains. (p. 3107)

The task force envisioned a system for state regulation of the health care work force for the 21st century that is "SAFE":

- Standardized where appropriate
- Accountable to the public
- Flexible to support optimal access to a safe and competent health care work force
- Effective and Efficient in protecting and promoting the public's health, safety, and welfare (Finnocchio et al., 1995).

Ten recommendations were offered, most of which addressed the need for restructuring and revising state and professional boards. The second and third address competence assessment and development:

> Recommendation 2. States should standardize entry-to-practice requirements and limit them to competence assessments for health professions to facilitate the physical and professional mobility of the health profession. (p. 5)
>
> Recommendation 3. States should base practice acts on demonstrated initial and

continuing competence. This process must allow and expect different professions to share overlapping scopes of practice. States should explore pathways to allow all professionals to provide services to the full extent of their current knowledge, training, experience and skills. (p. 9)

These two recommendations alone make it clear that the methods used to assess and develop competence must be tested for rigor, validity, and reliability. Only through continued experimentation, case study reports, and scientific problem solving will these staff development strategies become generally accepted principles.

The continued need to conduct research in the areas of the best methods to assess and develop competence in the health care professions is also evident as states pick up and drop legislation for mandatory continuing education requirements. There is no research that shows any connection between continuing education with license renewal and the continued competence of any licensed group. There is certainly an intuitive belief that the practice of any of the health care professions requires continued development and occasional skill monitoring; however, the best means and methods to measure those skills and developmental levels of health care providers remain unknown.

There is much to be done. Our job as SDSs is to focus on continuously evaluating the means and methods we use during the daily delivery of our services to the health care professionals and evaluate them against quality standards that usually go beyond public protection and toward service to patients, groups, and communities.

Research Priorities

Health care providers should identify research priorities relevant to their focus and scope of practice. What areas of inquiry should the SDS focus on? Depending on the scope of practice, the practice settings in health care are full of possibilities. For example, the novice SDS may want to collect data to evaluate his or her presentation style using a standardized form. The experienced SDS who needs to illustrate transfer of learning for clinical managers related to skillful monitoring of selected parameters may choose an instrument or tool to measure transfer of learning in a systematic and reliable way. This inquiry will provide data useful at many levels by many people interested in competence assessment. Yet another SDS may conduct in-depth interviews with former patients about their ability to cope with their chronic diseases, for the purpose of planning and improving the system of care for other patients like them. The scope of possibilities that SDSs can investigate is endless.

A few areas are reported regularly in the literature. I think we know that self-learning by package, module, or computer-assisted instruction is more efficient and that it costs less if one looks only at the classroom time "saved." I think we also know that clinicians, managers, and preceptors prefer preceptored experiences. I think we know that all the classic teaching strategies will work with clinicians when applied as recommended in the teaching, learning, education, and development literature. Finally, I think we also know that we can never evaluate enough and must continually challenge our habits of evaluation and attempt innovative evaluation strategies that are less costly, yield quality data, and are as accessible as we would like our health care system to be.

Thus, the research priority for clinical staff development and the groups that profess a commitment to it is simply this: What difference are we making in the health of the communities we serve? This simple question is actually full of complexities. We do not know how much assessment and development is enough to serve as evidence of competence, nor do we know the best strategies, the best technologies, or even the groups we should focus on. However, all of these strategies, and many more, are important in finding out what difference we are making in the health of the communities we serve.

LEADERSHIP FOR THE FUTURE

Leadership has gone through several developmental stages and phases during the past 50 years, from the "great man" theories, through charismatic and trait theories, to the more recent situational, contingency, and transformation models. As always, when many complexities, variables, and unknowns populate an idea or concept, conventional wisdom usually suggests blending, integrating, and using the ones that work best for you. Contingency theory is a favorite because it is based on the entire premise of "possibility" and recognizes that anything is possible.

Despite all these helpful theories and proposals about it, leadership remains an enigma. Many have offered explanations, and there will undoubtedly be more in the future. Kouzes and Posner (1993) explored credibility in leadership through surveys of more than 15,000 people, 400 case studies, and 40 in-depth interviews. The writers proposed that the key to effective leadership is credibility. Six key disciplines were identified:

- Discovering yourself
- Appreciating constituents
- Affirming shared values
- Developing capacity
- Serving a purpose
- Sustaining hope.

Each discipline was elaborately and richly supported, and first and next steps were advised. Similar to this work, but with its own twists, is Covey's (1989, 1994) challenge to leaders to practice principle-based leadership. Trust-based leadership grew out of the work of Shaw (1997), Whitney (1995), and others. Shaw said that following through on business commitments, behaving in a consistent manner, and respecting the well-being of others create a core of trust. Whitney proposed five trust-building premises:

- Establishing an aim, mission, vision, and values of the organization
- Creating a permeable organization structure and interactive management processes
- Understanding and communicating the interdependence of all components
- Conducting an audit of formal and informal measurements and controls
- Removing violators from the system.

Leider and Shapiro (1995) suggested that we repack our bags and lighten our load for the rest of our lives. Deming (1982) demanded that top management lead the way into quality. Burris (1993) urged using "technotrends" to revolutionize business and our lives, and Hammer and Champy (1993) said that corporate leaders must re-engineer.

What does all this mean to SDSs who take on the responsibility of competence assessment and development of clinical staff? It primarily means that there are a lot of people giving a lot of advice about the right way to lead. All of this advice is helpful to SDSs searching for increased understanding about leadership or practical models for leadership. I think leaders in staff development set an example by how they interact with others, help clinicians recognize and achieve their greatest potential, and understand and are committed to health care quality, cost, and access. Admired SDSs who are leaders in their organizations and elsewhere are honest, forward-looking, inspiring, and competent; when we learn and apply such leadership behaviors, we are demonstrating our competence. This is our work.

Vision

Senge et al. (1994) said it clearly when they advanced the notion of shared vision as a vehicle for building shared meaning. Every person, group, organization, and community has a destiny—that is, a deep purpose for its existence. In an organization, clues to the deeper purpose are often found in the founder's aspirations and the reasons the organization came into being. Today's health care environment, economically constrained and rapidly changing, creates a real challenge to those dreams and goals of the forebears of many hospitals, facilities, and health care systems. The need to build shared meaning among SDSs and clinical managers and administrators is key to the future of staff development work.

Mission

The word "mission" is not new to health care, but discussions about "what our organizational mission should be in the future" abound. Some such missions are held aloft in the form of a cross, a star, or even neon lights. Some hospitals engrave missionlike statements and symbols of the mission on entryway tiles, wood, and even concrete—and the symbols still get updated, refreshed, or redone to represent some new configuration. I believe it's a sign of great diplomacy in health care when the locally named Baptist, Lutheran, Methodist, Jewish, and Catholic hospitals merge and become some new religious-like name with the requisite symbol of the newly integrated health care system.

The symbols and the names of those symbols seem to change every few years. The processes of "re-engineer, reinvent, revise, review, and redo" still follow the classic scientific method for problem solving: assess, plan, implement, and evaluate are still the most sound approaches to continuous improvement of services. Some of the names may be new for the processes, and there may be subsets of processes described in very fine detail on flow charts, "fishbone" diagrams, and other tools designed to help us through the problem-solving process.

In clinical staff development, the mission is quite simple. The mission is toward quality care through competence. This is also the aim of all staff development activities. How you go about setting up those competence assessment and development activities is where the outcome of quality care is realized.

Goals

Choosing a simple term to describe the signposts you will use along the path toward quality care through competence can be difficult, given the plethora of advice available today. I will use the word "goals" here to represent what you identify you will do to create or develop your staff development practice within the scope of service of your organization. You need to set realistic goals that you can accomplish in service to people, the organization, and the community at large. This does not mean adding more to your "to do" list; it means that you must remain reality-based and work within your system to change and improve it.

Seligman (1993) provided good counsel about what we can change and what we cannot. Through his continued studies of animals under stress, he observed that some of the same breed of animals were more hardy than others and could deal with more stress. This finding led Seligman to consider the notion of "learning hardiness" or change capacity among humans. He theorized:

> It does not matter *when* problems, habits, and personality are acquired; their depth (and subsequent ability to change them) derives only from their biology, their evidence, and their power. (p. 252)

He provided a strong argument for learning optimism, or the conviction that you can change, as the necessary first step in the process of all change. Unwarranted optimism, or the conviction that you can change when in fact you cannot, is a tragic diversion. He proposed instilling a new, warranted optimism about the parts of your work and life you can change; this helps us focus our limited time, money, and effort on what we can change. SDSs will find this work useful as they seek understanding and perhaps new ways to manage change and help others learn about it.

In setting goals that will improve and change yourself, you may want to consider identifying several new skills that will be required of you in the next few years. If you are not sure what those skills might be, ask a trusted colleague or peer to provide input and get feedback from your superior. Because most health care systems still seem to have hierarchical structures, there may be several layers you will want to address. Other organizations structured in weblike arrangements provide you with other care providers and managers to ask for input, suggestions, and advice.

Nowicki (1996) listed 21 predictions for the future of hospital staff development. You can select one (or more) of the predictions and make it happen. Nowicki spoke from her experience in a health care system that underwent massive change with noticeable measures of improvement. Other SDSs who have also lived through that experience would agree that these predictions are a splendid way to generate conversations and thinking among SDSs and others and to continue the forward movement and development of this discipline and the specialists who practice it.

Another goal that an SDS can consider is the integration of various competency portfolios for people, groups, and even single systems. Methods of record-keeping and showing evidence of individual competence are becoming more complex and less integrated; this makes no sense given the mobility of clinical staff within systems. Records of patient care have probably achieved the greatest level of complexity possible before a major system change will need to occur—the movement toward computerized patient record systems, which are already a reality at several facilities.

In staff development, we have an opportunity to model a simple but effective approach to a professional portfolio that can, at the very least, serve to inform other SDSs about competence assessment and development activities. It is portable, accurate, and easy to understand. The work of the National Council of State Boards of Nursing (1997), regarding their commitment to develop personal accountability profiles to develop a practical how-to approach for the implementation of the regulatory role in continued competence, is a place for the SDS to begin.

The SDS who, as a leader, is responsible for organizing and developing other staff development personnel, can use several of the developmental models described in this text. Lane (1996) recently provided another one. Using the novice-to-expert conceptual model, she suggested various activities and topics for three levels of SDSs (novice, intermediate, and expert) that can be used to design a developmental program for others.

STRATEGIC THINKING

I believe the beauty of the work of clinical staff development is its unending possibilities. I sometimes view this as job security, although I've been laid off through reduction in force and terminated myself rather than another manager in another situation. The beauty of the practice is that you can do it in so many different settings within so many different clinical areas, and you can practice with others who have a mutual interest. Whether your role is full-time and dedicated to staff development or is voluntary because you are drawn to it and "there's no position for that here," you can still experience its pleasures and outcomes. Nonetheless, some strategic thinking is in order.

Strategic thinking grew out of the strategic planning literature, which grew out of the long-range planning literature. Although strategic planning implies design, schemes, and systems to accomplish stated goals, strategic thinking attempts to add the element of continual assessment of the situation, environment, or context of the plan. As mentioned earlier, planning processes may wear many new cloaks and coverings, but they are still the same scientific method for problem solving that we know: assessing, planning, implementing, and evaluating.

Campbell and Alexander (1997) provided insights about the "value creation" that must emerge from strategic planning. They proposed that the problem may not rest with the strategy itself (or implementation phase); rather, the problem lies with the formal planning processes used by so many organizations. They believe that the key to strategic thinking is to discover insights about how to create value, and then to focus planning on turning those insights into action. The SDS can use insights gained during assessment and development activities and create value for the contribution of the staff development department. The various stakeholders—our organizations, our groups of care providers, our individual clinicians, and our communities—can all provide us with data that can be used to demonstrate added value or reduced cost.

Strategic thinking requires the SDS to look at much larger pictures, even universes, than most direct care clinical practices. For example, the clinician who manages a caseload of patients may or may not appreciate how that caseload and the care given affects the entire system. SDSs should continually improve their strategic thinking skills by using the techniques of critical thinking development. Identifying the obstacles to high-quality thinking, such as habits, ruts, and anxiety, is a beginning (Rubenfeld & Scheffer, 1995). A second level of development is recognizing the uniqueness of individual thinking related to consistency, organization, memory, feelings, intuition, experience, and self-perception of intelligence. Reading, thinking, and doing are the hallmarks of high-level thinkers who consistently and persistently think about improving their daily practice and strategic thinking skills. SDSs can become well tuned into the real world of staff development when they adopt this circular (and never-ending) mode of reading, thinking, and doing in their practice.

Another goal that will contribute to the continuous improvement of care is to select a quality indicator from a professional organization and engage in measurement activities to find out how your organization scores. For example, the ANA (1997) has seven quality indicators relating to nosocomial infection rate, patient injury rate, patient satisfaction in four areas, maintenance of skin integrity, nurse staff satisfaction, staffing mix, and total nursing care hours provided per patient-day. Its recommended definitions can be used to set up measurement strategies with other clinicians, and then action planning begins.

For SDSs interested in developing their strategic thinking skills, Shoemaker (1995) suggested planning for the future by engaging in a formal activity called scenario planning. This steps of this process are listed on Display 15-1. The idea of this process, which seems similar to other strategic thinking and planning steps, is to use alternative scenarios. For instance, ask: "What if all perinatal patients were treated in a continuum of care in one place? What competencies would we need of what care providers?" Other scenarios can be envisioned by asking other "what if" questions. Using the steps individually and in groups will help SDSs plan well for their future in a continually changing health care environment.

Some final thoughts about complexity are relevant here. Waldrop (1992) addressed complexity in his report about the work of the Santa Fe Institute (1997), a place where

---

(D)ISPLAY 15-1

Steps in the Scenario Planning Process to Help Strategic Thinking With Change

1. Define the scope.
2. Identify the major stakeholders.
3. Identify basic trends.
4. Identify key uncertainties.
5. Construct initial scenario themes.
6. Check for consistency and plausibility.
7. Develop learning scenarios.
8. Identify research needs.
9. Develop quantitative methods.
10. Evolve toward decision scenarios.

Adapted from Shoemaker, P. J. (1995). Scenario planning: A tool for strategic thinking. *Sloan Management Review, 36*(2), 25–40.

artists and scientists from many disciplines converge to seek an understanding of the world. Their research agenda is focused on simplicity, complexity, complex systems, and particularly complex adaptive systems. This new kind of scientific research community is pursuing emerging synthesis in science and is conducting and fostering research that is transdisciplinary, excellent, fresh, and catalytic. The emerging science thus far is called complexity and points to numerous examples of complex systems that have somehow acquired the ability to bring order and chaos into a special kind of balance. "This balance point, called the edge of chaos, is where the components of a system never quite lock into place but never dissolve into turbulence either" (p. 12). They adapt; they change; they don't die. The edge of chaos is where new ideas and innovation are forever nibbling at the status quo; it is a constantly shifting battle zone between stagnation and anarchy. The edge of chaos is where a complex system can be spontaneous, adaptive, and alive. These findings are supported in the fields of economics, ecology, biology, mathematics, chemistry, sociology, psychology, and more. Adopting this refreshing view of change will create new ideas, opinions, beliefs, and strategies for those who choose to practice clinical staff development.

SUMMARY

This chapter—indeed, the whole second edition of this book—is intended to continue a dialogue about issues involved in initiating a clinical staff development program and practice within the health care environment. This edition is a collective reflection of the ideas and values of people deeply involved in staff development and is intended to build a community of clinicians with a common concern. It is also intended to sustain a journey that the contributors to this book and I believe is meaningful, worth the effort, and not yet complete.

I hope your journey is as much fun as mine and that you can do work that you love with good people. The work of staff development and the nature of the people who do staff development are found in this book. Reading the book will ease your journey. The sustained effort of leadership in staff development is about hard work, and it's about time and love. Enjoy your tour, and balance your life.

Leadership

DAVID MASELLO

Some years ago, when I was senior vice president and chief financial officer for a hospital in Ohio, I was asked to speak to a group of MBA students at Kent State University. One student asked me what leaders do. I responded that they intervene, manage, direct, control, teach, coach, educate, mentor, and observe the world around them. This story of leadership presents two ideas that are more powerful and more global than most ideas. First, leaders always influence the world around them. Second, the teaching model is the most powerful intervention through which to influence.

As president and chief operating officer of a hospital, I had to learn some very hard lessons about influence and the teaching model. My relations with the medical staff were a never-ending series of twists and turns—friends one day and adversaries the next. Money, power, fear, politics, and egos of megalomaniac proportions were the fuel for this tempest. One physician took me aside and told me that I had great influence with the medical staff, and he attributed this to the "mellifluous tones" in my speaking voice. I'll admit this is a term I had to look up! More importantly, he wanted me to think more appropriately about taking responsibility for the influence I had with other people. I remember arguing that how other people responded to me was not totally my issue, and that some of them would just have to deal with it. I'm not that codependent!

Sad to say, I should have paid more attention, and I wish someone had taught me how to be more responsible. It was the skill set for leadership I needed, not just the concept. I left that hospital on less-than-excellent terms with members of the staff. I started a career in consulting and discovered the answers to some of my questions about leaders and the teaching model. I participated in a training program—27 days over 6 months—to become certified as a practitioner in neurolinguistic programming (the study of models of human expert behavior).

During this study, I became acquainted with the work of Milton Erickson and his philosophy. He believed that all had the capability to work with people. His business was psychotherapy, and his reputation was one of respect and influence. He taught many to be more capable. Through Erickson's work, I discovered powerful concepts and skills for teaching others. I learned how to discover how people are already capable, and then to teach them how to use what they already know to be more successful. This creates a person who is more flexible and more resilient.

The wife of a physician and a close friend taught me the toughest lesson of all. She suggested—with much force of personality—that I see the film "Leap of Faith," starring Steve Martin as a flimflam preacher. Martin's character refuses to take responsibility for the influence he has on the people who attend his revivals. He discounts the effect of his efforts and ignores the evidence around him as he creates powerful change in people. Finally, one event, a crippled boy who walks again during a revival, proves too great to be ignored. Rather than continuing his ministry with this new-found understanding of his value and impact, the preacher leaves all of it behind.

I have learned in more powerful ways that leaders are responsible for the influence they have with others. It is impossible not to influence, and each leader must acknowledge this as accurate and reliable. Teaching people new skills and how to use what they already know in new ways is the most persuasive influence I can have with another person.

I teach now at every opportunity and try to create teaching moments from everyday encounters. I reread Erickson's writings repeatedly to enrich my understanding and capability. To teach is to influence, and when you influence you teach powerfully. I want to do each of these with a respect for people that helps them become even more capable than they already are.

REFERENCES

ANA. (1997). Nursing quality indicators for acute-care settings. *The American Nurse, 29*(5), 10.

Block, P. (1993). *Stewardship: Choosing service over self-interest.* San Francisco: Berrett-Koehler.

Burris, D. (1993). *Technotrends: How to use technology to go beyond your competition.* New York: HarperBusiness.

Campbell, A., & Alexander, M. (1997). What's wrong with strategy? *Harvard Business Review, 75*(6), 42–51.

Covey, S. R. (1989). *The 7 habits of highly effective people.* New York: Simon & Schuster.

Covey, S. R., Merrill, A. R., & Merrill, R. R. (1994). *First things first: To live, to love, to learn, to leave a legacy.* New York: Simon & Schuster.

Deming, W. E. (1982). *Out of the crisis.* Cambridge, MA: MIT Press.

Drucker, P. F. (1989). *The new realities.* New York: Harper-Row.

Finocchio, L. J., Dower, C. M., McMahon, R., Gragnola, C. M., and the Taskforce on Health Care Workforce Regulation. (1995). *Reforming health care workforce regulation: Policy considerations for the 21st century.* San Francisco: Pew Health Professions Commission.

Haller, K. B. (1998). Leadership and management in patient care delivery systems. In Dienemann, J. A. (Ed.). *Nursing administration: Managing patient care* (2nd ed.). Stamford, CT: Appleton-Lange.

Hammer, M., & Champy, J. (1993). *Reengineering the corporation: A manifesto for business revolution.* New York: HarperBusiness.

Kouzes, J. M., & Posner, B. Z. (1993). *Credibility: How leaders gain and lose it, why people demand it.* San Francisco: Jossey-Bass.

Lane, A. J. (1996). Developing healthcare educators: Application of a conceptual model. *Journal of Nursing Staff Development, 12*(5), 252–257.

Leider, R. J., & Shapiro, D. A. (1995). *Repacking your bags: Lighten your load for the rest of your life.* San Francisco: Berrett-Koehler.

Munhall, P. L. (1994). *Revisioning phenomenology: Nursing and health science research.* New York: National League for Nursing Press.

National Center for Health Statistics. (1997). *Health, United States, 1996–97.* (Table 104, p. 235). Hyattsville, MD: Public Health Service.

National Council of State Boards of Nursing. (1997). National council studies continued competence: Committee develops personal accountability profile. *Issues, 18*(2), 8–10.

Nowicki, C. R. (1996). Twenty-one predictions for the future of hospital staff development. *Journal of Continuing Education in Nursing, 27*(6), 259–266.

Porter-O'Grady, T. (1995). Creating a new system of health care. In Blancett, S. S., & Flarey, D. L. (Eds.). *Reengineering nursing and health care: The handbook for organizational transformation.* Gaithersburg, MD: Aspen.

Rubenfeld, M. G., & Scheffer, B. K. (1995). *Critical thinking in nursing: An interactive approach.* Philadelphia: Lippincott-Raven.

Safriet, B. J. (1994). Impediments to progress in health care workforce policy: License and practice laws. *Inquiry, 31*(3), 3107.

Santa Fe Institute. (1997). *Santa Fe Institute Home Page.* Retrieved from the World Wide Web on March 21, 1997: http://www.santafe.edu.

Schorr, T., & Zimmerman, A. (1988). *Making choices, taking chances: Nurse leaders tell their stories.* St. Louis: C. V. Mosby.

Seligman, M. E. (1993). *What you can change and what you can't.* New York: Fawcett Columbine.

Senge, P. M., Roberts, C., Ross, R. B., Smith, B. J., & Kleiner, A. (1994). *The fifth discipline fieldbook: Strategies and tools for building a learning organization.* New York: Doubleday.

Shaw, R. B. (1997). *Trust in the balance: Building successful organizations on results, integrity, and concerns.* San Francisco: Jossey-Bass.

Shoemaker, P. J. (1995). Scenario planning: A tool for strategic thinking. *Sloan Management Review, 36*(2), 25–40.

Tannen, D. (1990). *You just don't understand: Women and men in conversation.* New York: Ballantine.

Tecker, G. H., Eide, K. M., & Frankel, J. S. (1997). *Building a knowledge-based culture.* Washington DC: American Society of Association Executives.

Waldrop, M. M. (1992). *Complexity: The emerging science at the edge of order and chaos.* New York: Simon & Schuster.

Whitney, J. O. (1995). *The trust factor: Liberating profits and restoring corporate vitality.* New York: McGraw-Hill.

ANA's Standards and Criteria for Staff Development

ANA Standard 1. Administration

Administration of the provider unit is consistent with the organization's mission, philosophy, purpose, and goals. The organizational structure facilitates the provision of learning activities for nurses.

	Criteria
1. Organization mission, philosophy, and purpose	• The organization's mission, philosophy, and purpose contain statements that support the professional development of nurses.
2. Provider unit identified	• There is an identifiable education department responsible for nursing staff development and/or continuing education functions.
3. Provider unit philosophy and purpose	• The education department has a written philosophy, purpose, and goals that are congruent with ANA standards.
4. Goals and objectives	• The goals and objectives of the education department are written, reviewed annually, and revised as needed.
5. Educational activities consistent with philosophy	• There is documentation and record-keeping that verifies that educational activities are consistent with the education department's stated philosophy, purpose, and goals
6. Organizational chart	• The organizational chart shows lines of authority and communication within the organization, which includes the education department.
7. Provider unit administrator and educators	• The education department administrator and educators are involved in organizational activities through participation on committees, task forces, and organizational projects.
8. Policies and procedures	• There are written policies and procedures that guide the operation of the education department.
9. Financial management	• The education department is guided by cost/benefit principles in order to achieve optimal effectiveness and efficiency.
10. Financial planning	• The education department has an identifiable budget and the administrator prepares and manages this budget that supports the goals of the department.
11. Total program evaluation	• The overall evaluation of the education department includes learner feedback and measurement of outcomes as they relate to the philosophy, purpose, and attainment of the goals of the education department.

APPENDIX A (Continued)

	Criteria
12. Quality management	• The education department monitors its performance through the department's and organization's quality management program.

ANA Standard 2. Human Resources

Qualified administrative, educational, and support personnel are responsible for achieving the goals of the provider unit.

	Criteria
1. Financial planning for human resources	• The number of educational staff and support personnel is adequate to meet the needs and goals of the education department.
2. Staff development administrator	• The education department administrator has a baccalaureate or higher degree in nursing, and a graduate degree in nursing or a related field. The administrator consistently demonstrates managerial and educational knowledge and skills.
3. Members of the educational staff	• Educators within the education department have a baccalaureate or higher degree in nursing and have demonstrated relevant educational, content, and clinical expertise in addition to interest and the ability to provide education to adult learners. Preference is given to those with graduate degrees in nursing or a related field.
4. Position descriptions	• The position descriptions of the education staff, support staff, and administrator delineate the qualifications, responsibilities, authority, and accountability of all members of the education department.
5. Hiring and evaluation	• The hiring criteria and evaluation criteria for each staff member within the education department are clearly written.
6. Administrator competence	• The educational and management expertise of the education department administrator is developed, maintained, and enhanced through orientations, self-evaluation, and ongoing professional development.
7. Educational staff competence	• The educational and clinical expertise of the educators and support staff within the education department is developed, maintained, and enhanced through orientation, self-evaluation, and ongoing professional development.

ANA Standard 3. Material Resources and Facilities

Material resources and facilities are adequate to achieve the goals and implement the functions of the provider unit.

	Criteria
1. Financial planning for material resources	• There is an identifiable budget for meeting the goals and objectives of the education department.

	Criteria
2. Facilities, materials, equipment, and educational technologies	• There are adequate and appropriate facilities, materials, equipment, and educational technologies provided for the educational activities offered by the education department.
3. Support services	• Support services which are necessary for nursing educational activities are readily available to the education department—*e.g.*, library information services, printing, and audiovisual equipment.
4. Environment conducive to learning	• The physical facilities used by the education department are selected to accommodate various teaching methods, provide environmental comfort, and to allow accessibility for the target audience.
5. Evaluation of learning environment	• The learners evaluate the appropriateness and effectiveness of material resources and facilities as part of their evaluation of each educational activity.
6. Planning for material resources	• Annually the adequacy of space, materials, equipment, and budget that are necessary for the implementation of the goals of the education department is evaluated and documented.

ANA Standard 4. Educational Design

Principles of education and adult learning are used to design educational activities.

	Criteria
1. Learner participation in educational design	• The learner/participant is involved in assessing, planning, implementing, and evaluating educational activities.
2. Assessment	• The education department ensures that educational activities reflect the identified needs of the participants and/or organizational priorities, and that these activities relate to current nursing knowledge or nursing practice.
3. Planning for new competencies	• The education department plans activities that are designed to support critical thinking, new ideas, professional growth, open communication, and collaborative relationships
4. Planning for educational activity	• The education department includes in its design of every education program or activity documentation of a needs assessment, description of the target audience, educational objectives, content outline, teaching methods, evaluation strategies, and a designation of appropriate physical facilities and resources.
5. Educational direction	• The presenters and representatives of the target audience have input concerning the purpose, objectives, content, teaching methods, materials, and evaluation of each educational activity developed by the educators in the education department.

APPENDIX **A** (Continued)

	Criteria
6. Presenters	• The presenters are qualified in the content area being taught through education and experience.
7. Content, teaching methods, and evaluation strategies	• The education activity content, teaching methods, and evaluation strategies are consistent with the written objectives.
8. Marketing educational activities	• Publicity reaches the intended audience in a timely manner.
9. Educators as facilitators	• Educators within the education department assume a facilitator/consultant role in all aspects of the educational process.
10. Program evaluation	• Each educational activity is evaluated and changes made based on the analysis of the evaluation results.
11. Learner outcomes	• The evaluation design chosen by the education department includes a mechanism for feedback to the learner when appropriate.
12. Presenter feedback	• The presenters in each educational activity receive evaluative feedback for their component of the educational activity.

ANA Standard 5. Records and Reports

The provider unit establishes and maintains a record-keeping and report system.

	Criteria
1. Education activity documentation	• Documentation and records are maintained for all aspects of the educational activities of the department in compliance with departmental, organization, and external agency requirements.
2. Data retrieval	• Systematic, easy retrieval of data on educational activities and the participants in these activities is available.
3. Confidentiality	• Records are kept confidential and available only to authorized individuals.
4. Periodic reports	• Regular reports are made to organizational and/or agency representatives to document and evaluate the progress of the education department toward attainment of the goals of the department as well as the organization's goals.

ANA Standard 6. Professional Practice

The professional development educator role is practiced in a manner that enhances learners' competence to provide quality health care and enhance their contributions to the profession.

	Criteria
1. Lifelong learning	• Educators within the department promote lifelong learning as an essential and integral component of professional practice.
2. Educators as role models	• Educators and support staff model behaviors that reflect personal and professional growth within their education specialty.

APPENDIX A (Continued)

	Criteria
3. Educators as facilitators of competence	• Educators facilitate the process for learners to assume responsibility for maintaining competency in practice.
4. Educators as fiscally responsible stewards	• Management principles are applied in the design and delivery of learning activities by the educators.
5. Educators as promoters of diversity	• The understanding of cultural differences that affect health care consumers and learners is promoted by the educators.
6. Educators as agents for change	• The initiation and adoption of changes in health care are facilitated by educators.
7. Educators as systems thinkers	• Educators use and promote the use of a systematic analysis of issues in health care.
8. Educators as consultants	• Educators assume the role of consultant and assist individuals, departments, organizations, and other entities in the design and facilitation of professional development educational activities.
9. Educators as resources for current information	• Educational activities reflect current issues and trends as well as facilitate appropriate change in practice.
10. Educators as research utilization agents	• Research and current literature is integrated into educational activities.
11. Educators as promoters of research-based practice	• Learning opportunities are provided that enable nurses to utilize research findings in practice.
12. Educators as researchers	• Educators participate in research activities that target topics such as health care outcomes, issues, concepts and theories, and the learning process.
13. Educators as promoters of ethical practice	• Ethical principles are integrated into the practice of continuing education and staff development.

Reprinted with permission from *Standards for Nursing Professional Development: Continuing Education and Staff Development,* © 1994 American Nurses Publishing, American Nurses Foundation/American Nurses Association, 600 Maryland Avenue, SW, Suite 100W, Washington, DC 20024-2571, pp. 7–12. To order call, 800/637-0323, publication code COE-17.

University of Minnesota Hospital and Clinic Philosophy and Model for Competence Assessment

Philosophy Regarding Competence Assessment

At the University of Minnesota Hospital and Clinic, we have a responsibility to ensure that there are an appropriate number of qualified people to fulfill our mission and meet the needs of the patients we serve. Therefore, we believe the assessment of staff competence is applicable to all individuals who touch our organization, including employees, volunteers, and contractual staff.

We believe in a dynamic process for the assessment of competence. We acknowledge that competencies change over time based on patient and family needs, new technology, performance improvement activities, research, changes in care and practice, and organizational goals and directions.

We also believe in a developmental process for competence assessment. The process is effective when it provides opportunities to develop and maintain core competencies as well as to develop and achieve critical competencies on an ongoing basis.

We believe in universal critical competencies that help us to achieve organizational goals and directions. We also believe in role-specific and area-specific critical competencies that ensure our staff are prepared and able to function within their respective roles and responsibilities.

We believe in a shared responsibility for the assessment of competence. Organizational leaders create the environment that ensures staff have the ability to develop, maintain, and demonstrate competence. The Organizational Learning Team provides the overall direction and management of the competence assessment model and related developmental activities. Managers identify, assess, and evaluate the competence of staff within the work settings. And finally, each employee, volunteer, or contractual staff member meets competence standards as defined by role and work setting.

Philosophy Regarding Staff and Organizational Development

At the University of Minnesota Hospital and Clinic, we believe the development of staff is essential to the success of the organization.

We believe development is the process of enhancing one's present state of being. It includes the recognition of opportunities for growth and a planning process to bring oneself to a fuller state. It is an ongoing process.

We believe development is synonymous with learning. It occurs when the organization creates an environment for learning and facilitates ongoing development of individuals and groups. Therefore, we believe:

- learning occurs when employees can learn what they want to learn
- the environment provides the impulse for learning
- learning is inseparable from action; it is experience
- learning is the process of continually moving between action and reflection
- learning occurs when the motivation to learn comes from within the individual
- and, learning is lifelong.

We believe the responsibility for staff development is shared. The organization creates the environment for lifelong learning by supporting collaborative growth and development opportunities that enhance the organization's capacity to recreate its future. Leaders create the environment for learning by identifying competencies for roles, providing opportunities to achieve and demonstrate the competencies, tapping aspirations within employees, and encouraging further growth and development opportunities. Employees meet competence standards identified by role and unit. They initiate a personal development plan and actively participate in the development of others.

Model for Staff Assessment

This philosophy for competence assessment is based on an operating definition of competence as *the ability to perform a role with desirable outcomes under varied circumstances in the real world.* We believe this definition of competence assumes three domains of practice: cognitive, psychomotor, and affective. Therefore, we integrate technical, interpersonal, and critical thinking skill acquisition into our competence assessment process.

Our competence assessment model has four primary elements:

- The competence of new staff is assessed as part of the initial employment and orientation process.
- The competence of experienced staff is assessed on an annual basis.
- Staff have opportunities to develop and maintain competencies.
- The competence of staff is analyzed and reported on an annual basis to the governing board.

Initial Competence Assessment

At the time of employment, an initial assessment of competence for role and work area is completed by the employee and manager, with consultation as appropriate from the Organizational Learning Team. This assessment includes a review of performance standards and expectations for the role, identification of core competencies to be achieved, and an assessment of individual learning needs. This information forms the basis for an individualized orientation plan.

New staff are assisted in developing and demonstrating the identified core competencies through centralized and decentralized learning activities. Progress toward achievement of the core competencies is monitored by leadership staff and mentors. Successful achievement of the core competencies is documented on the competency assessment form and recorded within the computerized tracking system.

Ongoing Competence Assessment

On an annual basis, each work area develops appropriate role-specific or area-specific critical competencies. Additionally, organizational leaders identify universal competencies that are applicable to all staff. These annual competencies are identified based on changes in patient populations, changes in patient and family needs, new technology, research, new practice or care guidelines, quality improvement findings, and organizational goals and directions. The competencies address the three domains of practice and therefore reflect the integration of technical, interpersonal, and critical thinking skills.

Also on an annual basis, competencies are developed to respond to regulatory agency expectations regarding annual retraining. These competencies typically address the safe and effective use of equipment, infection control practices, and other safety expectations.

Staff are assisted in developing and demonstrating the identified critical competencies through centralized and decentralized learning activities. Progress toward achievement of the critical competencies is monitored by the employees and the leadership staff. Successful achievement of the critical competencies is documented on the competency assessment form and recorded within the computerized tracking system.

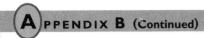

APPENDIX **B** (Continued)

Developing Competence

Staff members participate in formal and informal activities designed to maintain and improve their competence. The Organizational Learning Team, working in conjunction with area leadership staff, create opportunities to develop and demonstrate competencies. All activities are based on adult learning principles and include a variety of modalities such as skills fairs, case studies, self-learning packets, posters, didactic presentations, critical incident debriefing sessions, and peer review approaches. The learning methods are determined based on the most efficient and effective means to achieve the desired competencies.

Operational Responsibilities

Employee

The employee presents evidence of his/her competence to the manager. This evidence typically comes from a variety of competence assessment methods such as quality improvement monitors, continuing education activities, skill demonstrations, peer review processes, case study analyses, patient surveys, or self-assessments. The methods of assessment vary with the competencies to be measured.

The employee meets with the manager to discuss his/her competency achievement and overall performance. Based on the information presented, the manager deems the employee "competent" or "not competent" in the given role and work setting. If the employee is deemed "not competent," the employee develops an immediate action plan with the manager to address the deficiencies.

Manager

The manager records and reports on the competence of all staff within the work area. This information is recorded on the Competency Assessment Supervisor Documentation form and submitted for entry into the centralized tracking system. The information includes a listing of staff employed on the work area as well as which staff members have been deemed competent and which have not yet been deemed competent. The manager stores the individual competence assessment documentation forms in the respective personnel files within the work setting and gives the employee copies of all information verifying his/her competence.

The manager ensures that any employee deemed "not competent" has an immediate action plan to address deficiencies, and that work assignments are modified accordingly. The manager monitors progress toward competence until such time the competencies are demonstrated. Failure to prove ongoing competence is handled through the disciplinary process.

Organizational Learning Team

The Organizational Learning Team enters all competence assessment data into the computerized tracking system, archives the annual competency information, determines area-specific and organization-wide compliance data, analyzes the data, and reports the data to the governing board. The Organizational Learning Team also oversees the competence assessment model, identifies annual competencies, develops learning activities to achieve the competencies, and evaluates the competence assessment system to identify process improvement opportunities.

Operational Guidelines

Specific operational guidelines have been identified to address unique employment situations:

- Employees routinely assigned to, or employed by, more than one work unit complete the competence assessment process for each work unit.
- Employees hired into the float pool meet the competencies identified for float pool staff. These competencies are based on broad service delivery needs. If a float pool employee is expected to provide care to patients with specific needs for which the staff member has not demonstrated competence, either the care is provided by another staff member deemed competent in that skill, or direct supervision is provided by a competent staff member.

- Employees on leave of absence demonstrate competence within 3 months of return to work.
- Contractual staff demonstrate role-specific core competencies as well as requirements for licensure and/or certification. The respective agency ensures the competence of the contractual staff.
- Volunteers demonstrate core competencies based on role responsibilities.

Integration of Competence Assessment Into Practice

In any given setting, competence assessment data are used to make decisions regarding how care and service are provided. The responsibility for making these decisions rests with an identified person. This person may be called *shift supervisor, clinical coordinator, charge nurse,* or other such title. These individuals possess the necessary clinical and supervisory skills and abilities to competently make decisions within their respective work setting.

To make decisions regarding care and service delivery, these individuals consider factors related to the patient, the environment, and the competence of the staff. For instance, within clinical settings, assignments are made with consideration of at least the following elements:

1. The complexity of the patient's condition and care requirements,
2. The dynamics of the patient's status, including the frequency with which the need for specific care changes,
3. The complexity of the assessment required by the patient, including the knowledge and skills required to effectively complete the required assessment,
4. The type of technology required to provide care, with consideration given to the knowledge and skill required to effectively use the technology,
5. The degree of supervision required by each staff member, based on previously assessed levels of competence and current competence in relation to the needs of the patients,
6. The availability of supervision appropriate to the assessed and current competence of the staff members being assigned responsibility for providing care to the patients, and
7. Relevant infection control and safety issues.

Licensure, Registration, Certification

In addition to demonstrating competence, some employees are required by role to have evidence of current license, registration, or certification. This is verified at the time of initial employment and thereafter at designated intervals. Failure to prove current license, registration, or certification is handled through the disciplinary process.

Frequency Distribution, Central Tendency, Variability

DESCRIBING A SET OF SCORES: CENTRAL TENDENCY

Test-taker	Test 1 Score	Test 2 Score
Donna	97	95
Peggy	96	95
George	94	88
Cassandra	90	97
Sean	87	93
Connie	85	89
Keisha	84	98
Frank	82	91
Mary	79	86
Margaret	75	90

Mean—Arithmetic average of scores

$$\text{Mean} = \frac{\text{Sum of all scores}}{\text{Total \# of scores}}$$

$$\text{MEAN OF TEST 1 ABOVE} = \frac{869}{10} = 86.9 \qquad \text{MEAN OF TEST 2 ABOVE} = \frac{922}{10} = 92.2$$

Median—The score that divides a set of scores exactly in half; half the scores are below the median, half are above

$$\text{Median} = \frac{\text{Real lower limit}}{\text{of median interval}} + \left[\frac{\dfrac{\text{Total \# of scores}}{2} - \dfrac{\text{Total \# of scores below the real}}{\text{lower limit of median interval}}}{\text{\# of scores in median interval}} \times \frac{\text{Size of}}{\text{class interval}} \right]$$

Real Lower Limit of Class Interval

Although the limits of class intervals as shown in the distribution below are whole numbers, the *real* lower limit of the interval is a point halfway between the higher limit of one interval and the lower limit of the next. For the purposes of computing the median, the real lower limits of the distribution below are: 85.5, 88.5, 91.5, 94.5, 97.5. For example, a test score of 91.6 would be counted in the 92–94 interval.

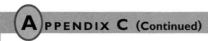

The Median Interval

The median divides the distribution exactly in half so that one half of the scores falls below the median and one half of the scores falls above the median. To identify the median interval, divide the total number of scores in half and count that number of scores from either end of the distribution.

In the example below: The total number of scores is 10, and one half of the total number of scores is five. The fifth score is one of the scores in the 89–91 interval. Therefore, the 89–91 interval is the median interval.

Because the 89–91 interval contains three scores, the *number of scores in the median interval* is 3. The *real lower limit of median interval* is 88.5.

Total number of scores below the real lower limit of median interval are counted from the lowest score to the last score before the lower limit of the median interval. In the example below, 2.

MEDIAN TEST 2

```
                o                    o
   o            o                    o
   o            o        o           o            o
  86–88       89–91    92–94       95–97        98–100
```

KEY:
o = SCORES ON TEST 2

Real lower limit of median interval = 88.5

Total number of scores = $\dfrac{10}{2}$ = 5

Total number of scores below real lower limit of median interval = 2

Number of scores in median interval = 3

Size of class interval = 3

$$\text{MEDIAN} = 88.5 + \left[\frac{\frac{10}{2}-2}{3} \times 3\right] = 88.5 + \left[\frac{5-2}{3} \times 3\right] = 88.5 + [1 \times 3] = 91.5$$

Mode—The score that has highest frequency (the score that the greatest number of students obtained). The mode is not meaningful with Test 1 results. The mode of Test 2 is 95.

DESCRIBING A SET OF SCORES: VARIABILITY

Range—The span that the lowest and highest score cover

TEST 1 RANGE = 75–97   TEST 2 RANGE = 86–98

Standard deviation—The average difference between the mean of a group of scores and the actual scores; the extent to which the group of scores deviates from the mean

$$\text{Standard deviation} = \sqrt{\frac{\text{Sum of squared deviations from the mean}}{\text{\# of scores}}}$$

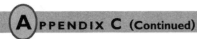

APPENDIX **C** (Continued)

Test 1

Test-taker	Test 1 Score	Mean Test 1	Difference From Mean	Difference From Mean Squared
Donna	97	86.9	10.1	102.01
Peggy	96	86.9	9.1	82.81
George	94	86.9	7.1	50.41
Cassandra	90	86.9	3.1	9.61
Sean	87	86.9	0.1	0.01
Connie	85	86.9	−1.9	3.61
Keisha	84	86.9	−2.9	8.41
Frank	82	86.9	−4.9	24.01
Mary	79	86.9	−7.9	62.41
Margaret	75	86.9	−11.9	141.61

Sum of differences squared = 484.9

$$484.9/10 = 48.49$$

$$\sqrt{48.49} = 6.96$$

STANDARD DEVIATION OF TEST 1 = 6.96

Description of Test Results

	Test-taker	Test 1 Score	Test 2 Score
	Donna	97	95
	Peggy	96	95
	George	94	88
	Cassandra	90	97
	Sean	87	93
	Connie	85	89
	Keisha	84	98
	Frank	82	91
	Mary	79	86
	Margaret	75	90
MEAN		86.9	92.2
MEDIAN		85.5	91.5
MODE		N/A	95
RANGE		75–97	86–98
STANDARD DEVIATION		6.96	3.82

FREQUENCY DISTRIBUTION

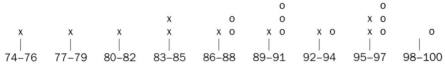

KEY:
x = TEST 1
o = TEST 2

Index

References with "t" denote tables; "f" denote figures; "d" denote displays